Speech Disorders in Children

Recent Advances

Editor in chief, Speech, Language, and Hearing Disorders Series
William H. Perkins, PhD

Speech Disorders in Children

Recent Advances

edited by

Janis M. Costello, PhD
Speech & Hearing Center
University of California, Santa Barbara

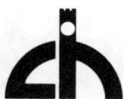

COLLEGE-HILL PRESS, San Diego, California

College-Hill Press
4284 41st Street
San Diego, California 92105

Library of Congress Cataloging in Publication Data

Costello, Janis M.
  Speech disorders in children.

  Bibliography: p
  Includes index.
    1. Speech disorders in children. I. Title. [DNLM: 1. Speech disorders—In infancy and childhood. WM 475 S7425]
RJ496.S7C66   1983   618.92'855   83-23141
ISBN 0-933014-90-2

Printed in the United States of America

Publisher's Note

These volumes were developed under the supervision of a group of leading scientists charged with the responsibility of assessing the most critical book needs of the speech-language-hearing profession. In consultation with William H. Perkins and Raymond G. Daniloff, serving as editors in chief of the ensuing volumes on speech, language, and hearing disorders (Perkins) and speech, language, and hearing science (Daniloff), the publisher planned a series of nine mutually independent texts covering the entirety of state-of-the-art knowledge in these disciplines, with contributions by respected, productive, and current scholars known for their expertise as specialists in key areas.

Each contribution has been stringently refereed for content, pedagogy, and practical value for students and practitioners by the individual volume editors, Charles Berlin, Janis Costello, Raymond Daniloff, Audrey Holland, James Jerger, Rita Naremore, and their designated reviewers, in close consultation throughout with the editors in chief and the publisher. Users are thus assured that their needs for accurate, timely information, reflecting the highest standards of scholarship and professionalism, have been faithfully met.

On behalf of the speech-language-hearing profession, its researchers, teachers, practitioners, and students, present and future, the publisher thanks the more than 100 authors and editors who have given generously of their time and knowledge to produce this magnificent contribution to the literature.

Speech Disorders in Children edited by Janis M. Costello, is one of nine state-of-the-art volumes comprising the College-Hill Press series covering the current body of knowledge in speech, language, and hearing.

Volume Titles:	Editors:
Speech Disorders in Children	Janis M. Costello
Speech Disorders in Adults	Janis M. Costello
Speech Science	Raymond Daniloff
Language Disorders in Children	Audrey Holland
Language Disorders in Adults	Audrey Holland
Language Science	Rita Naremore
Pediatric Audiology	James Jerger
Hearing Disorders in Adults	James Jerger
Hearing Science	Charles Berlin
Editor in chief, Speech, Language, and Hearing Disorders Series:	William H. Perkins
Editor in chief, Speech, Language, and Hearing Science Series:	Raymond G. Daniloff

Contents

Contributors

Martin R. Adams, PhD
Program in Communication Disorders
North Office Annex
University of Houston
Houston, TX 77004

Nicholas W. Bankson, PhD
Department of Communcative Disorders
Boston University
Boston, MA 02215

John E. Bernthal, PhD
Department of Speech Pathology &
Audiology
University of Nebraska at Lincoln
Lincoln, NE 68508

Elizabeth Cole, EdD
School of Human Communication
Disorders
McGill University
Montreal, Quebec
Canada H3G 1A8

Janis M. Costello, PhD
Speech & Hearing Center
University of California,
Santa Barbara
Santa Barbara, CA 93106

Richard F. Curlee, PhD
Department of Speech & Hearing Sciences
University of Arizona
Tucson, AZ 85721

Barry Guitar, PhD
Department of Communication Sciences &
Disorders
Allen House
University of Vermont
Burlington, VT 05405

Roger J. Ingham, PhD
School of Communication Disorders
Cumberland College of Health Sciences
P.O. Box 170
Lidcombe, New South Wales
Australia 2141

Mata B. Jaffe, PhD
Rehabilitation Institute
6301 North Umberland Street
Pittsburgh, PA 15217

Betty Jane McWilliams, PhD
Division of Speech Pathology–Audiology
Department of Speech
& Theater Arts
Cleft Palate Center
University of Pittsburgh
Pittsburgh, PA 15260

Marietta M. Paterson, MA
School of Human Communication
Disorders
McGill University
Montreal, Quebec
Canada H3G 1A8

Dennis M. Ruscello, PhD
Department of Speech Pathology &
Audiology
805 Allen Hall
West Virginia University
Morgantown, WV 26505

Richard G. Schwartz, PhD
Department of Audiology & Speech Science
Purdue University
West LaFayette, IN 47907

Frederick F. Weiner, PhD
Speech Pathology & Audiology
110 Moore Building
Pennsylvania State University
University Park, PA 16802

Foreword

From 1977 to 1982, while editing the *Journal of Speech and Hearing Disorders,* I became increasingly aware of the rate at which information about communication disorders was expanding. Not only was it an information explosion, it was a conceptual explosion as well, particularly in the area of children's language. We are departing rapidly from a relatively insular profession in which clinical practice has been based largely on what we could learn from our own experience. What we are moving toward is a theory-based profession in which we are open to broad-ranging conceptions, most notably from linguistics, medicine, and psychology.

It was against this background that *Recent Advances: Speech, Language, and Hearing Pathology* was spawned. In accepting the responsibility of being Editor-in-Chief, I saw several opportunities. Above all, it offered a vehicle by which the profession could remain current. Some areas have moved so rapidly that they bear little resemblance to what they were even a decade ago. Not only has information proliferated, but so have the journals and texts in which it has been preserved. Here, then, in *Recent Advances,* was an opportunity to organize a coherent and comprehensive account of the current state of affairs in all clinical aspects of speech, language, and hearing.

A price paid for advancement of knowledge is not only inability to consume the increasing glut, but even to comprehend it. One must almost be a specialist to understand what other specialists are talking about. To chronicle the state of the art across all areas of communication disorders, and still make responsible statements, would require the best minds available in each area. To know who the experts in these areas are, and to obtain their participation, would require scholars of such stature as to attract them. Hence, my most important responsibility in this project was the selection of volume editors. I take great pride that Janis Costello, Audrey Holland, and James Jerger agreed to participate.

With their respective editorships established, my remaining responsibility was to consult with them in determining the chapters needed to report the state of the art in their areas, and in selecting authors most qualified to prepare the chapters. We sought authors who not only are established scholars, but who also write with clarity. We were as concerned that anyone in the profession be able to read and understand what is going on in any area as we were with assembling the best information available. Aside from nudging the project along occasionally and final editing, I can claim little credit for the sterling quality of these texts. That credit belongs to the editors.

William H. Perkins
Editor in chief

Preface

While planning the organization and scope of this volume, the growth of information—paralleled unmercifully by the growth in new questions—taking place today in speech pathology became strikingly clear to me. With the assistance of the series' editor in chief, William H. Perkins, and our publisher, Sadanand Singh, I began to review the progress made in recent years in research and clinical practice. Occasionally, I was dismayed to note that seemingly little action and, therefore, few new developments, had occurred in a given area (hence, some areas are not addressed in this volume). For the most part, however, I was pleased to realize that new developments were taking place at nearly every turn and to observe that many of those advances stemmed directly from an increasing alliance between rigorous scientific method and important clinical pursuits.

The best people to write about recent advances are those who are making them, and this volume is filled by the writings of such persons. Their experiential and experimental knowledge of their topics is obvious in the content of each of these chapters, and I am exceedingly grateful for their willingness to contribute and for the patience they displayed with an everlengthening time line.

This volume is divided into separate sections on recent advances in child phonology and in stuttering. Each section is introduced by a chapter which provides an overview of the major developments in the area in order to set the scene and provide a framework for the description of recent advances in specific areas. Each of the recent advances chapters concentrates on major work, published and unpublished, carried out within the last few years, although the classic studies which often served as the impetus for work being produced now are generally described as well.

It is hoped that this volume and its companions in the *Recent Advances* series will help researchers and clinicians fill a major portion of the gap created by the fast-moving pace of speech pathology today.

Janis M. Costello
Editor

PHONOLOGY AND ARTICULATION

John E. Bernthal
Nicholas W. Bankson

Phonologic Disorders: An Overview

Introduction

Among the communication disorders which speech-language pathologists treat, it is probably safe to say that most clinicians feel more comfortable and competent when dealing with disorders of phonology than with other types of speech and language impairments. There are several factors that may be related to this proposition. First of all, articulatory behavior can be broken down into perceptually identifiable segments and, thus, may be considered more discreet in nature than certain other aspects of communication such as voice, fluency, or language. Second, a hierarchy of linguistic complexity is readily apparent, i.e., isolation, syllables, words, phrases, sentences. Third, clinicians have developed treatment procedures which, at least at an empirical level, have been demonstrated to modify target behaviors, especially with the less severe phonologically disabled individual. It is probable that these factors are related to the observation that clinicians are relatively confident when confronted with articulation impairments. In spite of this confidence, the theoretical constructs and data base supporting clinical decisions have been relatively lacking. Recent developments, however, have begun to bring about changes in this regard.

The past decade witnessed an unprecedented influence of psychology and linguistics on articulation assessment and management. In recent years, some speech scientists have focused their attention on articulatory phenomena. Such influences have served to encourage speech-language clinicians to take a critical look at our knowledge, practice, and research in this area.

The purpose of this chapter is to present an overview of where we have been and where we are going in articulation assessment and management and to identify strands of knowledge that have led to the current state of the art.

It is hoped that the reader will sense that recent advances in the field have led to a better understanding of phonologic disorders, and that such knowledge is establishing a data base that will result in more enlightened clinical decisions.

Functional-Organic Dichotomy

One aspect of articulation of continuing interest among investigators and clinicians is the specific influence of certain etiological factors which have been shown to relate to articulatory events and patterns. Since the early days of speech-language pathology, the terms *functional* and *organic* have often been ascribed to disorders in order to differentiate causal factors. In this book, organically based articulation disorders, such as those associated with neurologic, craniofacial, and hearing impairments, will be discussed in chapters by Jaffe, McWilliams, and Cole and Paterson, respectively. In addition, chapters by Ruscello and Weiner will discuss disorders that have been identified in the literature as nonorganic, functional, and developmental. As a prelude to further discussion of articulation impairments, it may be helpful to consider the background and current status of the functional-organic dichotomy.

In tracing the speech-language pathology literature, the terms "functional" and "organic" have been present for a long time. These terms were originally used in the field of medicine; and since the medical model of diagnosis had such a pervasive effect on the field in the early days, it seems only natural that such usage was adopted by speech-language pathology. As was customary with the medical model, attempts were made to determine the *cause* of the problem or disorder. It was recognized that some problems were related in an obvious way to neurologic, structural, and perceptual factors. It was also recognized, however, that not all disorders were organic in nature, but, rather, some were nonorganic, or to borrow a medical term, "functional." While the term functional was originally synonymous with nonorganic, its meaning was soon broadened to include all disorders of "unknown" causation.

Early writers in the field, such as West, Ansberry, and Carr (1937), cautioned the profession about problems inherent in the use of the term "functional." Such problems, however, are not unique to speech-language pathology. A report from the New York Milbank Medical Conference in 1950 stated the following:

> The semantic difficulty that kept cropping up during the conference was the confusion consequent upon the use of such terms as "organic," "functional," "mental," "physical," and "purely psychological." This confusion was enhanced by the apparently irresistible temptation of even superior scientists to dichotomize phenomena into "organic or functional," "mental or physical."

In spite of the inherent problems with this term, it would appear that practitioners of various disciplines who employ the medical model have a propensity to dichotomize disorders as either functional or organic.

Let us consider the meanings ascribed to the term "functional." The most frequently used definition has focused on an organic/nonorganic dichotomy. Travis (1931) indicated that in the absence of determined or inferred organic pathology, an articulation disorder may be classified as functional. More recently, however, Emerick and Hatten (1974) stated that some children identified as having functional articulation disorders, in which no readily discernible organic basis for the sound errors is found, may "possess subtle neurological impairments." They were especially concerned with children who seem to have difficulty modifying sound productions and who persist in the production of speech sound errors even after instruction. They reported preliminary data which indicate that children who have such persistent articulation disorders show more signs of possible organic impairment, including mild or marginal motoric disability, than either children without articulatory impairment or children who made improvement during the first year of intervention.

Other speech-language pathologists have extended or broadened the definition of "functional" and have indicated that the term should carry no inference of either organic or nonorganic cause, but should simply indicate that there are no obvious signs of structural, perceptual, or neurologic deviations. Some writers have used other labels to replace the term "functional"—such as "developmental errors" or "developmental delay." Powers (1957) has criticized our labeling of functional articulation disorders on the premise that it has constituted "diagnosis by default." Shelton (1978) also pointed out that the term has often served as a "waste basket" category for articulation problems of unknown causation. The lack of etiological and behavioral specificity that characterizes the category has caused some to question whether the term "functional" is even an appropriate or helpful label to be used in identifying articulation disorders.

It would appear that those clients considered to have functional disorders are a very heterogeneous group who might be better labeled as individuals with articulation disorders of *unknown etiology*. Behaviorally, this group varies in severity from those with a single sound in error to those with multiple errors. We would propose that the term "unknown etiology" is a more appropriate descriptor of this population than the term "functional." Not only does "functional" have a variety of meanings, it is also difficult to define on other than a "default" basis.

Factors Related to Phonologic Disorders of Unknown Etiology

Historically, investigators have spent a great deal of effort exploring possible factors related to "functional" articulation disorders. Such variables have included speech sound discrimination, intelligence, dentition, oral sensory perception, laterality, motor skills, personality, educational achievement, and language skills, among others. The types of research designs employed in such studies have typically been either correlational studies of the status of articulation and other variables within individuals or comparisons between nonimpaired subjects and subjects with disorders of articulation on one or more of these variables. As we know, correlational studies do not allow cause-effect statements. Similarly, a functional relationship between variables is not obtained through group comparisons. Thus, studies concerned with disorders of unknown etiology have not, for the most part, been successful in identifying possible causal factors. Shelton and McReynolds (1979) indicated that this may be true because (1) a common factor is not operating across all articulation-impaired individuals, (2) the factors may be too subtle to be identified with the methods used, (3) research methodologies have been inadequate, or (4) the wrong variables have been studied. At best, studies of status relationship have identified only a few variables worthy of further investigation as factors that may contribute to the presence of phonologic disorders. It has been suggested that rather than studying individual variables that relate to disorders of unknown etiology, we might better study a collection of variables simultaneously in order to discover possible relationships between clusters of factors and articulation.

The few studies of this nature (Arndt, Shelton, Johnson, & Furr, 1977; Prins, 1962) that have been done, however, have not been very successful in identifying distinct subgroups of the articulation-impaired population. One such subgroup is children who have been identified as syllable reducers because their speech sound error pattern is characterized by the reduction of CCV or CVC syllables to the CV or VC form. Compared to children whose errors are primarily substitutions, children with syllable reduction errors have a higher total number of articulation errors and make more extensive use of /ʔ/, /h/, and other sounds unlike the "intended" phonemes. Syllable reducers tend to be slower to respond to articulation remediation and have different patterns of transfer and generalization when compared to substituters (Elbert & McReynolds, 1978; Panagos, 1974; Prins, 1962; Renfrew, 1966). They have also been found to have lower IQs, to have more associated neurologic abnormalities, to repeat syllables at slower rates, to be from families rated as lower in socioeconomic status, and to perform more poorly on measures of linguistic ability when compared to substituters (Frisch & Handler, 1974; Prins, 1962). In order to subcategorize a group of children with articulation disorders of unknown etiology, it is necessary to demonstrate in some meaningful fashion that the behaviors seen are reflective of a particular cluster of characteristics. The meaningfulness of such differentiation will be strengthened if a functional relationship can be demonstrated between a change in one or more critical variables and a change in articulatory performance.

Articulation Patterns Associated with Second Language Learning

It seems appropriate in this discussion of factors associated with the presence of articulatory differences to make a statement about the unique problems associated with learning the phonologic system of a second language. Categorically, we must say that phonologic differences associated with second language learning, as well as those associated with geographic or social/dialect, are not appropriately viewed as articulation impairments. It is important to make the point that phonologic differences related to dialect or second language learning are not considered functional or organic impairments.

Etiology and Treatment Models

A wide variety of treatment approaches have been employed with those clients with articulation problems of unknown etiology. Shelton and McReynolds (1979) have delineated the following models:

1. Discrimination model   emphasis on external and internal monitoring, matching one's own productions to a standard model, using auditory,

	proprioceptive, and tactile feedback to control productions automatically.
2. Sensory-motor model	emphasis on production of sounds in various and increasingly complex contexts, with repetition of the motor skills involved in articulation.
3. Operant conditioning model	emphasis on shaping behaviors, programming, contingency management as a means of establishing new behaviors.
4. Phonologic disorders model	emphasis on teaching the phonologic contrasts of a language with efforts to increase the complexity of such contrasts.

All of these models approach articulatory disorders without specific evidence of the cause of the problem, yet there are particular etiologic biases that might be ascribed to the different models (e.g., perceptual deficiency, faulty learning). These models are not mutually exclusive, and, in reality, many clinicians tend to be eclectic in their use of treatment models. It should be pointed out that such models are also used in the treatment of clients whose articulation impairment has an organic base. This observation then raises the whole question of how important etiology is in the treatment of articulation disorders.

While treatment models used in the management of functional and organic articulation disorders are similar, an understanding of the organic basis underlying some articulatory/phonologic impairments is critical for the speech-language clinician. The child without an intact mechanism with which to develop speech and language frequently requires different or even unique assessment and treatment procedures as compared to a child with an intact speech mechanism. For example, the child who is not able to close the velopharyngeal valve adequately—with the result that the nasal cavity is coupled to the oral cavity during production of stops, fricatives, and affricates—may require physical management in order to produce appropriate levels of intraoral air pressure for such consonants. An understanding of which speech errors can be attributed to such a physical impairment and which can be attributed to learning or cognitive factors may be important considerations in management. Likewise, the child whose articulation impairment can be partly attributed to a perceptual deficit caused by a hearing loss will have certain error patterns and problems which can be explained by the hearing loss.

A similar statement can be made relative to the dysarthrias seen in children with neurological impairment in which a child with a moderate to severe motor involvement may display articulation deviations that result not only in unique management procedures but in reduced expectations for change.

The chapters in this book dealing with neurologic speech disorders in children by Jaffee, craniofacial anomalies by McWilliams, and hearing impairment by Cole and Paterson are intended to give the reader current information regarding the types of speech impairments associated with such organic problems. These chapters also discuss why such articulatory characteristics occur and provide management suggestions for individuals with such disorders.

Phonologic Development

The nature of phonologic development has long been of interest to speech scientists, linguists, and speech-language pathologists. For purposes of organization, investigations of phonologic development will be discussed from linguistic and motor-acoustic perspectives.

Schwartz points out in his chapter that child phonologists have not only looked at surface structures (observable phonetic events), but have also made inferences concerning children's underlying representations for sounds produced at the surface level, identified phonologic processes, and discussed the relationship between perception and production. Theories and models of phonologic development from a linguistic perspective have typically focused on phonologic universals (the child's theoretically innate ability to passively acquire a phonologic system). More recently, constructionist theories have emerged in which the child is assumed to take an active role in the construction of his phonologic system.

A second perspective related to phonologic development has been an emphasis on phonetic (surface level) or motor development of speech sounds. This research has focused on the phonetic inventories, coarticulation, and the effects of phonetic context.

The need exists for investigators to study phonologic development from both a linguistic as well as a phonetic perspective in order to obtain a more comprehensive understanding of phonologic development. Such studies require that investigators employ methods typically used in both linguistic and phonetic approaches.

Articulatory-Phonologic Disorders

Research in disordered articulation can also be viewed from motor-acoustic and linguistic perspectives. It has long been recognized that children's misarticulations reflect phonetic and phonemic error types even within the same child. In some instances, speech-language pathologists have viewed articulation errors as motor production problems with remediation focusing on motor practice. The chapter in this volume by Ruscello reflects a bias that remediation of many children's articulation errors can be approached from a motor learning perspective and that motor learning theory can serve as a model for articulatory training. A second type of articulation problem emanates from a linguistic perspective. Sound changes (errors) are described as phonemic or pattern based. The assumption by some speech-language pathologists has been that such phonemic productions reflect factors other than the child's ability to produce a sound at the motor level. In other words, children who substitute /θ/ for /s/ and then substitute /s/ for /ʃ/ are considered to have the necessary phonetic skills in their response repertoires to produce the /s/. Instead, the /θ/ for /s/ substitution probably reflects a phonologic rule operating on a child's phonologic output.

Since the publication of Ingram's monograph *Phonological Disability in Children* (1976), the emphasis on the linguistic aspects of children's speech sounds has been considerable. Weiner makes this observation as well in his chapter in this volume. The emphasis on patterns of sound production and the systematic nature of speech sound errors has resulted in the publication of several evaluation procedures which reflect this linguistic emphasis in the assessment of speech sound errors in children.

Perhaps it is appropriate at this point in the chapter to address the notion of how these disorders which reflect speech sound changes should be labeled. There have been suggestions that individuals with speech sound changes which deviate from the norm for a given age should be identified as having a phonologic disorder rather than an articulation disorder. It is our position that to a considerable extent this argument is a semantic one. There is no doubt that since the publication of Ingram's book in 1976, the focus of what has traditionally been called articulation disorders has been broadened to include a strong phonologic or linguistic emphasis. Some investigators have suggested that the term "articulation disorders" is too restrictive in that it suggests only concern for the motor and acoustic aspects of speech sounds involving just the peripheral aspects of the speech mechanism. On the other hand, it is argued that the term "phonologic disorders" encompasses not only the surface or motor aspects of production but also the underlying adult form, as well as phonologic rules and processes. From this perspective, "phonologic disorders" is a broader, more encompassing, and thus, more appropriate term than articulation disorders. However, some individuals seem to use the term "phonologic disorders" so that it does not include the motor aspects of sound production. When the term "phonologic disorders" is used in such a restrictive sense, it does not encompass the range of problems seen in the children who are the focus of this book. In the chapters which follow, the editor has chosen to employ the term "phonologic disorders" to refer to all children with speech sound errors, thereby using the term in a broad or generic sense to include not only the phonemic aspects of articulation, but also the motor and surface forms of sound productions. When the term articulation appears, it is meant to signify the exclusively perceptual-motoric aspects of phonologic performance.

Trends in Assessment

Since one section of this volume is designed to review recent advances in phonologic disorders, it is appropriate to review past and current practices in assessment of such disorders. Since the 1960s, the traditional assessment battery for articulation status has consisted of the following: (1) a connected speech sample, usually a spontaneous speech sample, (2) a phonetic inventory evoked by a picture-naming task, (3) a measure of articulatory consistency (deep testing), and (4) a measure of imitation or stimulability of segments produced in error. Before discussing the state of the art of each of these aspects of assessment, perhaps it would be helpful to briefly discuss the evolution of the test battery.

Historical Review

It goes without saying that spontaneous or connnected speech samples have always been of critical importance to clinicians, for that is the format in which appropriateness of speech sound production is ultimately judged. Thus, from the beginning of the profession, articulation evaluation has included listening to a talker's connected speech. Reading samples are one method that has often been used in order to obtain a sample of this speech. It should be recognized that reading samples are more artificial than true spontaneous speech, and thus, at the present time, clinicians are more interested in hearing a client produce sounds in a spontaneous situation. As audio tape recorders became widely available, clinicians recorded connected speech samples and used the recordings for more careful analysis than is possible with live online transcription. While the techniques for evoking connected speech samples have been fairly similar throughout the years (e.g., telling stories, answering questions), in recent years published articulation tests have included more formalized methods for obtaining these samples (e.g., pictures designed to evoke story telling responses, repeating a story after the examiner). The use of spontaneous speech samples as a primary data base for analysis has received increased emphasis since the late 1970s due to interest in a more linguistically based assessment of children's phonologic patterns.

As with spontaneous speech samples, phonetic inventories have been used in the assessment of articulatory status almost from the beginning of the profession. Phonetic inventories were developed in order to assess the sounds of the language in a relatively short period of time. In the late 1950s and early 1960s there was a feeling among many speech-language clinicians that since there was a relatively high correlation between overall intelligibility of spontaneous speech samples and the number of errors identified by a phonetic inventory, phonetic inventories could provide an accurate picture of a child's speech sound patterns. Many clinicians even came to use the phonetic inventory as their primary assessment instrument. Since the 1970s, however, there has been increased interest in connected speech samples as a primary sample for analysis, and thus, inventories have come to be used as only one measure in an articulation battery. The shift away from phonetic inventories to connected speech samples as the primary data base was related to the observation that within individuals there is frequently variation in performance between these two measures.

While clinicians have always been interested in clients' abilities to imitate the correct form of their misarticulations, imitative or stimulability testing as a potential prognostic tool was not examined systematically until the late 1950s and early 1960s. Several investigators demonstrated that a child's performance on stimulability tasks was related to the probability for correcting a sound without intervention. This measure continues to be used to determine if clients have the appropriate motor gestures to produce sound segments judged to be in error and to help determine the rate at which remediation can be expected to progress.

A major contribution to the methodology for assessing articulation was the appearance of contextual or "deep testing" of sounds. The prototype for such testing was *The Deep Test of Articulation* (McDonald, 1964). Such instruments allowed for an in-depth analysis of a particular segment by varying the phonetic contexts which preceded and followed a target sound. This addition to the traditional articulation battery provided clinicians with more systematic data regarding variation in sound productions than were typically available through inventories or spontaneous speech samples.

In the following paragraphs each of these elements of a traditional battery will be discussed. The point should be made that interactive variables affect speech samples, since phonologic behaviors are sensitive to linguistic and extralinguistic factors associated with the mode of evocation. However, such factors will not be elaborated in this chapter.

Review of Traditional Test Battery

Connected speech sample

The major advantage of a spontaneous or connected speech sample is its inherent face validity, since correct productions in conversational speech represent the terminal behavior of articulation instruction. In addition, spontaneous samples allow for a judgment of the client's overall intelligibility and may also be used to determine consistency of speech sound productions. Shriberg and Kwiatkowski (1980) suggested that a connected speech sample yields more stable data than alternative measures and recommended its use for their natural phonologic process analysis. The spontaneous speech sample also has the potential to be used for related language analyses, thus enabling an integrated speech-language assessment.

A limitation of spontaneous speech samples is observed in the case of individuals with severe articulation problems when responses are unintelligible and the intent of the message is unknown. Not knowing what a child is attempting to say is a significant problem, not only in transcription, but also in subsequent interpretation of error patterns. Most clinicians recognize this difficulty and use a gloss (an indication by the clinician of what the child attempted to say) in order to insure that the child's intended sounds are part of the data collection procedure.

A second limitation of spontaneous speech samples is the difficulty encountered in obtaining a representative sample of the speech sounds of a language, since the lexicon obtained in a particular sample may not contain an adequate sample of these. However, it may be that if a sample is of sufficient size, the problem of a nonrepresentative sample may not be a critical issue because a child's preference for certain sounds will be revealed, the sounds missing in his repertoire probably reflecting a selective avoidance on his part. Further, since the important sounds will be produced a number of times in such a spontaneous sample, a general picture of a child's phonologic system will be obtained. It is possible that apparent sound preferences may be as much or more a reflection of word preferences as they are of sound preferences. Conversely, the absence of sounds may reflect a selective avoidance or simply a difference in the frequency of occurrence of sounds in the language. Even if the assumption of selective avoidance is valid and a reasonable description of the child's phonology can be inferred from the speech sample, clinicians will typically still desire a more representative and systematic sample of the speech sounds in the language than can be obtained from a spontaneous connected speech sample.

At this time, most investigators and clinicians would agree that a spontaneous speech sample should be included as a routine procedure during the assessment of children with articulation disorders. The issue for which there is still disagreement is the extent to which a spontaneous speech sample should serve as the primary data base of the evaluation. Speech-language clinicians are aware that in the case of many children, the responses obtained from a spontaneous sample may be different from those obtained from other sampling procedures (Shriberg & Kwiatkowski, 1980). With other children, it has been shown that similar results may be obtained in a much shorter time with these alternative methods (DuBois & Bernthal, 1978). In summary, since spontaneous or connected samples have the best face validity, most speech-language pathologists agree that such samples should serve as the primary basis for the assessment and analysis of children's articulation. The second advantage in using continuous speech samples to assess children's articulation/phonologic status is that other language and linguistic analyses can be performed on the same corpus.

Phonetic inventory

The nature of sound inventories has changed little over the past four decades. The number of items, the order of items, vocabulary used, whether or not one or more sound segments are tested in a single item, and size and color of stimulus pictures are some of the minor types of changes seen in these instruments in the past two decades. The major changes have been in the scoring and analysis of such inventories. There has been a definite shift toward more phonetic detail in scoring, and conversely, a moving away from the more traditional scoring system of recording responses as correct or incorrect or even of classifying errors as substitutions, omissions, and distortions. The reason for this change is that clinicians are looking more carefully at error productions so that feature and process errors that may be present are identified. Only through detailed transcriptions do some of these errors surface.

The second major change associated with inventories has been a shift from sound-by-sound analysis to pattern analysis. *The Fisher-Logemann Test of Articulation Competence* (1971) was a notable attempt toward this emphasis on the identification of error patterns across sound segments. A third change which has emerged since 1950 is the collection of normative data which allowed clinicians to compare a child's performance at a particular age to norms for the instrument. These changes have served to increase the versatility of inventories.

Despite the criticism in the literature directed toward picture-naming articulation tests, they continue to enjoy widespread use as a clinical tool. Phonetic inventories allow the clinician to control the sample obtained and thereby assure sampling of all items of interest. In addition, such tests may be administered rather quickly, are convenient to transport, and provide the examiner with an easy-to-analyze sample of speech sound productions.

The most obvious disadvantage of single word inventories is that frequently segments produced in citation form (single words) are produced differently than they are in connected speech samples. It is well known that single word responses do not adequately reflect the effects of coarticulation or the effects of context which in many instances transcend syllable and lexical boundaries. Factors such as syllable structure, stress, and phonetic environment frequently affect production but are not controlled in such tests.

A second criticism is that most speech sound inventories contain only a single utterance of each target sound in each word position. Inconsistency of articulatory productions seen in children during phonological acquisition, as well as in children with articulation disorders, cannot be adequately assessed through such limited sampling. In addition, it is a reasonable speculation that word familiarity may also affect production of individual segments, although we are not aware of data to support this view. Nonetheless, phonetic inventories continue to serve a role in the clinical assessment of the articulation status of children and provide useful information despite their shortcomings.

Stimulability testing

Stimulability testing, advanced by Milisen (1954) in early treatment research, is assessment of the client's ability to imitate at a motor level the adult form of a misarticulated sound but does not provide information about phonemic competence. The unit to be imitated may include isolated sounds, syllables, or words, and usually involves the presentation of visual and auditory cues. The clinician can assume that the subject who is stimulable on an error sound has the motoric skills required to make the articulatory gesture for the target sound. It has been suggested that segments that can be produced via imitation can be corrected more rapidly through intervention than those sounds which cannot be imitated (Winitz, 1975). In recent years, it has been reported that once a sound can be imitated in a syllable or word context, response generalization to nontrained words and syllables begins to occur (McReynolds, 1972). Investigators have also reported that children with the poorest test scores on stimulability tests are most likely to benefit from intervention (Sommers, Leiss, Delp, Gerber, Fundrella, Smith, Revucky, Ellis & Haley, 1967). Other investigators have reported that children aged 5 through 7 who are able to correctly imitate syllables or words containing an error sound have a higher probability for self-correction of those sounds than those who are not stimulable (Carter & Buck, 1958; Farquhar, 1961). A clinical guideline might be that if a child has a mild articulation problem but can imitate the target sound(s) at the syllable level, then remediation may not be indicated. For those with more severe problems, however, sounds that can be imitated may represent a good beginning point for treatment. In summary, stimulability testing provides data that are useful in determining the need for intervention and in making treatment decisions.

Contextual testing

The notion that children's articulation productions are inconsistent (sometimes target sounds are produced correctly, sometimes they are not) is well documented in the literature, and thus some form of contextual or in-depth testing of error sounds has been suggested as part of the traditional articulation test battery. Van Riper (1939) stated long ago that the search for contexts in which an error sound is produced correctly is well worth the investment of time. He suggested that such key words can serve as a place to initiate instruction. Contextual testing is typically done with the *The Deep Test of Articulation* (McDonald, 1964), or the *Sound Production Tasks* (Elbert, Shelton & Arndt, 1967; Shelton, Elbert & Arndt, 1967), or in a connected speech sample. Many clinicians look upon such contextual testing as an initial step in the remediation process. Contextual or deep testing is most important for the clinician who samples the articulation of a given sound only in a limited number of contexts. Such testing can be used to get an idea of consistency of target production or to identify facilitating phonetic contexts. The selection of facilitating contexts also involves other factors (e.g., stress, word position, allophonic variation, frequency of occurrence) in addition to the influence of adjacent sounds. It is a reasonable speculation that the higher the percentage of correct to incorrect utterances identified in contextual testing, the more likely the child will self-correct the error and make progress in remediation. Although Lapko and Bankson (1975) reported a significant correlation between the *The Deep Test of Articulation* for the /s/ sound and the Carter-Buck task for speech sound stimulability for /s/, specific data to support the above speculations are lacking.

Scoring and Analysis

Traditionally, speech-language clinicians have scored responses as substitutions, distortions, omissions, or insertions. While there have been a number of different definitions for sound "omissions," or deletions, this term seems to be a useful concept and has remained in the literature across time, and in recent years omissions have come to be identified with more specificity, e.g., deletion of final consonants, deletion of unstressed syllables, and cluster reductions.

As well, the designation of substitutions and/or additions also seems to be a useful notion, since transcription of such segments is similar across most scoring systems except for the amount of phonetic detail included. On the other hand, use of the term "distortion" is a curious one, since it is really better described as a substitution in which the replacement segment is an incorrect variation within the perceptual boundary of the target sound.

Notation used to transcribe children's utterances will vary with the way the data are to be analyzed. In general, transcription and an analysis of the speech of a child with defective articulation requires use of the International Phonetic Alphabet and some system of diacritics.

The ways in which speech samples have been analyzed are: (1) judgment of overall intelligibility, (2) sound-by-sound analysis, and (3) pattern analysis. In sound-by-sound analysis, the emphasis is on individual segments and the number and type of errors. Typically, such analyses examine the stimulability of individual segments, the consistency of individual segments in a variety of phonetic contexts, comparison with developmental norms of the acquisition data for individual segments, and average number of errors for children of a given age. The third type of error analysis is a pattern analysis in which the examiner focuses on patterns of errors. One error pattern or simplification strategy may account for the sound changes seen across several segments.

The traditional pattern analysis usually consists of reviewing errors for commonalities in terms of place, manner of production, and voicing. The lack of specificity in the manner and place categories have limited their clinical use. The recent trend toward phonologic process analysis partially overcomes this limitation because of its increased specificity. Process labels such as *stopping, gliding for liquids, cluster reduction, final consonant deletion, fronting, backing* all provide specificity to place and manner categories.

We wish to point out that in the paragraph above, these terms only describe errors in the surface structure of the child's phonology and are not intended to make any inference concerning the child's underlying representations of the adult phonemic form. Use of the term "phonologic processes" to refer only to surface structures is not something all speech-language pathologists would agree upon. Authors, in describing procedures for phonologic process analysis, have used the term process differently. Weiner, in his chapter, defines a process by pointing out that the child is assumed to have an underlying phonologic representation nearly equivalent to the adult surface form. Shriberg and Kwiatkowski (1980) selected processes for their natural process analysis procedure that met additional criteria. These criteria specified that a proccess had to meet Stampe's (1973) criteria for a natural process, had to be observed frequently in the speech of young children with delayed speech, and further, had to be scored reliably by speech-language clinicians. In contrast, some investigators use the term "process" only as a label to describe surface patterns without any assumption about underlying representation.

In summary, the appealing notion of using linguistically based analysis procedures is that they facilitate a better understanding of the child's phonologic system and, one hopes, lead to more efficient clinical management. Khan (1982) furnished an example of how a process analysis can provide a better understanding of a child's phonologic system than the more traditional analysis. To describe the common replacement by children of /wawa/ for *water* as a /w/ for /t/ substitution with an omission for the final /ɾ/ does not reveal an accurate picture of the child's phonology. Rather, describing this "error" as an example of syllable reduplication reflects a better understanding of this child's phonology in that the child is repeating a syllable rather than replacing correct sounds with error sounds in the second syllable. Phonologic pattern analysis is not a replacement for traditional assessment procedures but rather, a supplementary tool. Recent recommendations for conducting a complete phonologic assessment include process analysis as but one of several recommended procedures.

Trends in Remediation

For the approximate half century that speech-language pathologists have sought to treat phonologic disorders, clinicians have moved from a point where they had to rely primarily on their own intuitions to the point where a clinical science data base for phonologic disorders has begun to emerge. From a retrospective view, it is possible to trace several trends that appear to reflect a greater sophistication in the management of phonologic disorders. In the following paragraphs we will trace some of the trends and influences in the area of remediation of phonologic disorders.

Historical Review

Traditional treatment

Early approaches to treatment emphasized a phonetic or motor approach to correcting sounds supplemented with perceptual or discrimination training. Sounds were taught one at a time with instruction focusing on "ear training" followed by phonetic placement cueing in order to evoke productions in isolation. Once a sound was established in isolation, production was shifted to increasingly complex contexts (i.e., syllables, words, phrases, sentences). Drill activities formed the heart of the treatment methodology. Such an approach had an inherent logic to it and was supported by early writers in the field.

Sensory-motor influence

In the early 1960s a new thought influenced remediation practices. McDonald (1964) described an approach to remediation that focused less on production of sound segments in isolation and more on syllable productions and the systematic production of sounds embedded in a variety of phonetic contexts. Specifically, McDonald suggested that remediation, based on prior assessment, should focus on sounds being produced in facilitating contexts and on increasing the number of contexts in which a sound was produced correctly. Practice in producing bisyllables and trisyllables with a variety of stress patterns was an integral part of this remediation approach. Thus, the attention of the clinician was directed to the importance of *phonetic facilitation*, which may be defined as improvement in the production of a target sound as a function of phonetic context. While it is probably accurate to say that McDonald's work had a greater impact on assessment procedures than on remediation procedures, nonetheless, his work added an important perspective to the process of making treatment decisions.

Behavioral influence

By the late 1960s and well into the 1970s, concepts from the field of behavioral psychology had a decided influence on the manner in which clinicians approached remediation, both in terms of instruction and the measurement of its effect. Concepts such as pinpointing behaviors, programming stimuli and responses, and controlling behavior by its consequences came into common understanding and application within the profession. In addition, the importance of repeated samplings of target behavior, both before and during treatment, was emphasized. In fact, measurement of responses was an integral part of this behavioral trend and served to foster a number of research studies concerned with articulation treatment (e.g., Bankson, 1974; Elbert & McReynolds, 1978).

It should be pointed out that this behavioral approach to management did not represent a completely novel approach to treatment; rather, in many instances it served as a framework or protocol in which existing intervention methodologies could be utilized. For example, a temporal sequence of clinical events might follow the (1) antecedent event, (2) response, and (3) consequent event paradigm with criterion levels established for progression from one level of instruction to another. Clinicians then inserted traditional as well as novel treatment techniques into this framework. Behavior modification, with its heavy emphasis on programmed instruction and the use of consequating events as a means for changing behaviors (see Costello, 1977) facilitated more sophisticated behavioral routines than had typically been practiced.

As stated above, not only did the behavioral movement serve to influence practices associated with clinical management, but it also served as an impetus for clinical research. Prior to this time there were few investigations which had specifically studied treatment approaches. Lack of interest in treatment research, coupled with the problems inherent in doing group studies (e.g., finding subjects who met similar selection criteria; running large numbers of subjects; and the masking of individual variation within the group mean) served to discourage treatment studies. The functional analysis of behavior, or within-subject experimental design, was perceived by speech-language clinicians as appropriate and convenient for study of the treatment of phonologic impairment (McReynolds & Kearns, 1982).

Behavioral studies have focused on the effect of particular treatment approaches including training sequences and aspects of articulation generalization. While investigations conducted thus far have only scratched the surface of research needed to develop a clinical science of phonologic remediation, efforts to develop a scientific base in the area of remediation have begun.

Linguistic influence

Concurrent with the influence of behavioral psychology on speech-language pathology was the influence which emanated from linguistics. This influence stemmed primarily from work in psycholinguistics, including child phonology, and was related to all aspects of language behavior. Linguists called the attention of speech-language pathologists to the notion that articulation behavior could be described within the framework of language behavior.

The work of Compton (1970) represented one of the early attempts to apply linguistic principles to disordered articulation. He proposed that when a child produced multiple articulation errors, such errors might be related. He demonstrated that a language corpus could be analyzed in such a manner that phonologic rules or patterns that were common across segments could be identified.

Interest in identification of patterns among misarticulations found increased focus through analyzing such errors via a distinctive feature analysis. Such analyses looked for distinctive feature commonalities among sound errors. While various methodologies for doing such analyses were developed, they have not been used widely by clinicians for two reasons: (1) the distinctive features borrowed from linguistic theory were sometimes ill-suited for clinical application and (2) the time required for most feature analysis systems was viewed as too lengthy by clinicians.

A rationale for use of a remediation approach based on distinctive feature analysis is the assumption that training of a feature in one segment will transfer to other segments where the feature is used inappropriately. Investigators have reported preliminary data which demonstrates that feature training in one or more sounds does, on occasion, transfer to other sounds (Costello & Onstine, 1976; McReynolds & Bennett, 1972). The degree of generalization, however, varies across segments, individuals, and linguistic units.

Phonologic process analysis procedures discussed earlier in this chapter were the next type of pattern analysis to emerge in the late 1970s. This type of pattern analysis was based on processes observed in young children developing phonology (Ingram, 1976). Such analyses describe simplification strategies—final consonant deletion, stopping, etc. Remediation that has been suggested for the elimination or suppression of selected processes focuses on targets such as establishing additional sound contrasts including the elimination of homonyms (e.g., [tu] for *two* and *tooth;* [wawa] for *water; waffle; wakeup*). Teaching techniques may also focus on perceptual tasks related to the training of various contrasts. At the present time data regarding the benefits of treatments derived from phonologic process analyses are only of a most preliminary nature, but it may turn out that such analyses lead to novel treatment procedures that are effective for certain clients with multiple errors.

Perhaps the major treatment contribution from linguistics has been in the nature of the target behaviors selected for remediation. For example, instead of treating an individual segment, a clinician may treat several sounds in an affected class or, at least, an exemplar of a class. An approach of this type assumes that generalization across phonemes within the affected class will occur and that the clinician will not have to teach all the segments that reflect the operation of a given phonologic process. If generalization of this type does not occur and a clinician must remediate all affected segments, there may be minimal efficiency in this approach.

When evaluating the current status of remediation, the following statements can be made. While the data base for making treatment decisions is still woefully lacking, nonetheless, the field has moved forward in developing such a base and can at least acknowledge an increase in applied research. Because of the great variability observed among clients, within-subject research designs, including replication with a small number of subjects, have been found particularly useful and have served to advance our data base. A related phenomenon has been the trend toward more precise and thorough measurement of progress in remediation employed by clinicians. Treatment methodologies have expanded in format and sophistication; however, in most instances these expansions have represented adaptations of traditional methodologies. Clinicians have become more interested in children with severe phonologic impairments, and target behaviors selected for treatment with this population have been more often based on pattern analysis, especially phonologic process analysis, than the traditional sound-by-sound analysis. In cases where only a few unrelated sounds are in error, more traditional analyses seem to be adequate.

In terms of those clients with organically based disorders, progress has been made in the identification of particular syndromes and subgroups. It is hoped that identification of such subgroups will lead to more appropriate treatment methodologies for these individuals.

References

Arndt, W., Shelton, R., Johnson, A., & Furr, M. Identification and description of homogeneous subgroups within a sample of misarticulating children. *Journal of Speech and Hearing Research*, 1977, *20*, 263-292.

Bankson, N. Assessment of the effectiveness of articulation therapy. *Journal of National Student Speech and Hearing Association*, 1974, *2*, 13-21.

Carter, E.T., & Buck, M.W. Prognostic testing for functional articulation disorders among children in the first grade. *Journal of Speech and Hearing Disorders*, 1958, *23*, 124-133.

Compton, A. Generative studies of children's phonological disorders. *Journal of Speech and Hearing Disorders*, 1970, *35*, 315-339.

Costello, J.M. Programmed instruction. *Journal of Speech and Hearing Disorders*, 1977, *42*, 3-28.

Costello, J., & Onstine, J. The modification of multiple articulation errors based on distinctive feature theory. *Journal of Speech and Hearing Disorders*, 1976, *41*, 199-215.

DuBois, E., & Bernthal, J. A comparison of three methods for obtaining articulatory responses. *Journal of Speech and Hearing Disorders*, 1978, *43*, 295-305.

Elbert, M., & McReynolds, L.V. An experimental analysis of misarticulating children's generalization. *Journal of Speech and Hearing Research,* 1978, *21,* 136-150.

Elbert, M., Shelton, R.L., & Arndt, W.B. A task for evaluation of articulation change. *Journal of Speech and Hearing Research,* 1967, *10,* 281-288.

Emerick, L., & Hatten, J. *Diagnosis and evaluation in speech pathology.* Englewood Cliffs, N.J.: Prentice-Hall, 1974

Farquhar, M.A. Prognostic value of imitative and auditory discrimination tests. *Journal of Speech and Hearing Disorders,* 1961, *26,* 342-347.

Fisher, H., & Logemann, J. *The Fisher-Logemann Test of Articulation Competence.* Boston: Houghton Mifflin, 1971.

Frisch, G.R., & Handler, L. A neuropsychological investigation of "functional disorders of speech articulation." *Journal of Speech and Hearing Research,* 1974, *17,* 432-445.

Ingram, D. *Phonological disability in children.* New York: American Elsevier, 1976.

Khan, L.M.L. A review of 16 major phonological processes. *Language, Speech, and Hearing Services in Schools,* 1982, *13,* 77-85.

Lapko, L., & Bankson, N. Relationship between auditory discrimination, articulation stimulability and consistency of misarticulation. *Perceptual and Motor Skills,* 1975, *40,* 171-177.

Milisen, R. and Associates. The disorder of articulation: a systematic clinical and experimental approach. *Journal of Speech and Hearing Disorders, Monograph Supplement 4,* 1954.

McDonald, E.T. *Articulation testing and treatment: A sensory-motor approach.* Pittsburgh: Stanwix House, 1964.

McReynolds, L. Articulation generalization during articulation training. *Language and Speech,* 1972, *15,* 149-155.

McReynolds, L., & Bennett, S. Distinctive feature generalization in articulation training. *Journal of Speech and Hearing Disorders,* 1972, *37,* 462-470.

McReynolds, L.V., & Kearns, K. *Single-subject experimental designs.* Baltimore: University Park Press, 1982.

Panagos, J.M. Persistence of the open syllable reinterpreted as a symptom of language disorder. *Journal of Speech and Hearing Disorders,* 1974, *39,* 23-31.

Powers, M.H. Functional disorders of articulation—Symptomatology and etiology. In L. E. Travis (Ed.), *Handbook of speech pathology.* New York: Appleton-Century-Crofts, 1957.

Prins, D. Analysis of correlations among various articulatory deviation. *Journal of Speech and Hearing Research,* 1962a, *5,* 152-160.

Renfrew, C. The persistence of the open syllable in defective articulation. *Journal of Speech and Hearing Disorders,* 1966, *31,* 370-373.

Report of the 27th Annual Conference of the Milbank Memorial Fund. New York: Hoeber-Harper, 1952.

Shelton, R.L. Disorders of articulation. In P.H. Skinner & R.L. Shelton (Eds.), *Speech, language and hearing.* Reading, Mass.: Addison-Wesley, 1978.

Shelton, R.L., Elbert, M., & Arndt, W.B. A task for evaluation of articulation change: II: Comparison of task scores during baseline and lesson series testing. *Journal of Speech and Hearing Research,* 1967, *10,* 578-585.

Shelton, R.L., & McReynolds, L.V. Functional articulation disorders: Preliminaries to therapy. In *Speech and language: Advances in basic research and practice.* New York: Academic Press, 1979.

Shriberg, L.D., & Kwiatkowski, J. *Natural process analysis.* New York: John Wiley, 1980.

Sommers, R.K., Leiss, R., Delp, M., Gerber, A., Fundrella, O., Smith, R., Revucky, M., Ellis, D., & Haley, V. Factors related to the effectiveness of articulation therapy for kindergarten, first, and second grade children. *Journal of Speech and Hearing Research,* 1967, *10,* 428-437.

Stampe, D. A dissertation on natural phonology. Unpublished doctoral dissertation, University of Chicago, 1973.

Travis, L.E. *Speech pathology.* New York: Appleton, 1931.

Van Riper, C. *Speech correction: Principles and methods.* Englewood Cliffs, N.J.: Prentice-Hall, 1939.

West, R., Ansberry, M., & Carr, A. *The rehabilitation of speech.* New York: Harper & Brothers, 1937.

Winitz, H. *From syllable to conversation.* Baltimore: University Park Press, 1975.

Richard G. Schwartz

The Phonologic System: Normal Acquisition

The translation of Jakobson's 1941 theory in 1968 seems to have been the point from which all recent advances in normal phonologic development emanate. The changes in our views of phonologic acquisition closely parallel the recent changes in our views of other aspects of language acquisition. Rather than viewing acquisition as simply the mastery of inventories of units (i.e., sounds, words, sentences), we have come to think of it as the development of a system in which units are but a single component. In reviewing these recent advances, some theoretical perspective is necessary as a framework for a subsequent discussion of recent issues which have arisen and of the information we have acquired over the last decade concerning phonologic acquisition.

Theoretical Advances

An acceptable theory of child phonology must simultaneously account for a number of aspects of children's speech sound behavior, including both the progression of development and adult phonology, since that is the child's ultimate achievement. Additionally a theory should: (1) account for the acquisition of phonology in any language, (2) be consistent with the amount and type of input received by the child, (3) be consistent with the time typically required for acquisition, and (4) be consistent with the child's abilities in other areas at given points in development (Pinker, 1979).

An ideal theory would also, at least indirectly, account for developmental and acquired disorders of phonology. These represent rather stringent and extensive requirements. Thus, it is not surprising that no current theory of acquisition meets all these requirements. In spite of this, a review seems in order to determine where we currently stand and what may be on the horizon in terms of a theoretical framework for better understanding of phonologic acquisition and disorders.

Structuralists

Jakobson (1968) viewed phonologic acquisition as involving two distinctly different periods, prelinguistic babbling and linguistic production. More recent observations and investigations have indicated that there are differences between these two periods. However, they have also revealed relationships between babbling and linguistic productions contrary to Jakobson's suggestion. It appears that at least in some respects developments in linguistic productions may depend upon developments during the prelinguistic period.

The second aspect of Jakobson's theory concerns what he viewed as the core of phonologic development—the acquisition of a phonemic system. He maintained that the child proceeds through an invariant, universal sequence, governed by a hierarchy of feature oppositions. The developmental sequence is based on a principle of maximum contrast with development moving from an undifferentiated to a differentiated and stratified system of phonemic contrasts. It is extremely important to note that the theory deals with the acquisition of contrasts, not individual sounds. The first contrast throught to be acquired is between what is termed an optimum consonant and an optimum vowel, which contrast maximally (i.e., differ in many features rather than few features). Development proceeds with the acquisition of contrasts that are progressively less distinct in terms of the number of features that differ. Jackobson argued that at any given point in time a child has his own system, distinct from the adult system. However, the child's system is based on an unfolding of the contrast hierarchy rather than active acquisition on the part of the child.

The final aspect of Jakobson's theory involves what is commonly referred to as the regression hypothesis. This entails the notion that in an acquired phonologic disorder, such as in aphasia, the order of loss will be the mirror image of the order of acquisition. Those contrasts acquired latest will be lost first.

Moskowitz (1970, 1973) has added to and modified Jakobson's proposals by considering children's more general recognition of units of speech. She argued that children only gradually recognize and identify smaller units of speech, beginning with the sentence and proceeding to the word-syllable, word and syllable. Recognition of the distinction between word and syllable is a significant attainment and depends upon reduplication (e.g., [wɔwɔ] for *water*). Thus, the child realizes that a syllable is a separable component of a word. Contrary to Jakobson's position, Moskowitz argued that children acquire contrasts between syllables rather than phonemes. This is consistent with more recent views concerning the psychological reality of the syllable in phonologic acquisition (Bell & Hooper, 1978). Finally, Moskowitz observed in diary data reported by Leopold (1947) that some words may be initially acquired independent of a child's phonologic system. For instance, at a time when she was not producing consonant clusters or prevocalic or intervocalic voiceless consonants, Hildegard Leopold first produced the word *pretty* as [prʌti] and then as [prIti]. Over a period of approximately 6 months, her production of the word gradually deteriorated until it was consistent with the way she was producing similar words ([bIdi] for *pretty*). This observation is important for two reasons. It suggests that children have their own phonologic system into which some new words may be only gradually assimilated. Additionally, it demonstrates that the "errors" young children make in producing words are not solely attributable to motoric or perceptual limitations, since at one point in time the child is able to produce the word accurately.

Although these theories have made significant contributions in their focus on the acquisition or loss of a phonologic *system,* they appear to have many weaknesses (Ferguson & Garnica, 1975; Kiparsky & Menn, 1977). First, because of the limited nature of children's early lexicons, there are few minimal pairs (e.g., [kIt vs. bIt]) and many gaps in the sounds produced. Consequently, it is difficult to determine whether or not contrasts are actually present. Second, in spite of Moskowitz's focus on the syllable, the theories are still largely segmental in nature. Thus, they are unable to explain aspects of acquisition and behavior which involve larger units (e.g., words). Finally, since the theories place so much emphasis on the acquisition of contrast, many developmental phenomena such as phonological idioms and developmental error patterns remain unexplained.

Natural Phonology

Natural phonology has led to a somewhat different view of the substance and nature of phonologic acquisition (Stampe, 1973). It has served as the basis for a good deal of recent work concerning normal and disordered development. In the course of these applications, Stampe's theory has been modified and on occasion misrepresented. Consequently, some clarification seems in order.

Several premises form the basis of this theory. First, Stampe maintains that children's perceptions are completely accurate from the outset. Thus, the basis for a child's production is the accurate adult form of the word which is stored as a perceptual representation. All aspects of a child's "errors" are attributable to motor production abilities (e.g., *dog,* child's representation [dɔg], child's production [dɔ]). Second, a set of innate processes which reflect the limitations of the human speech mechanism determine the child's productions. These processes serve to eliminate contrast by leading to the merger of classes of sounds or word forms (e.g., both nasal and oral sounds are produced as oral; forms with and without final consonants are produced as forms without final consonants). Because these processes are supposed to be a natural reflection of the human speech mechanism, they are viewed as universal. This also means that the direction of sound class mergers are predetermined. For example, fricatives may be changed to stops, or obstruents (fricatives, stops, and affricates) may be devoiced, but the reverse of these changes does not typically occur. Evidence for these processes comes from their occurrence across languages, evidence concerning the structure and physiology of the speech mechanism, and inferences regarding ease of articulation.

At the outset of development, processes occur without restrictions of any sort; they are unordered and unlimited. Thus, there are no phonemic distinctions. The child's task in phonologic acquisition is to overcome the limitations caused by these processes by suppression (complete elimination), limitation (allowing them to occur only in certain contexts), or by order ing multiple processes (applying only one of two or more possible processes to a word or words, thereby "blocking" the occurrence of other processes). Individual variations may arise as the result of different courses a child may take in eliminating processes. In doing this, the child is not only overcoming processes, but is also resolving conflicts between processes (e.g., changing all nasal sounds to oral sounds versus changing oral sounds to nasal sounds when nasal sounds precede or follow them). What remains after the child completes acquisition are processes characteristic of that language.

Another important premise of Stampe's proposal concerns the distinction between rules and processes. The basic difference is that rules are learned while processes are innate. In addition, while processes may become limited in the contexts in which they apply, they cannot have formal morphological or lexical restrictions. Rules, though, can have these kinds of limitations, as in the case of velar softening in English which changes words like *electric* to *electricity.* Finally, rules cannot be based on phonetic or physiologic motivations.

Like Jakobson, Stampe maintains that phonologic acquisition is essentially predetermined. According to Jakobson, the phonologic system unfolds. However, according to Stampe, the inborn processes are discarded and the system remains. Neither really credits the child with an active role in constructing a phonologic system.

Stampe's proposal makes an important contribution in its attempt to explain the patterns of children's errors and in proposing a source for such errors. The weakest point in the proposal, however, concerns Stampe's insistence on the accuracy of perception and the use of the adult form as the child's representation. While there is no doubt that by the time the child begins to use language he can discriminate many or most of the speech sounds of English, that does not mean that a given word will be accurately perceived or represented. Additionally, although Stampe's distinction between rules and processes may be theoretically clear (there is some disagreement on this point), in practice it is not always clear. To date, no universally agreed-upon set of natural processes has been constructed. Ease of articulation has always been, and continues to be, an elusive notion. Furthermore, there appear to be patterns of errors in children's speech that are not natural or reflective of the limits of the speech mechanism. It is not clear from Stampe's proposal how such patterns should be regarded. Since they are errors, they would not be regarded as rules. Since they are not natural, the use of the term "processes" as Stampe describes it would seem inappropriate. Finally, other theorists have argued that children play a more active role in constructing a phonologic system.

Constructivists

Several more recent proposals have involved a very different perspective concerning the nature of phonologic acquisition (Ferguson & Macken, 1980; Kiparsky & Menn, 1977; Schwartz & Leonard, 1982; Schwartz & Prelock, 1982; Waterson, 1971; 1981; Menn, Note 1). In contrast to the preceding theories, these proposals all view the child as actively constructing a phonologic system.

Waterson's (1971) prosodic theory differs from previous proposals in its emphasis on individual differences and the role of developing perceptual abilities in determining the nature of children's early productions. According to this proposal, children selectively attend to adult utterances that are in some way highly salient. The focus of the child's perception is on a limited set of salient features of a word. Based on this set, the child constructs a representation, termed a "schema", which serves as the basis for his productions. A given schema may represent more than a single word, thus explaining some of the patterns in children's early speech. For example, the schema for the words *finger* and *window* may involve a palatal or alveolar nasal plus a vowel in a reduplicated form (two identical or nearly identical syllables), such as [ɲẽːɲẽ/nIːni:] for *finger* and [ɲeːɲeː] for *window*. Similarities and differences across children arise as the result of similarities and differences in input to children. More recently, Waterson (1981) has expanded her proposal to include one level of representation involving possible phonetic patterns of the language extracted and synthesized from perceptually salient features. Additionally, a second level of representation involves patterns specific to words along with their meanings. This model links input to these two levels of representation and ultimately to output.

Menn (Note 1) argues for a somewhat different view, emphasizing the role of output or articulatory constraints. Rules also seem to play a role in this model, but serve as a means by which the child can observe an output constraint. For example, a young child may have a constraint such as, "Don't produce any words with more than one consonant, unless the consonants are the same." A number of rules can help to keep the child within this constraint, such as eliminating consonants (e.g., *dog* [dɔ]) or whole syllables *kitty* [kI]), changing one of the consonants so that the consonants are the same (*boat* [boʊbo]), or taking one syllable of a word and duplicating it (*water* [wɔwɔ]). Additionally, this model involves a number of levels of phonologic representation and behavior including output, articulatory instructions, output lexicon (production store), input lexicon (recognition store), and an overall level of abstracted underlying forms. These levels are related by different types of phonologic rules. Similar to Waterson, and in contrast to Stampe, this proposal involves the notion that the child's underlying representation of a word is not necessarily just a copy of correct adult production.

A more recent proposal along the same lines suggests a more balanced view of perception and production in children's phonologic representation and acquisition (Schwartz & Leonard, 1982). Additionally, this proposal considers the role of a child's cognitive abilities in determining the type of representation attributed. The model proposed involves three general levels: phonetic, representational, and organizational. The phonetic level is comprised of two components: perceptual and motoric. The perceptual component involves the basic processes of audition, discrimination, and identification of a signal as speech. The motoric component is responsible for the execution of the motor movements for speech production.

The representational level also includes a perception component and a separate production component. The perception component is comprised of schemas, which are representations of the units of speech that the child has segmented from the adult's speech. While at the outset these may be rather large units, for most children at least some schemas represent words by about the age of 10 months. These, then, are the first words comprehended by the child. During the same period of time, the child is constructing schemes, or plans, for motor action. These also are initially large unstable units as characterized by the child's babbling, but are gradually stabilized and refined so that they, too, are word-like in structure. At both levels, perception and production begin as completely independent systems and maintain some degree of autonomy after acquisition. After the child has constructed a number of schemes and schemas, development proceeds with additions to these repertoires and coordinations between existing schemes and schemas. Once a schema is coordinated with a scheme, the child can both meaningfully produce and comprehend a word. Additionally, this coordination increases the likelihood that a child will attempt a given word.

This is essentially the whole of a child's phonologic representation during the period of sensorimotor intelligence (0-18 months), which roughly corresponds to the period of the first 50 words. During this period, the child, according to Piaget (1962), has limited representational abilities and is lacking any overall representations. Thus, the model is consistent with the child's overall cognitive abilities and with the observations that phonologic behavior during this period is variable, unsystematic, and apparently word-based. Once the child reaches the end of the sensorimotor period, he is able to construct overall representations at the organizational level. This leads to more stable phonologic behavior and more systematic behavior in his simplifications of sounds, syllables, and words. Attempts have been made to describe a number of developmental phenomena such as phonologic idioms and selectivity within the context of this model. Additionally, its implications for differential diagnosis and remediation of speech sound disorders have been specified (Schwartz & Prelock, 1982).

There is clearly a good deal of overlap among these three proposals and others (Ferguson & Macken, 1980; Macken, 1979). While a number of differences remain to be resolved (e.g., number of levels), they seem to represent a significant departure from previous proposals. In general, they are broader in their perspective and, thus, seem better able to deal with a wider range of facts concerning both child and adult phonology. They seem to be more generally consistent with the criteria mentioned earlier, such as time span of acquisition (without falling back on the notion of innateness), the type and nature of input to the child, and consistency with other aspects of development. Also, the last model may have some explanatory value for disordered development. Careful examination of these proposals reveals specific and testable predictions concerning the nature and progression of phonologic acquisition. One general weakness in all of these proposals is their failure to deal with the specific nature and development of motoric and perceptual mechanisms and processes. However, more recently some proposals have begun to address these issues (e.g., Locke, 1979a;

MacNeilage, 1980). Some integration of cognition-oriented and mechanism-oriented proposals may ultimately be required.

These advances in theory are exciting in that they suggest that we are close to having one or more detailed frameworks within which we can examine a wide range of aspects of children's phonologies. The significance of this should not be underestimated. Even though most theories are ultimately proved false, the existence of a theoretical framework can facilitate systematic experimentation (including therapeutic intervention) and consequently, in some cases, a more rapid acquisition of knowledge. While we await the further refinement of these proposals, we can consider the current empirical issues and recent advances in the data available concerning phonologic acquisition.

Current Issues

A number of issues remain unresolved even after many years and, thus, are not new. Others have simply been reformulated because of new information concerning acquisition. Finally, some issues are genuinely new, arising from recent investigations of acquisition. The purpose of this section is to provide a brief listing of those that seem most fundamental and which will consequently be addressed in the subsequent review of phonologic acquisition.

The issues seem to fall into four major areas: the nature of production; the nature of perception; the relationship between production and perception; and the relationships among phonologic acquisition, cognitive development, and other aspects of language acquisition. Issues concerning production include the most appropriate way of describing the nature of children's productions and their relation to the adult target form (features versus sounds versus syllables, versus various types of rules), the description of the course of development, the basis of developmental errors, the nature and sources of variability in production, individual differences in the course of acquisition, and the description and development of contrast. Because of less research activity in the area of perception, the issues have remained more general. Basically, they concern the nature, developmental progression, and description of perceptual abilities. An issue related to both perception and production concerns the roles of input and linguistic perception in phonologic acquisition.

The relationship between perception and production in phonologic acquisition is another topic of interest. The issues center on the developmental sequence in these two components (i.e., whether perception precedes production, follows it, or both) and the reciprocal influence of perception and production (e.g., whether production errors reflect errors in perception).

More recently, we have been increasingly aware of the fact that phonologic acquisition and behavior do not occur in isolation. Instead, other aspects of language (syntax, semantics, pragmatics) and cognitive abilities appear to influence and are influenced by phonologic abilities. Additionally, many aspects of communicative and cognitive development appear to be interrelated. The specific nature and extent of these relationships is an issue of some importance.

Although few if any of these issues have been resolved, recent research has greatly expanded our knowledge in these areas. A review of the current state of our knowledge base follows. Since these issues take somewhat different forms when applied to different levels of development, the remaining portion of the chapter is organized in a developmental sequence.

Prelinguistic Period

The prelinguistic period of development includes the ages from birth to approximately 12 months, when true words first appear. It should be noted that in many children this period may overlap with the beginning of the linguistic period (i.e., babbling may continue when real words emerge).

Perception

Over the last decade, interest in infants' perception of speech has grown at a phenomenally rapid rate. We have gone from a point of having little specific information concerning infant perceptual abilities to a point of having a large body of information concerning these abilities. Most recently, this has led to a shift in issues considered from simply the "what" of prelinguistic perception to examinations of its origins, its developmental progression in this period, the roles of input and experience, and the actual process of perception.

Three types of methodologies have been employed. Two of these procedures are based on some type of orienting response to a novel stimulus. They also depend upon the fact that infants will become habituated with repeated presentations of stimuli they perceive as similar. The first procedure has been termed the high-amplitude sucking procedure. It involves providing the infant with a non-nutritive nipple to be sucked. After a baseline sucking rate is established, the infant is presented with a sound (e.g., "ba") each time sucking occurs. Initially, because of an orienting response, the sucking rate increases to a peak, and then, because of habituation, begins to level off. At this point, infants in an experimental group are presented with a new sound (e.g., "pa") each time they suck, while infants in a control group continue to hear the same sound (i.e., "ba"). If the sucking rate of infants in the experimental group increases (dishabituates) relative to the rate for infants in the control group, this serves as evidence that the infants discriminate the two different sounds. More recently, an alternating pattern of the old and new stimuli has been employed to reduce the memory requirements of the procedure. This has been used with children ranging in age from 0 to 4 months.

The second procedure, the heart rate paradigm, involves presenting a stimulus (e.g., "ba") and measuring the infant's heart rate. In this case the infant does not control the presentation of the stimulus, and orienting is measured by a decrease in the heart rate. The initial stimulus is presented repeatedly in blocks until the child habituates and no longer exhibits an orienting response. Then a new stimulus is presented (e.g., "pa"). If the heart rate decreases, the infant is assumed to discriminate between the two sounds. More recently, Leavitt, Brown, Morse, and Graham (1976) modified this procedure by decreasing the interval between blocks so that memory requirements were reduced. These procedures have been used with infants from about 1 to 8 months of age.

The final procedure, visually reinforced infant speech discrimination, is an adaptation of an audiological procedure used to test children's hearing in a free field. One stimulus (e.g., "ba") is presented repeatedly as a background. Periodically, for a fixed period of time, this sound is changed to a second sound (e.g., "pa"). When this change occurs and the infant's head turns toward the sound, head turning is reinforced by the activation of a toy (e.g., a lit monkey banging cymbals). Subsequently, consistent head turns toward the reinforcer in anticipation of its activation during stimulus change, but not during periods when the change doesn't occur, indicate discrimination. This procedure has been altered to a perceptual constancy paradigm (Kuhl, 1976; 1977; 1980), which allows investigation of the boundaries of sound categories, rather than simply discrimination of two sounds. These procedures have been employed with infants in the 6- to 18-month-age range and may be applicable to somewhat older children as well.

To date, these procedures have yielded a large body of information concerning what infants can and cannot discriminate (Eilers, 1980). They have also been employed in examining a number of issues concerning the perceptual abilities of infants (Eilers, 1980). It appears that, while some aspects of these abilities are innate, other aspects may be dependent on experience or involve a complex interaction of environmental and genetic factors (Aslin & Pisoni, 1980). There also seem to be some rather interesting relationships between characteristics of adult speech to infants and infant perceptual abilities (e.g., Williams, Note 2). For example, infants seem to be able to discriminate differences in place in intervocalic position only when there is a period of silence during closure. Adults seem to make this modification in their speech to young children.

Some findings have been surprising in terms of our prior expectations. It has long been commonplace knowledge that infants may respond differentially to suprasegmental features before they respond in the same way to segmental features. While infants do respond differentially to some varying prosodic cues (Morse, 1972; Spring & Dale, 1977; Kaplan, Note 3), this may not always be the case. It appears that when segmental differences (e.g., /i/ vs. /a/) compete with suprasegmental differences (e.g., pitch differences), children do not evidence discrimination of pitch differences (Kuhl, 1976). Nor is there evidence that stress facilitates segmental discriminations (Jusczyk & Thompson, 1978; Williams & Bush, 1978). Equally surprising is the finding that—contrary to the suggestion that fricatives are among the later acquired sounds in production because they are not discriminated early in development due to late myelination of the auditory (VIII) nerve (Salus & Salus, 1974)—infants are able to discriminate a great many fricatives (Eilers, 1980).

Most investigations of infant speech perception have understandably focused on auditory aspects of these abilities. However, Kuhl and Meltzoff (1982) have employed an infant preference procedure in examining perception as a bimodal phenomenon involving both audition and vision. They found that when infants (18 to 20 weeks of age) are presented simultaneously with film loops of a face producing an /i/ and the same face producing an /a/ along with an auditory presentation of one of these vowels, they spend a longer period of time looking at the face corresponding to the vowel heard. Even more intriguing are their findings that when certain spectral information (i.e., formant frequencies) is removed from the auditory presentation, the infants do not demonstrate a preference for one face over the other. This suggests that, even at this early age, infants are responsive to a relationship between facial configurations or movements and certain auditory spectral characteristics. It also raises the possibility of some general, early link between audition and motor movements for speech. The subsequent translation of this information from infants' perceptions of others to their own motor movements may prove to be an important factor in the development of both speech perception and production.

The exact nature of the relationship between prelinguistic perception and linguistic perception and production remains unclear. However, it seems likely that, given the methods and information currently available, the beginning of an understanding of this relationship is relatively close at hand. For individual children we may ultimately be able to draw some inferences regarding later linguistic abilities from an examination of prelinguistic perception.

Production

We have known for some time that infants' vocalizations start out exclusively as reflexive and vegetative and gradually expand to include nonreflexive and nonvegetative sounds (i.e., speech). Additionally, it has long been known that infants proceed through a series of periods of speech production from cooing (predominantly back vowel-like sounds with some back consonants), to babbling (a wider variety of consonants and vowel strings along with variation in stress and intonation), to jargon (greater control over stress and intonation), to meaningful speech. Finally, as a result of the work of Orvis Irwin and his associates (see Winitz, 1969, for a complete review), we know that, in terms of the specific sounds infants produce, there is a progression from a low proportion of front and high proportion of back consonant-like sounds to a higher proportion of front sounds. Moreover, there is an opposite trend in vowel-like sounds, with a slight increase in back sounds over time.

In the last decade, however, through the use of instrumental analyses in addition to perceptually based examinations (i.e., phonetic transcription), our knowledge of infant vocalization has markedly expanded. The work of several investigators (Stark, 1980; Oller, Note 4; Zlatin, Note 5) seems to generally agree that there are five stages in the development of speech production prior to the emergence of true words or word-like forms.

The first stage begins at birth and lasts from 4 to 6 weeks. Vocalizations during this period are primarily reflexive, including crying, fussing, and primative vegetative sounds. Stark (1980) has characterized some of these sounds as exhibiting the first combination of vocalic and suprasegmental features of crying and consonantal features of vegetative sounds. Nasal and liquid sounds seem to result when the mouth is open during crying, the tongue returns to a position in opposition to the soft palate, and subsequent closure occurs while vocalization continues. There also appear to be some nonreflexive sounds produced during this period. These seem to be predominantly what Oller (Note 4) has termed quasi-resonant nuclei (QRN). Generally, these are vocalizations that involve normal phonation but do not involve clear contrast between an open and closed vocal tract and thus do not reflect the full range of resonance of the vocal cavity. Acoustically, QRNs are identified by a broad range of various low amplitude resonances predominantly below 1200 Hz (Oller, Note 4). Phonetically, these sounds are usually syllabic nasals ([ŋ] as in [bʌtṇ]) or high-mid, unrounded (the mouth is usually nearly closed), nasalized vowels (e.g., something like [Ĩ]). There may also be some seemingly random occurrences of fully resonant nuclei (FRN) which more closely resemble vowels or coos. QRNs, however, seem to predominate even into the next stage and are the most frequent vocalization during the first 4 months (Oller, 1980).

The second stage seems to cover the period from approximately 6 weeks to 4 months and to be generally characterized by cooing and laughter. More nasal consonant elements occur, and voicing may be combined with obstruent (stop, fricative, and affricate) sounds that were previously produced vegetatively without voicing. An important aspect of this is the infant's ability to produce voicing in nondistress states. These "goo" sounds have been observed to be repetitive, and perhaps reflect greater control on the part of the infant. Specifically, at around 3 months, greater control is gained over the tongue and lips which may give rise to some bilabial nasal sounds during play.

Further support for the assumption that infants have at least some control over aspects of their vocalizations during this period comes from early research concerning infant vocal conditioning (Rheingold, Gewirtz, & Ross, 1959; Weisberg, 1963). It has since been recognized that there are some serious weaknesses in this research (Bloom, 1979). However, there is evidence from more recent, better controlled research, that 3-month-old infants do respond differentially (in terms of the pattern or distribution rather than the frequency of vocalization) to contingent and noncontingent stimulation (Bloom, 1977; Bloom & Esposito, 1975). The differential responsiveness takes the form of differing pause times which occur prior to the infants' vocalizations following each type of stimulation. Further research is needed to determine the extent of infants' control over the content of such vocalizations.

Laughter may first appear at around 4 months. It is an important development because it often occurs in the course of interactions. As Stark noted, this involves rapid alteration of voiced and voiceless vocalization as well as a voiced inspiration.

Stage 3 has been referred to as exploratory phonetic behavior (Zlatin, Note 5), vocal play (Stark, 1980), and expansion (Oller, 1980). All three terms describe general characteristics of this period. By this time (4 to 7 months), infants have gained sufficient control over their speech mechanism to allow play with a wide range of speech sounds. Included among the vocalizations of this period are FRNs, vowel-like sounds with resonances above 1200 HZ (Oller, Note 4; Doyle, Note 6), raspberries (Doyle, Note 6), squeaking (Stark, 1980; Zlatin Laufer & Horii, 1977; Doyle, Note 6), growling (Stark, 1980; Zlatin Laufer & Horii, 1977), yelling and sequences of alternating vocalization on egressive and ingressive air (Zlatin Laufer & Horii, 1977; Oller, Note 4). Perhaps the most important aspect of this period is that infants seem to begin to sequence and resequence series of sounds in novel ways and begin to insert pauses into these sequences (Stark, 1980). This development leads to the marginal babbling at the end of this stage. Marginal babbling involves sequences of open vocal tract (FRN) and closed vocal tract sounds. The consistency, repetitiveness, and rigid timing of later babbling is not yet present.

Investigators report a fourth stage, reduplicated or canonical babbling, which lasts from approximately 6 to 10 months. This babbling includes consonant-like sounds and vowel-like sounds (FRNs) arranged in a rather standard timing sequence (e.g., CV or VC). In one sense, the infant seems more limited in this period than the previous period. In concentrated periods, infants seem to produce one specific syllable (e.g., *bababababa*). While many vocalizations are in this consonant-vowel reduplicated form, others (e.g., *imi*) may not be (Oller, 1980). As Stark noted, during this period children are increasingly likely to vocalize while looking at an adult rather than while handling objects or performing actions as in previous periods.

The final period is comprised of nonreduplicated or variegated babbling. The same types of timing sequences or alternations of consonant-like and vowel-like sounds are present. However, the sound content of the sequences is no longer restricted to a single sound or syllable. Additionally, other syllable sequences (CVC, VC) may appear. This period is also character-ized by the infant's more consistent control over stress and intonation. This leads to what has been traditionally referred to as jargon. Finally, this period may overlap with the beginnings of word-form production (see below).

With these advances, we now know a good deal about the general pro-gression and many specific details concerning what constitutes normal develop-ment. Furthermore, the fact that there is at least some relationship be-tween prelinguistic and linguistic productions seems well established (Oller, Wieman, Doyle, & Ross, 1975). These productions share many common characteristics. However, the ability to predict the specific nature of linguistic vocalizations from prelinguistic vocalizations has not yet been achieved. There are a number of other issues which remain unresolved.

While we focus on the surface nature of these vocalizations, there may be more general characteristics (pitch, vocal quality, voicing, resonance, timing, respiration, amplitude) which may provide direct evidence of the infant's motor speech capacity specific to certain components of the speech mechanism (Oller, 1980). The influence of the changing physical characteristics of the infant speech mechanism, linguistic experience and input, and the increasing association of vocalizations with objects and situa-tions all represent issues for further research (Kent, 1981; Netsell, 1981). As we learn more about this period and its relation to linguistic produc-tions, we come closer to understanding the nature of speech production development. Additionally, it may mean that we can evaluate the normalcy of prelinguistic productions.

Transition

The notion that prior to the production of real, recognizable words, children produce vocalizations that only superficially resemble words is not new. A number of diary studies (e.g., Halliday, 1975; Leopold, 1947) have included observations of isolated, segmental vocalizations (vowels, syllables, syllabic consonants) that have some relationship to context (i.e., meaning). More recently, such vocalizations have been described in greater detail (Carter, 1975; 1979; Dore, Franklin, Miller, & Ramer, 1976; Menn, Note 7). They have been referred to varyingly as sensorimotor morphemes, phonetically consistent forms (PCFs), and protowords. In general, these units are unlike babbling in that they are isolable, bounded by pauses, occur with sufficient frequency so as to be recognizable, seem to be related to some recurring aspect of context, and seem to be more phonetically stable than variegated babbling. They are not quite true words in that they are less clearly related to recurring aspects of context (i.e., they are not coherent in their use), and they are less phonetically consistent than true words. Menn employed these two criteria in describing protowords and added the criterion that protowords are less autonomous than true words in that they are tied to an action or a routine.

These forms are perhaps best explained by example. One type of PCF is illustrated by the observation of a child who said [gægi], [gaga], [gagi], [əgagi] on various occasions while chewing crayons, being dressed, and handling a toy (Dore et al., 1976), the common thread here being pleasurable affect on the part of the child. Carter reported the production of an initial [m] followed by a variety of vowels as an apparent request for an object along with a reaching gesture. Protowords, as described by Menn (Note 7), seem somewhat different than most sensorimotor morphemes or PCFs in that they apparently are not based on affect or internal states and they seem to be more object or action specific. Jacob, the one child studied by Menn, produced various versions of [ioio] while watching tape reels go around and while making objects rotate. It is clearly more externally coherent than the first example given above. Protowords have only been observed in one child, who did not exhibit anything more closely resembling PCFs. Consequently, it is unclear whether there is a developmental progression from sensorimotor morphemes or PCFs to protowords to true words. Phonetically consistent forms and protowords may simply prove to be two alternative transitions between babbling and words. Not surprisingly, these preword forms seem to be related both to babbling and to later words. Menn noted that [ioio] appeared first in strings of babble before it was produced as an isolated form. Some true words (e.g., *mine, my, more*) have been traced back to sensorimotor morphemes. There is still a need, however, for more detailed information concerning these relationships.

The most important aspect of these findings is the fact that there are structures which seem to bridge the gap between babbling and true words. Words then develop gradually rather than suddenly. These preword forms may be the child's first linguistic forms used communicatively. The vocalizations which Bates, Camaioni, and Volterra (1975) noted in children's performance of early communicative acts are likely to have been some type of preword form.

The Period of Prerepresentational Phonology

Although the dividing line between preword forms and true words is often somewhat fuzzy, at about 12 months of age children begin to produce their first true words. This represents the beginning of what various investigators have termed the period of the first 50 words (e.g., Nelson, 1973). Although in one study of phonologic development (Ferguson & Farwell, 1975) the decision to focus on children at this level of development was arbitrary, Ingram (1976) has characterized this as a separable period in phonologic acquisition. The basis for this argument is that it is roughly concomitant with the period of sensorimotor intelligence and the period of single word utterances. At around 18 months most children have acquired their 50th word, have begun using two-word utterances and, perhaps more importantly, have attained Stage VI of sensorimotor intelligence. Prior to this stage, children do not have a well-developed representational system according to Piaget (1962). This means that mental representations are isolated, often based on immediate perceptions, and somewhat unstable. Additionally, during this period children do not appear to have any overall representations. One implication for phonologic behavior during this period is that children are likely to be variable in their productions of given words because of unstable representations (e.g., *dog* may be produced on various occasions as [dɔ], [dɔg], [gɔ], [dɔd]). Additionally, because they have no overall representation, children will not exhibit a system of consistently applied rules or processes in their productions, nor will they exhibit a *system* of sound contrasts. In a recent investigation, Schwartz and Folger (1977) compared the phonologies of children who had attained Stage VI of sensorimotor intelligence with those of children who had not yet attained this stage. The pre-Stage VI children evidenced significantly more variability in word production, fewer systematic developmental errors, and fewer systematic contrasts. The authors suggested that prior to attainment of Stage VI of sensorimotor intelligence, it may be inappropriate to credit the child with a set of processes or rules (i.e., mental operations), and a system of sound contrasts. Additionally, rather than equating the boundary of this period with the acquisition of the 50th word (vocabulary size did not explain these differences), it seemed more appropriate to distinguish between representational and prerepresentational phonology.

A number of investigations have revealed some more specific facts regarding phonologic behavior during this general period (see Ingram, 1976 for a review of some early diary studies such as Leopold, 1947; and more recently Leonard, Newhoff, & Mesalam, 1980; Shibamoto & Olmsted, 1978; Menn, Note 7). In general, this period appears to be characterized by individual differences, variability, lack of sound contrasts, and the absence of consistent rules or processes.

Individual differences

One of the more striking observations in light of previous assumptions of universal orders of acquisition has been the seemingly large range of individual differences between children. These differences seem to center on two aspects of phonology: the sounds produced and the characteristics of the adult words attempted. The results of early investigations indicated that such differences were prevalent, but shed little light on their actual range. More recently, Leonard, Newhoff, and Mesalam (1980) examined the word-initial sounds (phones) of 10 children ranging in age from 1;4 to 1;10, for the purpose of specifying the extent of individual differences. In general they found that certain sounds were notably absent across most subjects [ɵ], [tʃ], [ð], [f], [I], [dʒ], [z], and [r]. Among the sounds produced by all or most subjects were [m], [b], [d], [kʰ], [g], [pʰ], [w]. Five of the children produced [n] and [h]. The remaining consonants were produced by only 2 or 3 children. It should be noted that while some of these represent accurate productions of target sounds, others represent errors. Additionally, in some cases sounds may be freely substituted for one another (see below). Thus, although there is variation in the sounds produced by children during this period, the variation seems to be limited by certain sounds which are produced by most or all children and by sounds that consistently do not appear in young children's productions.

Some investigators have suggested that input may play a major role in determining a child's early phonetic repertoire (e.g., Olmsted, 1971; Waterson, 1971). Although the distributional frequency of sounds may prove to have some general influence in determining the consistencies described above, there is some evidence to suggest that its influence is not absolute. In a second experiment reported by Leonard, Newhoff, and Mesalam (1980), the word-initial sounds produced by a set of twins were examined. These children were no more similar in the sounds produced than any 2 of the 10 children described above. In other words, there were sounds that both children produced, some that neither produced, and some that only one of the twins produced. Since we can assume that these children both received essentially the same input, it seems likely that individual differences are attributable to some other factor. The most logical candidate is the argument by several child phonologists (Kiparsky & Menn, 1977; Schwartz & Leonard, 1982) that each child individually constructs a phonology within some general limitations of the linguistic environment.

Another aspect of phonologic behavior during this period which is also subject to individual differences is selectivity. A number of phonologists have observed that children are selective in the words they attempt. They appear to select words with certain phonologic characteristics and do not attempt words with other characteristics following a variety of individual patterns. These patterns may be based upon the structure or syllable shape of adult words as well as the sounds of which they are comprised. For example, one child reportedly attempted words with an open syllable structure (CV or CVCV), but did not attempt adult words with other syllable shapes (Ingram, 1974). At a similar point in development, Hildegard Leopold (Leopold, 1947) only attempted adult words with initial labial and apical stop and nasal consonants, while another child primarily attempted words with initial fricatives (Ferguson & Farwell, 1975). In general, selectivity appears more likely to influence word-initial sounds (Shibamoto & Olmsted, 1978). It should be noted that Leonard, Newhoff, and Mesalam (1980) reported that, as in the case of production, there are some limitations in the extent of these individual differences. Most, if not all, of the 10 children they studied attempted words beginning with [m], [b], [n], [g], [k], [w], and [p]. None of the children attempted words beginning with [v], [θ], [l], [z], or [r]. Words beginning with other consonants seemed to involve individual differences in terms of whether they were attempted. While these differences might be attributed to differences in input, there is some convincing evidence that this is not a determining factor.

Two types of evidence bear on this issue. The first comes from the twin study reported by Leonard, Newhoff, and Mesalam (1980). In spite of the assumed identical input, these twins did evidence some differences in their pattern of selection of attempted words. Additionally, a series of investigations (Leonard, Schwartz, Chapman, & Morris, 1981; Leonard, Schwartz, Chapman, Rowan, Prelock, Terrell, Weiss, & Messick, 1982; Schwartz & Leonard, 1982) have involved use of a nonsense or unfamiliar word acquisition paradigm. In this general procedure children were presented over a period of time a set of words corresponding to unfamiliar referents (objects or actions), and the acquisition of the words was examined. The words were chosen or constructed individually so that half of the words had phonologic characteristics which were consistent with words the child was producing and attempting (IN), and half of the words had characteristics that were inconsistent with the child's existing phonology (OUT). Across all of these investigations, which collectively involved children with vocabularies between 5 and 75 words, the children consistently acquired more IN than OUT words. Because all of the experimental words were presented an equal number of times, it seems unlikely that input variations are the sole determiners of selectivity.

Two remaining findings concerning this phenomenon should be mentioned. At an early point in this period children are similarly selective in imitative and nonimitative productions (Schwartz & Leonard, 1982). However, toward the end of this period these patterns first begin to disappear. Children stop being selective in imitative productions, while they are still selective in spontaneous productions (Leonard, Schwartz, Folger, & Wilcox, 1978). Regardless of selectivity, the extent of errors in imitative and spontaneous productions is comparable throughout this period. Finally, it has been demonstrated that while selectivity strongly influences production, it has no effect on children's comprehension. Children comprehend words with characteristics that are "out" of their phonologies as readily as words with characteristics that are "in" their phonologies.

The phenomenon of phonological selectivity has both theoretical and clinical import. It provides evidence that children during this period have the perceptual abilities to discriminate between IN and OUT words. Additionally, it provides further evidence for the child's active role in constructing a phonologic system. There have been several suggestions concerning the basis for selectivity. Ferguson (1978) suggested that it serves to simplify the task of phonologic acquisition by allowing the child to focus on a limited number of word types (i.e., sounds and syllable shapes). Alternatively, it has been suggested that selectivity is one of several ways a child may observe certain output constraints or limitations (Menn, Note 1). For example, there may be a constraint in the child's system which "prohibits" the production of final consonants. The limitation may be observed either by omitting final consonants or, more simply, by not attempting to produce adult words with final consonants. Finally, the basis of selectivity may lie in the nature of children's initial perceptual representations (schemas) and their coordination with production representations (schemes) (Schwartz & Leonard, 1982). At the outset and through much of this period, children may only attempt words for which they have an established schema and a coordinated scheme. Other words similar in phonologic composition may also be attempted. These constraints relax gradually as the child's repertoire is expanded to include a greater variety of coordinated schemes and schemas. Ultimately the child may no longer be limited to pre-existing schemes and schemas, and selectivity largely disappears.

Phonologic selectivity may also have some important implications for determining the content of remediation for phonologic disorders. It has been demonstrated that older language-impaired children at this same level of development also exhibit this selectivity (Leonard et al., 1982). Consequently, to insure maximum initial success in a remediation program, one should choose words for training with characteristics that are consistent with the child's phonology.

One final aspect of individual differences during this period, individual learning strategies (Ferguson & Farwell, 1975), warrants consideration. Reduplication is one such strategy which has been observed in children at this point and seems to continue into the next period of phonologic acquisition. Some children frequently produce single syllabic (e.g., *boat*) as well as multisyllabic words (*water*) by producing two or more identical or nearly identical syllables ([boubo]; [wɔwɔ]). Other children rarely produce such forms. It appears that a reduplication strategy may be generally related to a child's ability to produce final consonants and more closely to the production of nonreduplicated multisyllabic forms (Fee & Ingram, 1982; Ferguson, 1983; Schwartz, Leonard, Wilcox, & Folger, 1980). Reduplicating a word helps the child avoid final consonant production, but, more importantly, it may be an easier way to produce words with 2 syllables. Other individual learning strategies which may serve similar functions include the use of [j] as a syllable-initial consonant (e.g., *panda* [pajan]) across various monosyllabic and multisyllabic words (Priestly, 1977), the production of diminutive forms [i] across a variety of words such as [auti] for *out* (Ingram, 1974), and, somewhat later in development, the production of a form *ri-* as a prefix for a variety of multisyllabic words, such as *attack* [ritæk] (Smith, 1973). More recently, Klein (1981) has identified two broader strategies that are related to children's productions of adult multisyllabic words at the end of this period and the beginning of the representational period. She observed that 2 children exhibited various syllable-maintaining strategies in attempting to produce multisyllabic words. The remaining 2 children primarily exhibited various forms of syllable-reducing strategies.

Such "strategies" or patterns in children's phonologic behavior may represent the first instances of their being systematic. However, their identification represents only a first step. We will ultimately need to determine the specific roles of these patterns in phonologic acquisition (see Ferguson, 1983). If this can be accomplished, it should markedly expand our understanding of the process of phonologic acquisition. It might also lead to modification in approaches to altering the phonologic systems of disordered children.

Variability and contrast

As was noted earlier, children seem to be more variable in their productions of words during this period. Specifically, they may produce a given word such as *moon* differently on various occasions (e.g., [bun] [mu] [mun]). Such variability has been measured by calculating a ratio between the total number of different forms produced and the total number of different words produced (Schwartz & Folger, 1977). This ratio was consistently higher, indicating greater variability, in prerepresentational than in representational children. The instability of the child's perceptual and motor representations may be only one source of such variability. During this period, as well as in later periods, variability may also be due to certain contextual factors, motoric factors, and the fact that a child's phonologic system is undergoing rapid change.

Variability has a significant impact on the establishment of contrast between sounds. If a child is producing the word *moon* as described above, he or she clearly does not have a contrast in production between /b/ and /m/ since they may vary without a change in meaning. Such examples are common in children's speech during this period. In fact, it is almost impossible to find what we have traditionally viewed as clear evidence of sound contrast, minimal pairs (e.g., *pit* and *bit*). Consequently, Ferguson and Farwell (1975) have argued that children at this point in development do not have production contrasts between sounds but, rather, between whole words. This has led to an alternate method of evaluating contrasts in children's speech involving the notion of a phone class. A phone class is a sound and all the other sounds with which it may vary in a given position. For example, a child may produce the following: *see* [ti] [di]; *sun* [dʌn] [sʌn] [ʌn]; *feet* [fit]; *play* [beI] peI]. Assuming this is the child's complete production repertoire, the word-initial phone classes would be [s~p~d ø(null)], [f], and [b~p].[1]

The degree of contrast may be measured by the number of phone classes, the number of single-member phone classes, and the mean number of members per class. No age norms are currently available. However, the extent of the child's contrasts may be compared with the adult system in which there would be approximately 24 single-member consonant phone classes. It should be remembered that even though these phone classes contain sounds, the contrast is between words. For example, *see* and *feet* may be considered to contrast because there is no overlap in their word-initial phone classes. Ferguson and Farwell (1975) found no clear evidence of contrast between sounds. Additionally, in an experiment with his son, Braine (1971) tried to teach the child two nonsense words, [ʔiː] and [daI], representing an apparent contrast in his own speech. The words were ultimately produced as [di:] and [da], or [dʌ], suggesting no true contrastive value between the [d] and [ʔ].

An aspect of phonologic behavior observed during this period, which is closely related to the lack of contrast, is homonymy. Homonymy occurs when a child produces two different words in the same way. It has been suggested that normally developing children have a tendency to avoid homonymy by not producing a potentially homonymous word or by altering one of the forms in some way (Ingram, 1975). For example, a child may produce *bow* and *boat* as [boʊ] and [boʊ:], respectively. While some children may avoid homonymy, others may "seek out" or "collect" homonyms to reduce the number of different forms they have to produce for different words (Vihman, 1981). However, even in instances that appear homonymous a child may make imperceptible distinctions between apparently homonymous forms (e.g., less distinct vowel length differences) or distinctions which have no measurable acoustic consequences, such as slight lip rounding versus no lip rounding (Priestly, 1980). Thus, there may not be as many instances of true homonymy as have been reported. One aspect of homonymy for which we have little evidence other than anecdotes is the child's awareness of instances of homonymy. Additionally, the extent of true homonymy (no difference between forms) versus pseudohomonymy (articulatory or acoustic differences between the forms) needs to be determined. Some attempts have already been made to examine the influence of the child's view of whether or not two productions are homonymous and the influence of the hearer's view (Locke, 1979a; 1979b). However, some further research which takes the possibility of pseudohomonymy into account is needed. Another issue concerning homonymy revolves around the possibility that older disordered children might be more "tolerant" of homonymy in their systems (Ingram, 1976). Two recent investigations, one based on diary data from a variety of sources (Ingram, 1981) and one on samples collected in a standardized fashion from normally developing and language-impaired children at the one-word stage, revealed no differences in the extent of homonymy (Leonard, Camarata, Schwartz, Chapman & Messick, Note 8). In both groups there was a wide range of individual variation in the number of homonyms. One final aspect of homonymy which has not been examined in detail concerns a potential relationship with semantic factors (Vihman, 1981). It may prove to be the case that at least some apparent homonyms are actually semantic overextensions. Similarly, some apparent overextensions may prove to be homonyms. Until recently (Smith & Brunette, Note 9) such possibilities have not been considered.

The most consistent observation concerning phonologic behavior during the prerepresentational period is that children's errors do not always follow consistent patterns (Ferguson & Farwell, 1975). Thus, they cannot be readily described in terms of processes or rules (although the notion of variable rules might have some application, cf., Sankoff, 1978). Furthermore, because of the child's cognitive abilities, imputing a system of rules or processes as mental operations may be inappropriate at this stage.

One phenomenon of phonologic behavior described earlier, which further suggests that children at this point in development do not have a rule system into which new words are automatically assimilated, is represented by phonological idioms (Moskowitz, cited in Ferguson & Farwell, 1975). An idiom occurs when a child produces a word accurately, or nearly accurately (as compared with productions of other similar words) when it is first acquired. The accuracy of that production may then "deteriorate" over time. This has also been termed recidivism (Smith, 1973). An example, cited earlier, was Hildegard Leopold's acquisition of the word *pretty* which was initially produced as [prʌti] at 10 months and [prIti] at 11 months. At this point Hildegard did not appear to be producing any other prevocalic or intervocalic voiceless stops. Nor was she producing any consonant clusters in other words. Gradually, the production changed to [pIti] or [pwIti] at 16 months, [pIti] at 21 months, and finally changed to [bIdi] at 22 months. At that point, Hildegard, across all of her words, consistently produced voiceless prevocalic and intervocalic stops as their voiced counterparts and consistently simplified consonant clusters.

Phonological idioms are important for two reasons. First, they indicate that children at this point in development do not have a systematic set of rules into which each newly acquired word is assimilated. Instead, each word seems to be dealt with individually, some being produced more accurately than others. It is only later, when a system of rules develops, that different words with similar characteristics may be treated consistently in the child's phonology (e.g., all pre- and intervocalic stops are produced as voiced; all clusters are simplified). Consequently, a word such as *pretty* may be produced quite accurately at the outset, but as the child develops systematic rules or patterns for simplifying words (errors), its production may deteriorate.

The second important aspect of this phenomenon is that it provides evidence that, at least at one time, the child perceived and produced a word accurately. Thus, later errors (e.g., [bIdi] for *pretty*) may not be attributable to basic perceptual or motoric limitations. Instead, these errors seem more appropriately attributed to some systematic set of patterns or rules for dealing with various characteristics of adult words.

There are two other similar phenomena which also may provide evidence that during the next period of development a phonologic system is operative. They warrant discussion here because of their similarity to phonological idioms. The first has been termed "puzzle phenomena" (Smith, 1973). At a given time a child produced the word *puzzle* as [pʌdl̩], while the word *puddle* was produced as [pʌgl̩]. This demonstrates that the child's inaccurate production of *puddle* was not due to a motor inability to produce this form. It has been argued that this error may be the result of some misperception (cf., Macken, 1980b). However, it might also be taken as evidence that the child's developmental errors are the result of patterns of change applied to the adult forms being attempted regardless of whether they apply to perceptual representations or production representations (e.g., "change voiced fricatives to homorganic stops," "change alveolar stops to velar stops"). A similar point has been made regarding the occurrence of alternation (Dinnsen, Elbert, & Weismer, Note 10). Evidence that a child omits or deletes a final consonant in *dog* [dɔ], yet at the same time produces [dɔgi] has been proposed as evidence that the child has an accurate, perception-based underlying representation of the word *dog* that includes a final /g/.

Thus, given such evidence, Dinnsen et al. argue that final consonant omission ([dɔ] for *dog*) can be assumed to result from the application of some rule. This particular type of evidence should be viewed as less conclusive than the evidence provided by idioms or puzzle phenomena. First, it is not clear that *dog* and *doggie* represent true alternate forms for a child in the same way that an adult recognizes *electric* and *electricity* as alternate forms of a single word. Second, the child's ability to accurately perceive (as well as produce) a [g] in [dɔgi] only ensures that the child can do so in syllable-initial position. The failure to produce this sound in syllable-final position might as readily be attributed to motor or perceptual limitations as to some mental operation or rule without additional evidence.

In summary, this period of phonologic acquisition has proved to be a rich source of observational, anecdotal, and experimental data which support the view of it as a somewhat separable period of development. Children's phonologic behavior during this period may be described as variable, individually different within certain limits, as well as generally unsystematic in terms of rules, patterns, and contrasts, and markedly different from the period to follow. To the extent that much of their behavior seems based exclusively upon individual words without more general patterns, this period could also be termed the period of word-based phonology. Clearly, a good deal of additional research is needed to confirm and further specify the aspects of phonologic behavior described in this section.

The most obvious omission in this discussion has been any information concerning children's perceptual abilities during this period. Some investigations have examined phonetic perception in children at this point in development (Kuhl, 1980). However, to date no investigation has examined phonologic perception (i.e., perception in meaningful units such as words) in these children. The greatest obstacle to such research seems to be methodological. Children of this age are not sufficiently passive to allow the use of heart rate procedures, nor are sucking procedures appropriate. Tasks employed with older children (see the following section) are unlikely to be successful. However, some procedures such as visually reinforced infant speech discrimination (Eilers, 1980) and perceptual constancy (Kuhl, 1980) have the potential for testing perception in meaningful units. The next few years should see some significant advances in our knowledge of perceptual abilities during the prerepresentational period.

The Period of Representational or Systematic Phonology

This period, extending from approximately 18 months to 7 years, incorporates what has been discussed elsewhere (Ingram, 1976) as the period of the simple morpheme and the completion of the phonetic inventory. Since the justifications for viewing these two developments as separable periods in terms of changes in the basic nature of phonologic, cognitive, and general linguistic behavior are significantly weaker than in the case of the preceding period, this division will not be made. The hallmark of the representational period is the apparent systematic nature of children's phonologic behavior. Specifically, children seem to follow fairly systematic patterns in their errors and acquisition. While individual differences may still exist, children appear to be less variable (except in cases where they may vary between correct and previously incorrect productions), become gradually more systematic in their correct or incorrect production of classes of sounds across words and across types of words, and seem to be developing a system of sound contrast in perception and production. In the course of these developments, children also appear to gradually master the phonetic inventory of their language. Finally, during this period the more complex system of rules governing the use of morphophonemics is initially acquired.

Traditionally, we have only considered the general articulatory (production) aspects of speech sounds during this period. Consequently, descriptions of development and clinical applications were limited to information concerning the mastery of the phonetic inventory. Although this is an important aspect of development, it is by no means the whole of phonologic acquisition. The focus of this section will reflect this view.

Production of segments

At the beginning of this period, children's speech can be readily characterized as exhibiting pervasive errors. By the end of the period, errors may be rare or nonexistent. It is what occurs in between these two points that is of interest. With the exception of a few scattered diary studies, until the years between 1930 and 1960, we had little specific information regarding the development of speech production. However, three cross-sectional studies of large numbers of children conducted during that period radically changed that situation (Poole, 1934; Templin, 1957; Wellman, Case, Mengurt, & Bradbury, 1931). The data they provided were almost seductive in their appeal. We were suddenly able to take a given chronological age, look at these data, and determine what sounds should be acquired and what sounds should not yet be acquired. However, while these data have provided some general developmental signposts, their use seems fraught with difficulties.

There are significant weaknesses in both the methods of data collection and data analysis (Bernthal & Bankson, 1981; Schwartz, in press; Shriberg & Kwiatkowski, 1980; Winitz, 1969). Overall, the bases of these norms may be extremely unrepresentative of the speech of individuals and groups. Furthermore, the criteria employed in determining ages of acquisition (e.g., 75% or 100% of the subjects correctly articulating a sound in initial, medial, and final position) may present an extremely distorted picture of development. For example, although the age of acquisition for /t/ is given as 6 years (Templin, 1957), it is likely that most, if not all, children produce this sound accurately in some context at a much earlier age. It is also possible that for a given sound 70% of the children tested were correct in their production at one age, and only a few children caused the age of acquisition to be set at a higher age.

One way in which these latter two difficulties may be partially ameliorated is by considering an average age or age of customary usage rather than an age of mastery. Age of customary usage may be defined as the age at which more than 50% of the children tested correctly produce a given sound in two positions (Sander, 1972). Although this does not compensate for weaknesses in the way such data were collected, it does provide a somewhat better balanced picture of speech sound acquisition. The point remains, however, that these data tell us little about the way in which development proceeds from the point of pervasive errors on a given sound to the points at which customary usage or mastery are reached. What is lacking is a detailed description of children's errors and the nature of their gradual approximation to correct productions. Although it is easy to argue that this is what we need, achieving an agreed-upon description is quite another matter.

Two more recent reports (Ingram, Christensen, Veach, & Webster, 1980; Macken, 1980a) have provided some of these details. Macken described the development of the voicing distinction in stops in 4 English-speaking (1;6 to 2;4) and 7 Spanish-speaking (1;7 to 4;0) children. She found that the ages of acquisition varied considerably, by as much as a year. However, in English there seemed to be 3 general stages: (1) no voicing contrast, (2) a consistent but not audible difference between voiced and voiceless stops, and (3) an approximation of adult VOT distinctions. Additionally, there seems to be a lexical bias in the early stages in favor of words beginning with /b/, /d/, and /k/.

Ingram et al. (1980) studied the acquisition of word-initial fricatives and affricates in 73 English-speaking children ranging in age from 1;10 to 5;11. In general, the order of acquisition was /f/ before /t∫/, /dʒ/, /∫/, before /s/, /v/, /z/, /ɵ/. However, a good deal of individual variation was noted. Additionally, individual children varied in their productions of given sounds across words and also varied in their productions of given words. They also noted some of the more common errors as [s], [p], or [b] for /f/; [b] for /v/; [f] for /ɵ/; [ɵ] for /s/; [x] or [s] for /z/; [s] for /∫/; [t], [s], or [ts] for /t∫/; [d], [ts], or [dz] for /dʒ/. Some allophonic ("distortion") errors were also noted.

Such investigations represent a beginning in obtaining a more complete picture of normal phonetic development. In particular, instrumental analyses and multiple contexts of testing may be critical in establishing the range of normal developmental errors and normal developmental sequences.

It is generally agreed that the most striking characteristic of children's errors during this period is that they appear to be systematic within a given child. Furthermore, although some individual differences exist, these error patterns seem generally consistent across children. Several different approaches have been employed in describing these error patterns. These have included distinctive features, generative phonological rules, and phonological processes. The use of distinctive features involves the application of a set of typically binary (+, −) articulatory and/or acoustic features of speech segments (i.e., consonants and vowels) in describing acquisition and developmental errors. There are a number of such feature systems available (e.g., Chomsky & Halle, 1968; Jakobson, Fant, & Halle, 1963), differing in their relative emphasis on articulatory and phonetic features. Using such a system to describe speech sound development, Menyuk (1968) found evidence for the following order of acquisition: nasal, grave, voice, diffuse, continuant, strident. However, these data are somewhat limited in that it may be difficult to determine precisely when a child acquires an isolated feature.

There are many other limitations in using distinctive features. The binary nature of these features (e.g., ±voicing) may not be an accurate representation of the dimensions of features such as voicing. There may be many values of a feature such as this, rather than simply voiced and unvoiced. Additionally, there is no general agreement as to the specific set of features that should be employed. However, some relatively recent advances in the use of multidimensional scaling procedures (Singh, 1976) or alternative feature values such as markedness (Toombs, Singh, & Hayden, 1981) may help in resolving this problem. Even with this work, questions remain concerning the psychological reality of these features for adults. In paradigms designed to encourage categorizations of sounds according to their features, adults seem unaware of some features commonly included in such systems (LaRiviere, Winitz, Reeds, & Herriman, 1974; Ritterman & Freeman, 1974). The fact that children only gradually acquire a given feature (e.g., voicing) across sounds and words raises further questions about the use of this descriptive device. Finally, the most serious weakness of distinctive features concerns their exclusive focus on segmental aspects of speech. They do not take into account the fact that a given sound may be produced differently in different phonetic contexts and the fact that many developmental errors may be context dependent.

The second major approach to the description of developmental error patterns involves the use of generative rules such as those described by Chomsky and Halle (1968). Such rules involve the assumption that the child has a single underlying form for each word which is then transformed into the surface form (i.e., the production) by the application of these rules. In most cases (Smith, 1973) the assumption is made that the underlying form is based on the child's accurate perception of the adult's production. The rules which are then written formally characterize the relationships between these assumed underlying forms and the child's productions. The rules may be written in terms of sound classes (e.g., consonants, fricatives), individual sounds (e.g., /s/), or features (e.g., $\left[\begin{smallmatrix} + \text{ continuant} \\ + \text{ strident} \end{smallmatrix}\right]$). These rules also can be written to be either context-free (e.g., fricatives → stops, s →t, $\left[\begin{smallmatrix} + \text{ continuant} \\ + \text{ strident} \end{smallmatrix}\right] \rightarrow \left[\begin{smallmatrix} - \text{ continuant} \\ - \text{ strident} \end{smallmatrix}\right]$) or context-sensitive by using a variety of symbols and conventions (e.g., C → Ø/__#, final consonants are deleted; s → t/__V, /t/ is substituted for /s/ prevocalically). The advantage of such rules is that they can be used to describe errors that are context-specific, unlike distinctive feature descriptions. The disadvantage of such rules is their level of formality and the potentially incorrect assumptions concerning children's underlying forms.

The final method employed in describing patterns of developmental errors involves the use of phonological processes based on Stampe's (1973) proposal. A number of investigators have employed these processes in describing error patterns in normal as well as phonologically impaired children. As mentioned earlier, there is no generally agreed-upon list of processes that can be used to describe these patterns. Investigators have suggested lists of as few as 8 (Shriberg & Kwiatkowski, 1980) up to as many as 40 or more (Ingram 1981; also see Edwards & Shriberg, 1983 for a more complete review). In using few processes, many unified patterns of errors may be overlooked. Using more may divide these patterns so finely that more general patterns may be missed.

Besides the unresolved issue of what specific set of processes should be considered, no resolution concerning the criteria for saying a process exists or quantifying the extent of processes has been reached. For instance, is it a process if a child substitutes /t/ for /s/, but produces other fricatives correctly? Is it a process if a child substitutes a stop for a fricative in only a single word? Is it a process if a child produces all final consonants except for /n/, which is deleted? Within the context of Stampe's theoretical proposal one could argue that all of these are in fact processes. From a more pragmatic standpoint, however, one might argue that these instances are quantitatively different from instances in which a child has an across-sound and an across-word pattern of errors, such as stopping or final consonant deletion. When this kind of distinction is made, it is in part with the intent of differentiating among idiosyncratic productions of words—isolated sound errors which might be attributable to misperceptions or inaccurate motor learning—and patterns of errors which may reflect some organizational aspect of the child's phonology (regardless of whether the origins of these error patterns are perceptual, structural, or motoric). To do this, then, we can require that for a process to exist, the pattern must affect more than a single sound in a sound class (e.g., more than a single fricative for it to be considered stopping) or more than a single sound regardless of class (e.g., more than /n/ deleted in final position). Using more stringent quantitative criteria (a minimum of 4 possible occurrences of a process and a minimum of 20% frequency of occurrence for the process), McReynolds and Elbert (1981) have demonstrated that a process analysis of disordered children's productions with these criteria differs markedly from one without any criteria. If some type of quantitative criteria is not employed, a process, on the surface, does little more than rename an individual error. The only thing it might imply in such instances is that the error is the result of the "natural limitations of the speech mechanism," which may or may not be accurate.

Other, qualitative, distinctions in error patterns may need to be drawn. Not all patterns identified perceptually by transcribers as the same process may be identical. For example, Weismer, Dinnsen, and Elbert (1981) have noted that in disordered children who appear to omit final consonants, the acoustic characteristics of the children's productions may differ significantly. Specifically, some children omit final consonants while maintaining a vowel length distinction between target words with voiced versus voiceless final consonants in the adult forms. Other children do not maintain this distinction. Consequently, it may be inappropriate to group both types of omission under the same process of final consonant deletion. Instead, as Weismer et al. suggest, these qualitatively different types of error patterns may need to be differentially labelled.

Finally, we will ultimately need to make quantitative distinctions among error patterns. Patterns may need to be distinguished in terms of the relative number of sounds affected (e.g., stopping for all fricatives versus stopping for only 3 fricatives). Patterns may also need to be distinguished on the basis of their within-sound, across-word consistency (e.g., stopping for /s/ and /z/ in all productions versus stopping for these sounds in some words, but not others).

The discussion of pattern analysis has thus far tended to focus on rather narrow patterns which, while consistent with the intuitions of some adults (i.e., child phonology researchers), may not have any psychological reality for the child. Instead, children's developmental sound error patterns may simply reflect much more general patterns. Some preliminary evidence for a more general view has recently become available. Menn (Note 1) suggested that in their error patterns, children follow more general constraints such as "don't produce final consonants" in a number of ways (e.g., final consonant deletion, syllable deletion, reduplication, failing to attempt to produce adult words with final consonants). Some diary evidence can be used to support this view. We may have sometimes missed such patterns in other children because our focus has been upon more narrow or isolated rules or processes. Also, in the last several years, evidence for such patterns in the phonologies of disordered children has been reported. Patterns have been observed such as consonant harmony involving the alteration of target words with more than one consonant to forms in which the consonants are similar or identical (Leonard, Miller, & Brown, 1980). Similarly, general patterns of sound preference in which a given consonant is substituted for a variety of consonants following no specific process or rule have been reported (Edwards, Note 11; Weiner, 1981).

While we may simply have missed many such general patterns in the errors of normally developing children, some such patterns have been discussed in terms of individual strategies of phonologic acquisition like those mentioned earlier (e.g., reduplication, syllable-maintaining vs. syllable-reducing). Other individual strategies have been described by Fey and Gandour (1982) and Priestly (1977). Recognition of these apparently individual paths and more general patterns in phonologic acquisition may aid in our understanding of the general process and nature of acquisition as well as in our understanding of phonologic disorders.

Another aspect of production during this period which has received little attention concerns phonetic development. While we have a good deal of information concerning the phonemes children acquire based on the perceptual judgments of transcribers, little information is available concerning aspects of production that are difficult, if not impossible, to perceive (e.g., voice onset time—VOT).

Some limited information has recently become available. Longitudinal data from 4 children suggest that the acquisition of the voicing contrast is gradual, occurring in 3 stages: (1) no contrast, (2) a contrast in VOT which falls within one of the adult categories—usually voiced, and (3) contrast resembling the adult contrast (Macken & Barton, 1980a). In Spanish, where the contrast is between lead voicing and short-lag VOT, the acquisition of this contrast is even more gradual with a mastery occurring after age 4 (Macken & Barton, 1980b). Other features, such as aspiration and spirantization, which add to the voicing contrast in English and Spanish, respectively, also may play a role in this aspect of development. Another such instance involves the earlier mentioned finding that some disordered children maintained a distinction in vowel length (longer vowel length associated with voiced final consonants; shorter vowel length associated with voiceless final consonants) even though the final consonant was not actually produced (Weismer et al., 1981). A similar distinction among children who are not disordered may prove to have some developmental significance. Along the same lines, it was also noted earlier that children's productions of what are perceived to be homonyms may not be truly homonymous (Priestly, 1980). Children may make articulatory distinctions between such words which do not have significant acoustic consequences. There may also be acoustic distinctions that are not perceptible to adult listeners. In all of these cases some instrumental analysis would reveal significant information not apparent in the perceptual judgments of transcription. Thus, the further use of such analyses is critical for more complete understanding of phonetic and phonologic development.

Production of suprasegmentals

Virtually all of the preceding information has focused exclusively on segmental phonology. Until recently, little attention has been directed toward the development of suprasegmentals (intonation, duration, stress, rhythm) and the influence of suprasegmental factors on segmental phonology (see Crystal, 1973; 1975). In a series of studies (Allen, in press; Allen & Hawkins, 1978), the discrimination and production of various aspects of suprasegmentals have been examined in French- , German- , English- and Swedish-speaking children ranging from 2 to 5 years of age. The discrimination and production of lexical stress patterns by these children from differing linguistic environments seems to gradually improve through 4 years of age. The abilities of the children seem to be similar in spite of differences in the stress patterns of the languages they are acquiring. After 4 years of age, however, the children appear to take on patterns characteristic of their native language. In some cases this involved the inability of 5-year-olds to produce and discriminate a pattern of stress that can be produced and discriminated by 4-year-olds.

These findings have been explained in terms of an "attunement" view of language acquisition (Aslin & Pisoni, 1980). Such a view suggests that certain abilities may be "lost" over time because the child only maintains those that are relevant to his or her native language. Further development of stress production and perception occurs through age 12. Atkinson-King (1973) demonstrated that only by age 12 do children accurately discriminate and perceive contrastive stress differentiating compound nouns (*greenhouse*) from noun phrases (*green house*).

Another aspect of suprasegmental phonology that has been examined developmentally is duration. Duration has been examined primarily in terms of the length of individual segments (i.e., vowels and consonants) within words (Gilbert & Purves, 1977; Hawkins, 1979), syllables (Oller & Smith, 1977; Smith, 1978), and larger units (Tingley & Allen, 1975). By 18 months, there is some differential duration of vowels and consonants with vowels reaching adult norms by 4 or 5 years of age. There is greater variability across consonants, with maturity being attained at 10 years of age or later. The relative and absolute duration of two-syllable words appears to approximate adult values by 2 years of age. However, the duration of syllables seems greater than that of adults and decreases only gradually. The results of a more recent investigation (Kubaska & Keating, 1981) suggest that developmental decreases in duration are not related to word familiarity. In fact, when utterance position is controlled, there is no decrease in some cases. The most significant factor in duration appears to be utterance position; nonfinal words are shorter in duration.

There is a need for further research in this area. Specifically, investigations involving greater control of familiarity and experience—perhaps employing nonsense or unfamiliar word/unfamiliar referent paradigms— might yield more conclusive results. A more complete understanding of this aspect of production may provide some clues regarding the child's developing motor control for speech.

A final aspect of suprasegmental phonology which has been considered is the acquisition of intonation. Intonation may be viewed as the prosodic use of tone or changes in fundamental frequency (Allen & Hawkins, 1980). Tone, as it is used in tone languages such as Gã (Kirk, 1973) or Mandarin Chinese (Clumeck, Note 12), functions almost segmentally in contrasting meaning at a word level. However, intonation affects much larger units of speech. Therefore, it should not be surprising that these two types of tone are acquired somewhat differently. In general, it appears that tone contrasts are acquired before rhythmic contrasts and segmental contrasts. The use of pitch for intonational features appears prior to the emergence of language and is gradually used in a systematic fashion (affirmative-negative and falling-rising contrasts). Tone, however, seems tied to the emergence of words; and while some tone characteristics are mastered at a very early age, other characteristics may emerge much later (Clumeck, 1980).

One of the more intriguing aspects of recent research concerning suprasegmental aspects of speech involves the apparent relationships among suprasegmental factors and segmental behavior. For example, unstressed or light syllables are likely to be deleted in initial position and in positions adjacent to another unstressed syllable (Allen & Hawkins, 1980). Similar findings have been reported by Klein (Note 13) regarding the influence of stress as well as serial position of a syllable in determining whether it is produced. She found that final unstressed syllables are most often produced when preceded by another unstressed syllable. In other environments such syllables are more often omitted. A major stress level (primary or secondary) in combination with a later occurring syllable was found to be the most likely situation in which a consonant was retained in multisyllabic words (e.g., *spaghetti* [gɛ]). Such findings represent an important first step in understanding the basis of developmental segmental errors. In the past we have focused largely on segmental aspects of phonology, and suprasegmental aspects were considered separately. Examination of the relationships between segmental and suprasegmental factors may serve to better explain patterns of production in both normally developing and disordered children.

Production of morphemes

The final aspect of speech production which begins to develop during this period is the system of bound morphemes. While such morphemes comprise only a small portion of the child's production, they represent an important advance in the child's phonologic abilities. Ultimately, this is the first clearly generative, rule based aspect of the adult phonologic system acquired by the child. Much of the research has focused on English morphophonology including plural, present progressive, past tense, and third person singular. However, this provides a somewhat limited picture since adjectival (comparative and superlative forms) and adverbial (e.g., -*ly*) inflections also occur in English. Additionally, some other languages (e.g., Hungarian) have extensive inflectional systems that indicate other linguistic information, such as case. In spontaneous speech, inflectional endings may begin to appear as early as 2 years of age, but the first which seems to be acquired (90% correct in obligatory contexts) is the present progressive (Brown, 1973; deVilliers & deVilliers, 1973). This is followed by plurals, possessives, past tense, and third person singular endings. However, even when children master such inflectional endings, we cannot be certain that their use is a reflection of generative rules.

The first evidence we have of the existence of generative morphophonological rules is children's overgeneralizations (e.g., *goed*). Another type of evidence for the generative nature of these rules is provided by studies that have employed Berko's (1958) now classic "Wug" procedure. In this procedure, children are presented with a novel nonsense word in a situation that encourages the use of an inflectional ending (e.g., "Here is a wug. Now there are two _____."). Because such words are novel, if they are inflected in the same way as familiar words, we have evidence for general morphophonological principles or rules. According to Berko's findings many of these rules are acquired by approximately age 5. However, the study did not provide much information concerning the developmental sequence in the acquisition of specific rules.

A subsequent study represented an attempt to provide such information for plural forms (Innes, Note 14). Using a task similar to that used by Berko, the following developmental sequence was found: (1) no extension of a plural rule to novel words, (2) use of rules to pluralize novel words except those ending in fricatives and affricates, (3) use of these rules with all words except those ending with sibilants, (4) use of these rules with all words except those ending in /z/, and (5) complete mastery. This suggests a gradual, phonetically based extension of a morphophonological rule. It remains to be seen whether a similar sequence occurs in the acquisition of rules governing other bound morphemes.

A more recent and extensive experimental study of the relative ease of morpheme acquisition by children between 3 and 9 (Derwing & Baker, 1977) has revealed a pattern similar to the order of acquisition in spontaneous speech mentioned earlier. Children made fewest errors on progressive endings, a greater number of errors on plural and past tense endings, followed by possessive endings and, finally, third person singular endings. The basis for this apparently consistent order and ease of acquisition is still a matter of some debate. In a lengthy disussion of this issue Brown (1973) considered grammatical complexity, semantic complexity, perceptual saliency, and frequency of occurrence. He rejected perceptual saliency and frequency of occurrence as possible determinants and suggested that semantic and grammatical complexity in combination may determine the order of the acquisition.

Still more recently, debate has surfaced concerning the influence of frequency of occurrence on input. When input data are analyzed in certain ways, there appears to be a relationship (Derwing & Baker, 1979; Moerk, 1980; 1981). However, when input data are analyzed differently, there seems to be no relationship between input frequency and the order of morpheme acquisition (Pinker, 1981). The problem centers on the issue of how one compares input with the child's usage of these morphemes in order to infer a causal relationship. To date, there are no satisfactory solutions. New experimental methodologies may be required to resolve this issue.

Further research (Cousins, Note 15) has also raised the possibility that, contrary to Brown's conclusion, perceptual saliency may have a role in determining the order of morpheme acquisition in one aphasic child. While the apparent influence of this factor cannot be generalized to normally developing children, further investigation seems warranted.

An exciting new direction in the study of morpheme acquisition involves the application of information-processing principles to construct a model of morphophonological behavior and acquisition (MacWhinney, 1978). MacWhinney considers three types of abilities as underlying this and other aspects of language acquisition: rote memorization, productive combination, and analogy formation. These are considered to be processes within a more general cyclical process of learning. In learning, acquisition leads to a process of application, which in turn leads to a correction process and then further acquisition. MacWhinney has employed morphophonologic data from various languages and some preliminary computer simulation to explore the nature of these processes. While the simulation is not an exact replication of children's acquisition of bound morphemes, it forces us to think about the specific components and processes that are required. This approach seems to hold a great deal of promise for this and other aspects of language acquisition.

Perception

This section on the representational period of phonologic acquisition has, to this point, focused almost exclusively on production. From the perspective of some child phonologists such an imbalance is perfectly acceptable. Such phonologists might argue that since perception is essentially accurate from the outset of development, no developmental changes would occur during this period (e.g., Smith, 1973; Stampe, 1973). Although data concerning infant speech perception indicate extensive abilities shortly after birth, it must be remembered that this involves perception of segments and acoustic features in the context of nonmeaningful syllables. This does not guarantee that children will accurately perceive aspects of a meaningful word. Nor does it guarantee that, even if "lower level" perception is accurate, the word (or larger unit) will be accurately represented and stored (cf. Braine, 1974). Finally, it has been argued that perception is generally an active rather than a passive process (Bryant, 1974). Many instances of anecdotal evidence can be provided to argue that, in spite of the actual physical characteristics of a stimulus and the actual physical information received by the sensory mechanism, perception involves the interpretation of this information in the context of existing knowledge. It is perhaps a common occurrence for adults to fail to notice or attend to speech errors in conversational speech. In fact, the word in which such an error occurs may be "heard" as a correct production, both because of expectancy and because it is heard and interpreted through the "filter" of the adult's representations and phonologic system. It would not, therefore, be surprising if children's perceptions were altered in some way by their own phonologic representational and organizational systems.

Even though there may be good reason to suspect that young children's perception may only gradually approach that of adults', we still do not have solid empirical evidence to support this view or to describe the actual course of development. A number of studies of phonemic perception in children under 4 years of age have been reported (Edwards, 1974; Garnica, 1971; 1973; Shvachkin, 1973; Strange & Broen, 1980; Barton, Note 16). However, some of these investigations are methodologically or statistically flawed (see Barton, 1975); and others, for pragmatic reasons, have focused on very specific aspects of perception during this period. Thus, we do not yet have a complete picture.

Shvachkin's (1973) investigation of 18 Russian children led to the proposal of an order of acquisition for perception of phonemic contrasts. The method employed involved teaching children nonsense CVC names for objects and then testing their ability to discriminate among these names. In each discrimination item the children were presented with three objects, two of which had names that differed by only one sound (e.g., *bak* and *dak*) and the third differed in all three sounds (e.g., *mup*). A similar procedure employed with English-speaking children yielded a generally comparable order of acquisition (Garnica, 1971). However, in these investigations a criterion of 7 correct out of 10 trials was employed in determining ages of acquisition. Such a criterion is too low because too often it may be reached by chance (Barton, 1975). When a more stringent criterion is employed, these orders of acquisition do not hold true. Apparent differences in ages of acquisition disappear.

More recently, Barton (1975; Note 17) has reported two investigations in which discrimination was examined in children ranging in age from 18 to 24 months in the first, and 27 to 35 months in the second. Minimal pair discriminations were employed using slightly different tasks than those described above. However, the child's response still was to point to a picture or pick up an object when given its name. Most of the younger children were able to discriminate at least *goat/coat* or *bear/pear*. The older children performed far better than Garnica's data indicated, with many instances of errorless discriminations. Consequently, it appears that phonemic discrimination abilities emerge quite early, although some cautionary notes are in order. Barton found that the extent to which the child knew the words being tested had a significant influence on the child's response. Additionally, particularly in the case of the younger children, task difficulty may have impinged on and distorted the results.

A number of earlier investigations examined the accuracy of children's discriminations after age 3 (Graham & House, 1971; Koenigsknecht & Lee, Note 18; Templin, 1957; Wepman, 1958). These investigations have involved a variety of methodologies, including same/different judgments of minimal pairs (real words and nonsense words), word monitoring, and selection of a picture(s) from an array of "minimal pair referents" in response to a word. In general, error rates appear to decrease with age, but children as old as 8 years continue to make some errors. Additionally, it appears that discriminations between stimuli differing by a single feature are more difficult than discriminations between stimuli differing by more than one feature. Few other generalizations are possible because of differences in stimuli and methodologies. The implications of these differences (e.g., real versus nonsense words; relative task difficulty type of response) are not yet fully understood (Barton, 1980).

More recently, some alternate methodologies for examining children's perception have been suggested (Locke, 1980a; 1980b). These alternatives have been drawn from procedures that have been used for some time in examining adult speech perception. They differ significantly in the tasks and types of responses involved from the procedures that have thus far been employed with children. For example, one alternative method involves asking a child if a given stimulus (word or syllable) is more like a second or a third stimulus. Another procedure involves asking a child to judge which one of three stimuli is different from the other two. However, even these tasks may be too difficult for children who are between 2 and 4 years of age. For these children, alternative procedures are needed. Promising sources for such procedures may be conditioning and habituation paradigms used in concept research with infants (e.g., Ross, 1980) as well as the visually reinforced head turn paradigms that have been used with younger children.

A final aspect of perceptual development during this period is the relationship between perception and production. Intuitively, it would seem as though perception and production would be closely related and that, in general, perception abilities at a given point in development would be advanced relative to production. However, these assumptions may not always be accurate. A first indication of their inaccuracy is provided by the somewhat analogous relationship between the production and comprehension of various aspects of language. Although, in general, comprehension is in advance of production, in some aspects of language the reverse appears to be true (Chapman & Miller, 1975). Additionally, very different strategies and processes may be involved in these systems. The same may well be true in the perception and production of speech.

Unfortunately, relatively few investigations have provided conclusive information regarding this relationship. Menyuk and Anderson (1969) found that children identified and categorized /l/, /r/, and /w/ more accurately than they were able to repeat these sounds. However, Zlatin & Koenigsknecht (1976) found comparable levels of behavior in children's identification and production of word-initial voiced and voiceless stops. Using the Schvachkin-Garnica technique, Edwards (1974) found that the phonemic perception of glides precedes their correct production. However, for other sounds, perceptual and productive abilities may appear simultaneously and, in rare instances, production may precede perception. A more recent investigation focusing on the perception and production of approximant consonants (specifically, /r/, /l/, and /w/) supports Edwards' conclusion that both perception and production develop gradually, with perception usually in advance of production (Strange & Broen, 1980). Finally, in findings analogous to those reported by Chapman and Miller (1975), Greenlee (1980) has observed that young children consistently maintain a distinction in vowel duration, but are unable to use this particular cue perceptually in distinguishing voiced from voiceless stops.

The literature concerning the relationship between perception and production seems to be somewhat contradictory, although some general conclusions can be drawn. There are differences as well as similarities in the development of perception and production abilities. Perceptual abilities seem to be generally more advanced than production abilities, with some clear exceptions. This suggests the existence of two separate but related systems. The exact nature of the relationship, however, is still unclear. One of the most important concerns for clinicians and researchers interested in speech sound disorders is the relationship between production errors and perceptual abilities. Such a relationship has yet to be established. Further research is needed involving converging methodologies to clarify these relationships.

Phonology and other aspects of language

Throughout this chapter the phonologic system has been discussed largely in isolation from other language components. This represents a distortion generally accepted for pragmatic reasons. In reality, phonologic behavior and development seem to be intimately related to other aspects of language. The relationship between phonologic and other components may take two forms: (1) the reciprocal influences of phonologic, syntactic, semantic, and pragmatic factors, and (2) the general developmental relationship between phonologies and other linguistic components.

It has long been commonplace knowledge that children make fewer errors producing words in isolation than producing words in sentences. In a series of studies involving children with phonologic and syntactic disorders, Panagos and his colleagues (Panagos & Prelock, 1982; Panagos, Quine, & Klich, 1979; Schmauch, Panagos, & Klich, 1978) have demonstrated that increases in the length and syntactic complexity of utterances led to an increase in speech sound errors. Similarly, they have demonstrated that increases in phonologic complexity (increased numbers of syllables) led to increases in syntactic errors. More recently, Prelock (Note 19) has demonstrated similar effects of increases in complexity on the speech and language of normally developing and disordered children. However, it should be noted that in somewhat younger children, ranging in age from 23 to 34 months, the effects of increases of syntactic complexity on phonologic production are not consistent (Kamhi, Catts, & Davis, Note 20). Kamhi et al. suggest that at some points in development other factors, such as representational abilities, may have a stronger influence on phonologic and phonetic behavior. It may also be true that while phonology is related to other aspects of language, language components remain, to some extent, autonomous. At some point in development there may be a relationship among these components, but not a one-to-one correspondence.

There appear to be other factors which influence speech sound behavior. For instance, Campbell and Shriberg (1982) found fewer instances of phonological processes in words encoding new, as opposed to old or shared, information. The influence of phonologic factors on lexical acquisition was discussed earlier in the chapter in terms of selectivity. Speech perception may be subject to the influence of semantic predictability (e.g., Cole & Jakimik, 1978; Morton & Long, 1976). It has also been demonstrated that in normally developing and language-impaired children at the one-word utterance level, both word type (object vs. action words) and extent of comprehension influence accuracy of production (Camarata & Schwartz, Note 21; Messick & Schwartz, Note 22). Children at this level produce object words more accurately than action words, perhaps because of differences in the conceptual or semantic complexity of these words. Words for which children have demonstrated comprehension tend to be produced less accurately than those for which the child has not demonstrated this degree of understanding. It may be that the child's increased knowledge of a word indicates that the word has been integrated into a phonologic system and is then subject to simplification rules that do not affect it before such integration occurs. Other potentially influencing factors, such as propositional complexity, have yet to be examined.

The other aspect of the relationship between phonology and other components of language is the development of these domains. This issue has been addressed within the context of phonologic disorders and more general linguistic disorders. It appears that, in at least some children, disorders of the phonologic system and disorders of syntax may be concomitant (Menyuk & Looney, 1972; Panagos, 1974; Shriner, Halloway, & Daniloff, 1969; Whitacre, Luper, & Pollio, 1970). Additionally, when language-disordered children are compared with normally developing children at a comparable level of syntactic development, their phonologies are very similar (Schwartz, Leonard, Wilcox, & Folger, 1980). This suggests that, at least during early stages in development, the development of phonology and syntax are closely related. Moreover, when specific disorders of language occur, they may affect phonology as well as other language components. Thus, there appears to be a synergistic relationship among the components of language which needs to be recognized in both discussions and future investigations of phonologic acquisition.

Formal Phonology

By approximately 7 years of age, children appear to be able to produce all the sounds of their language correctly in most, if not all, contexts. Typically, no processes remain other than those that might be characteristic of the child's dialect. However, phonologic acquisition is not yet complete. There are several aspects of phonology, primarily those thought to depend on generative rules, that are not mastered until after age 7. Seven years of age seems to be a landmark of sorts with respect to several aspects of development bearing some relationship to phonologic acquisition. At approximately age 7, children enter what Piaget (1970) has termed "the period of concrete operations." With this attainment, children are able to perform what he has called "mental transformations." A hallmark of this ability is the mental operation of reversibility. Although no direct relationship has been established (cf., Beilin, 1975), it has been suggested that children's understanding and use of active and passive forms of sentences are related to this ability. Similarly, Ingram (1976) has posited that these cognitive abilities may be important to those phonologic developments of this period that require more complex operations.

Another change which takes place during this period involves the child's schooling. By age 7, most children are enrolled in first grade and are beginning to learn to read and spell. The translation of their phonetic system into an orthographic system is likely to have significant effect on the child's whole phonologic system.

In spite of the important changes that occur during this period, we know little about the simultaneous changes in phonologic behavior. This is simply the result of a greater focus on early periods of development in recent research. However, several investigations have provided some preliminary information regarding the developments of this period.

In one study, Moskowitz (1973) examined children's rules concerning vowel shifts (alterations) in different forms of a given word (e.g., *divine-divinity; profane-profanity; serene-serenity*). A nonsense word task required the child to add an *-ity* ending to words that would, and words that would not, require a vowel alteration. Five-year-olds generally made no alterations. The 7-year-old children and some of the children ranging in age from 9 to 12 made alterations, but the correct vowel was not always used. The remaining 9- to 12-year-olds made only the correct vowel change. So the vowel-shift rule appears to be acquired gradually beginning at age 7. Moskowitz suggested that the source of the children's understanding of this shift is their spelling knowledge.

The same source of knowledge may account for another set of findings concerning children's understanding of contrastive stress differentiating nouns from verbs (*'convict* vs. *con'vict*) and compound nouns from noun phrases (e.g., *greenhouse* vs. *green house*). Atkinson-King (1973) found that while 5-year-olds had little or no understanding of this feature, by age 12 children had mastered these distinctions.

The fact that learning to read, learning to spell, and learning a phonology are related is not at all surprising. The specific nature and extent of these relationships are unknown. A study by Read (1971) of preschool children's early spellings suggests that their naive views of spelling are largely influenced by their phonologic knowledge and their rote knowledge of letter names. Other research has indicated that speech processes play an important role in learning to read (Hogaboam & Perfetti, 1978; Lesgold &

Curtis, 1981) but not necessarily in later "skilled" reading (Coltheart, Besner, Jonasson, & Davelaar, 1979). However, a good many issues concerning these relationships remain unresolved (see Lesgold & Perfetti, 1981 for an extensive review). Further research might aid speech-language pathologists in dealing with older impaired children. Additionally, it might enable us to provide reading instructors with more efficacious methods of aiding children in the translation of an oral and auditory phonologic system into an orthographic system (cf., Chomsky, 1970; 1972).

Conclusion

It should now be clear that we have made significant advances in our knowledge of phonologic acquisition since Jakobson's work was first translated in 1968. However, like so many young fields, this geometric expansion of knowledge has led to an exponential increase in the number of questions for which we do not yet have answers. Perhaps in the next decade some research will be conducted within the frameworks of new theories or more refined versions of the theoretical models discussed in this chapter. Such focused research, in conjunction with research conducted outside these frameworks, will provide some of the answers to these questions and, in turn, lead to further refinement of existing theories. Ideally, researchers will also provide clinicians with the specific developmental data they need to plan diagnosis and remediation.

Reference Notes

1. Menn, L. Towards a psychology of phonology: Child phonology as a first step. Paper presented to the Michigan State University Conference on Metatheory: Applications of Linguistic Theory in the Human Sciences, East Lansing, 1978.

2. Williams, L. The effects of phonetic environment and stress placement on infant discrimination of the place of stop consonant articulation. Paper presented to the Boston University Conference on Language Development, 1977.

3. Kaplan, E. The role of intonation in the acquisition of language. Unpublished doctoral dissertation, Cornell University, 1969.

4. Oller, K. Analysis of infant vocalizations: A linguistic and speech science perspective. Miniseminar presented to the American Speech and Hearing Association, Houston, 1976.

5. Zlatin, M. Explorative mapping of the vocal tract and primitive syllabification in infancy: The first six months. Paper presented to the American Speech and Hearing Association, Washington, 1975.

6. Doyle, W. On the verge of meaningful speech. Unpublished master's thesis, University of Washington, 1976.

7. Menn, L. Pattern, control and contrast in beginning speech: A case study in the development of word form and word function. Unpublished doctoral dissertation, University of Illinois, 1976.

8. Leonard, L., Camarata, S., Schwartz, R., Chapman, K. & Messick, C. Homonymy in the speech of children with specific language impairment. Unpublished paper, 1983.

9. Smith, M., & Brunette, D. Homonymy as a strategic conspiracy in phonological and lexical development. Paper presented to the American Speech-Language-Hearing Association, Toronto, 1982.

10. Dinnsen, D., Elbert, M., & Weismer, G. On the characterization of functional misarticulations. Paper presented to the American Speech-Language-Hearing Association, Detroit, 1979.

11. Edwards, M.L. Velar preferences in phonologically disordered children. Paper presented to the American Speech-Language-Hearing Association, Los Angeles, 1981.

12. Clumeck, H. Studies in the acquisition of Mandarin phonology. Unpublished doctoral dissertation, University of California, Berkeley, 1977.

13. Klein, H. The relationship between perceptual strategies and productive strategies in learning the phonology of early lexical items. Unpublished doctoral dissertation, Columbia University, 1978.

14. Innes, S. Developmental aspects of plural formation in English. Unpublished master's thesis, University of Alberta, 1974.

15. Cousins, A. Grammatical morpheme development in an aphasic child: Some problems with the normative model. Paper presented to the Boston University Conference on Language Development, 1979.

16. Barton, D. The role of perception in the acquisition of phonology. Unpublished doctoral dissertation, London, Indiana University Linguistics Club, 1976.

17. Barton, D. The discrimination of minimally different pairs of real words by children 2;3-2;11. Paper presented at the Third International Child Language Symposium, London, 1975.

18. Koenigsknecht, R., & Lee, L. Distinctive feature analysis of speech-sound discrimination in children. Paper presented to the American Speech and Hearing Association, 1968.

19. Prelock, P. Cumulative effects of syntactic and phonological complexity on children's language production. Unpublished doctoral dissertation, University of Pittsburgh, 1983.

20. Kamhi, A., Catts, H., & Davis, M. The effects of increases in language complexity on children's word productions: Evidence for the autonomy of language and phonology. Unpublished paper, 1982.

21. Camarata, S., & Schwartz, R. Phonological production of action words and object words. Paper presented to the American Speech-Language-Hearing Association, Toronto, 1982.

22. Messick, C., & Schwartz, R. Does imitation or comprehension affect phonological production in stage I children? Paper presented to the American Speech-Language-Hearing Association, Toronto, 1982.

References

Allen, G. Linguistic experience modifies lexical stress perception. *Journal of Child Language,* in press.

Allen, G., & Hawkins, S. The development of phonological rhythm. In A. Bell & J. Hooper (Eds.), *Syllables and segments.* Amsterdam: North Holland, 1978.

Allen, G., & Hawkins, S. Phonological rhythm: Definition and development. In G. Yeni-Komshian, J. Kavanaugh, & C. Ferguson (Eds.), *Child phonology Vol. I - Production.* New York: Academic Press, 1980.

Aslin, R., & Pisoni, D. Some developmental processes in speech perception. In G. Yeni-Komshian, J. Kavanaugh, & C. Ferguson (Eds.), *Child phonology. Vol. II. Perception.* New York: Academic Press, 1980.

Atkinson-King, K. Children's acquisition of lexical stress contrasts. *Working Papers in Phonetics,* UCLA Phonetics Laboratory, 1973.

Barton, D. Statistical significance in phonemic perception experiments. *Journal of Child Language,* 1975, *2,* 297–298.

Barton, D. Phonemic perception in children. In G. Yeni-Komshian, J. Kavanaugh, & C. Ferguson (Eds.), *Child phonology. Vol. II. Perception.* New York: Academic Press, 1980.

Bates, E., Camaioni, L., & Volterra, V. The acquisition of performatives prior to speech. *Merrill-Palmer Quarterly,* 1975, *21,* 205–224.

Beilin, H. *Studies in the cognitive basis of language development.* New York: Academic Press, 1975.

Bell, A., & Hooper, J. (Eds.) *Syllables and segments.* Amsterdam: North Holland, 1978.

Berko, J. The child's learning of English morphology. *Word,* 1958, *14,* 150–177.

Bernthal, J., & Bankson, N. *Articulation disorders.* Englewood Cliffs, N.J.: Prentice-Hall, 1981.

Bloom, K. Patterning of infant vocal behavior. *Journal of Experimental Child Psychology,* 1977, *23,* 367–377.

Bloom, K. Evaluation of infant conditioning. *Journal of Experimental Child Psychology,* 1979, *27,* 60–70.

Bloom, K., & Esposito, A. Social conditioning and its proper control procedures. *Journal of Experimental Child Psychology,* 1975, *19,* 209–222.

Braine, M. The acquisition of language in infant and child. In C. Reed (Ed.), *The learning of language.* New York: Appleton-Century-Crofts, 1971.

Braine, M. On what might constitute learnable phonology. *Language.* 1974, *50,* 270–299.

Brown, R. *A first language: The early stages.* Cambridge, Mass.: Harvard University Press, 1973.

Bryant, P. *Perception and understanding in young children: An experimental approach.* New York: Basic Books, 1974.

Campbell, T., & Shriberg, L. Associations among pragmatic function, linguistic stress and natural phonological processes in speech-delayed children. *Journal of Speech and Hearing Research,* 1982, *25,* 547–553.

Carter, A. The transformation of sensorimotor morphemes into words: A case study of the development of "more" and "mine." *Journal of Child Language,* 1975, *2,* 233–250.

Carter, A. The disappearance schema: Case study of a second-year communicative behavior. In E. Ochs & B. Schieffelin (Eds.), *Developmental pragmatics.* New York: Academic Press, 1979.

Chapman, R., & Miller, J. Word order in early two and three word utterances: Does production precede comprehension? *Journal of Speech and Hearing Research,* 1975, *18,* 355–371.

Chomsky, C. Reading, writing and phonology. *Harvard Educational Review,* 1970, *40,* 307–308.

Chomsky, C. Write now, read later. In C. Cazden (Ed.), *Language in early childhood education.* Washington: National Association for the Education of Young Children, 1972.

Chomsky, N., & Halle, M. *The sound pattern of English.* New York: Harper & Row, 1968.

Clumeck, H. The acquisition of tone. In G. Yeni-Komshian, J. Kavanaugh, & C. Ferguson *Child phonology. Vol. I. Production.* New York: Academic Press, 1980.

Cole, R., & Jakimik, J. Understanding speech: How words are heard. In G. Underwood (Ed.), *Strategies of information processing.* London: Academic Press, 1978.

Coltheart, M., Besner, D., Jonasson, J., & Davelaar, E. Phonological encodings in the lexical decision task. *Quarterly Journal of Experimental Psychology,* 1979, *31,* 489–507.

Crystal, D. Non-segmental phonology in language acquisition: A review of the issues. *Lingua,* 1973, *32,* 1–45.

Crystal, D. *The English tone of voice*. London: Edward Arnold, 1975.

deVilliers, J., & deVilliers, P. A cross-sectional study of the acquisition of grammatical morphemes in child speech. *Journal of Psycholinguistic Research*, 1973, *2*, 267-278.

Derwing, B., & Baker, W. The psychological basis for morphological rules. In J. Macnamara (Ed.), *Language learning and thought*. New York: Academic Press, 1977.

Derwing, B., & Baker, W. Recent research on the acquisition of English morphology. In P. Fletcher & M. Garman (Eds.), *Language acquisition*. Cambridge: Cambridge University Press, 1979.

Dore, J., Franklin, M., Miller, R., & Ramer, A. Transitional phenomena in early language acquisition. *Journal of Child Language*, 1976, *3*, 13-28.

Edwards, M. L. Perception and production in child phonology: The testing of four hypotheses. *Journal of Child Language*, 1974, *1*, 205-219.

Edwards, M. L., & Shriberg, L. *Phonology: Applications in communicative disorders*. San Diego: College-Hill Press, 1983.

Eilers, R. Infant speech perception: History and mystery. In G. Yeni-Komshian, J. Kavanaugh, & C. Ferguson (Eds.), *Child phonology. Vol. II. Perception*. New York: Academic Press, 1980.

Fee, J., & Ingram, D. Reduplication as a strategy of phonological development. *Journal of Child Language*, 1982, *9*, 41-54.

Ferguson, C. Learning to pronounce: The earliest stages of phonological development in the child. In F. Minifie & L. Lloyd (Eds.), *Communicative and cognitive abilities—Early behavioral assessment*. Baltimore: University Park Press, 1978.

Ferguson, C. Reduplication in child phonology. *Journal of Child Language*, 1983, *10*, 239-244.

Ferguson, C., & Farwell, C. Words and sounds in early language acquisition: English initial consonants in the first fifty words. *Language*, 1975, *51*, 419-439.

Ferguson, C., & Garnica, O. Theories of phonological development. In E. Lenneberg & E. Lenneberg (Eds.), *Foundations of language development (Vol. I)*. New York: Academic Press, 1975.

Ferguson, C., & Macken, M. Phonological development in children: Play and cognition. *Papers and Reports on Child Language Development*, 1980, *18*, 138-177.

Fey, M., & Gandour, J. Rule discovery in phonological acquisition. *Journal of Child Language*, 1982, *9*, 71-81.

Garnica, O. The development of the perception of phonemic differences in initial consonants by English-speaking children. *Papers and Reports on Child Language Development*, 1971, *3*, 1-29.

Garnica, O. The development of phonemic speech perception. In T. Moore (Ed.), *Cognitive development and the acquisition of language*. New York: Academic Press, 1973.

Gilbert, J., & Purves, B. Temporal constraints on consonant clusters in child speech production. *Journal of Child Language*, 1977, *4*, 103-110.

Graham, L., & House, A. Phonological oppositions in children: A perceptual study. *Journal of the Acoustical Society of America*, 1971, *49*, 559-566.

Greenlee, M. Learning the phonetic cues to the voiced/voiceless distinction: A comparison of child and adult speech perception. *Journal of Child Language*, 1980, *7*, 459-468.

Halliday, M. *Learning how to mean: Explorations in the development of knowledge*. London: Edward Arnold, 1975.

Hawkins, S. Temporal coordination of consonants in the speech of children: Further data. *Journal of Phonetics*, 1979, *7*, 235-267.

Hogaboam, T., & Perfetti, C. Reading skill and the role of verbal experience in decoding. *Journal of Educational Psychology*, 1978, *70*, 717-729.

Ingram, D. Phonological rules in young children. *Journal of Child Language,* 1974, *1,* 49–64.

Ingram, D. Surface contrast in phonology: Evidence from children's speech. *Journal of Child Language,* 1975, *2,* 287–292.

Ingram, D. *Phonological disability in children.* New York: Elsevier, 1976.

Ingram, D. *Procedures for the phonological analysis of children's language.* Baltimore: University Park Press, 1981.

Ingram, D., Christensen, L., Veach, S., & Webster, B. The acquisition of word-initial fricatives and affricates by children between 2 and 6 years. In G. Yeni-Komshian, J. Kavanaugh, & C. Ferguson (Eds.), *Child phonology. Vol. I. Production.* New York: Academic Press, 1980.

Jakobson, R. *Child language, aphasia and phonological universals.* The Hague: Mouton, 1968.

Jakobson, R., Fant, G., & Halle, M. *Preliminaries to speech analysis: The distinctive features and their correlations.* Cambridge: MIT Press, 1963.

Jusczyk, P., & Thomson, E. Perception of a phonetic contrast in multi-syllabic utterances by 2-month old infants. *Perception and Psychophysics,* 1978, *23,* 105–109.

Kent, R. Articulatory-acoustic perspectives on speech development. In R. Stark (Ed.), *Language behavior in infancy and early childhood.* New York: Elsevier North Holland, 1981.

Kiparsky, P., & Menn, L. On the acquisition of phonology. In J. Macnamara (Ed.), *Language learning and thought.* New York: Academic Press, 1977.

Kirk, L. An analysis of speech imitations by Gã children. *Anthropological Linguistics,* 1973, *15,* 267–275.

Klein, H. Productive strategies for the pronunciation of early polysyllabic lexical items. *Journal of Speech and Hearing Research,* 1981, *24,* 309–405.

Kubaska, C., & Keating, P. Word duration in early child speech. *Journal of Speech and Hearing Research,* 1981, *24,* 615–621.

Kuhl, P. Speech perception in early infancy: Perceptual constancy for vowel categories. *Journal of the Acoustical Society of America,* 1976, *60,* Supplement 1, S90.

Kuhl, P. Speech perception in early infancy: Perceptual constancy for the vowel categories /a/ and /ɔ/. *Journal of the Acoustical Society of America,* 1977, *61,* Supplement 1, S39.

Kuhl, P. Perceptual constancy for speech-sound categories in early infancy. In G. Yeni-Komshian, J. Kavanaugh, & C. Ferguson (Eds.), *Child phonology. Vol. II. Perception* New York: Academic Press, 1980.

Kuhl, P., & Meltzoff, A. The bimodal perception of speech in infancy. *Science,* 1982, *218,* 1138–1141

LaRiviere, C., Winitz, H., Reeds, J., & Herriman, E. The conceptual reality of selected distinctive features. *Journal of Speech and Hearing Research,* 1974, *17,* 122–133.

Leavitt, L., Brown, J., Morse, P., & Graham, F. Cardiac orienting and auditory discrimination in 6-week-old infants. *Developmental Psychology,* 1976, *12,* 514–523.

Leonard, L., Miller, J., & Brown, H. Consonant and syllable harmony in the speech of language-disordered children. *Journal of Speech and Hearing Disorders,* 1980, *45,* 336–345.

Leonard, L., Newhoff, M., & Mesalam, L. Individual differences in early child phonology. *Applied Psycholinguistics,* 1980, *1,* 7–30.

Leonard, L., Schwartz, R., Chapman, K., & Morris, B. Factors influencing early lexical acquisition. *Child Development* 1981, *52,* 882–887.

Leonard, L., Schwartz, R., Chapman, K., Rowan, L., Prelock, P., Terrell, B., Weiss, A., & Messick, C. Early lexical acquisition in children with specific language impairment. *Journal of Speech and Hearing Research,* 1982, *25,* 554–564.

Leonard, L., Schwartz, R., Folger, M., & Wilcox, M. Some aspects of child phonology in imitative and spontaneous speech. *Journal of Child Language,* 1978, *5,* 403–416.

Leopold, W. *Speech development of a bilingual child: A linguistic record* (4 vols.). Chicago: Northwestern University Press, 1939–1947.

Lesgold, A., & Curtis, M. Learning to read words efficiently. In A. Lesgold & C. Perfetti (Eds.), *Interactive processes in reading.* Hillsdale, N.J.: Lawrence Erlbaum, 1981.

Lesgold, A., & Perfetti, C. Interactive processes in reading. Hillsdale, N.J.: Lawrence Erlbaum, 1981.

Locke, J. The child's processing of phonology. In W. A. Collins (Ed.), *Minnesota symposium on child psychology* (Vol. 12). Hillsdale, N.J.: Lawrence Erlbaum, 1979. (a)

Locke, J. Homonymy and sound change in the child's acquisition of phonology. In N. Lass (Ed.), *Speech and language: Advances in basic research and practice.* New York: Academic Press, 1979. (b)

Locke, J. The inference of speech perception in the phonologically disordered child. Part I: A rationale, some criteria, the conventional tests. *Journal of Speech and Hearing Disorders,* 1980, *45,* 431–444. (a)

Locke, J. The inference of speech perception in the phonologically disordered child. Part II: Some clinically novel procedures, their use, some findings. *Journal of Speech and Hearing Disorders,* 1980, *45,* 445–468. (b)

Macken, M. Developmental reorganization of phonology: A hierarchy of basic units of acquisition. *Linga,* 1979, *49,* 11–49.

Macken, M. Aspects of the acquisition of stop systems: A cross-linguistic perspective. In G. Yeni-Komshian, J. Kavanaugh, & C. Ferguson (Eds.), *Child phonology. Vol. I. Production.* New York: Academic Press, 1980. (a)

Macken, M. The child's lexical representation: The 'puzzle-puddle-pickle' evidence. *Journal of Linguistics* 1980, *16,* 1–17. (b)

Macken, M., & Barton, D. The acquisition of the voicing contrast in English: A study of voice onset time in word-initial stop consonants. *Journal of Child Language,* 1980, *7,* 41–74. (a)

Macken, M., & Barton, D. The acquisition of the voicing contrast in Spanish: A phonetic and phonological study of word-initial stop consonants. *Journal of Child Language,* 1980, *7,* 433–458. (b)

MacNeilage, P. The control of speech production. In G. Yeni-Komshian, J. Kavanaugh, & C. Ferguson (Eds.), *Child phonology. Vol. I. Production.* New York: Academic Press, 1980.

MacWhinney, B. The acquisition of morphophonology. *Monographs of the Society for Research in Child Development,* 1978, *43,* (174), 1–2.

McReynolds, L., & Elbert, M. Criteria for phonological process analysis. *Journal of Speech and Hearing Disorders,* 1981, *46,* 197–204.

Menyuk, P. The role of distinctive features in children's acquisition of phonology. *Journal of Speech and Hearing Research,* 1968, *11,* 138–146.

Menyuk, P., & Anderson, S. Children's identification and reproduction of /w/, /r/ and /l/. *Journal of Speech and Hearing Research,* 1969, *12,* 39–52.

Menyuk, P., & Looney, P. Relationships among components of the grammar in language disorder. *Journal of Speech and Hearing Research,* 1972, *15,* 395–406.

Moerk, E. Relationships between parental input frequencies and children's language acquisition: A reanalysis of Brown's data. *Journal of Child Language,* 1980, *7,* 105–118.

Moerk, E. To attend or not to attend to unwelcome reanalyses? A reply to Pinker. *Journal of Child Language,* 1981, *8,* 627–632.

Morse, P. The discrimination of speech and non-speech stimuli in early infancy. *Journal of Experimental Child Psychology,* 1972, *14,* 718–731.

Morton, J., & Long, J. Effect of word transitional probability on phoneme identification. *Journal of Verbal Learning and Verbal Behavior,* 1976, *15,* 43–51.

Moskowitz, A. The two-year stage in the acquisition of English phonology. *Language,* 1970, *46,* 426–441.

Moskowitz, B. On the status of vowel shift in English. In T. Moore (Ed.), *Cognitive development and the acquisition of language.* New York: Academic Press, 1973.

Nelson, K. Structure and strategy in learning how to talk. *Monographs of the Society for Research in Child Development,* 1973, *38,* (149) 1-2.

Netsell, R. The acquisition of speech motor control: A perspective with directions for research. In R. Stark (Ed.), *Language behavior in infancy and early childhood.* New York: Elsevier North Holland, 1981.

Oller, D. The emergence of speech sounds in infancy. In G. Yeni-Komshian, J. Kavanaugh, & C. Ferguson (Eds.). *Child phonology. Vol. I. Production.* New York: Academic Press, 1980.

Oller, D., & Smith, B. The effect of final-syllable position on vowel duration in infant babbling. *Journal of the Acoustical Society of America,* 1977, *62,* 994-997.

Oller, D., Wieman, L., Doyle, W., & Ross, C. Infant babbling and speech. *Journal of Child Language,* 1975, *3,* 1-11.

Olmsted, D. *Out of the mouths of babes.* The Hague: Mouton, 1971.

Panagos, J. Persistence of the open syllable reinterpreted as a symptom of language disorder. *Journal of Speech and Hearing Disorders,* 1974, *39,* 23-31.

Panagos, J., & Prelock, P. Phonological constraints on the sentence productions of language disordered children. *Journal of Speech and Hearing Research,* 1982, *25,* 171-177.

Panagos, J., Quine, M., & Klich, R. Syntactic and phonological influences on children's articulation. *Journal of Speech and Hearing Research,* 1979, *22,* 841-848.

Piaget, J. *Play, dreams and imitation in childhood.* New York: Norton, 1962.

Piaget, J. Piaget's theory. In P. Mussen (Ed.), *Carmichael's manual of child psychology* (Vol. I). New York: John Wiley, 1970.

Pinker, S. Formal models of language learning. *Cognition,* 1979, *7,* 217-283.

Pinker, S. On the acquisition of grammatical morphemes. *Journal of Child Language,* 1981, *8,* 477-484.

Poole, E. Genetic development of articulation of consonant sounds in speech. *Elementary English Review,* 1934, *11,* 159-161.

Priestly, T. One idiosyncratic strategy in the acquisition of phonology. *Journal of Child Language,* 1977, *4,* 45-65.

Priestly, T. Homonymy in child phonology. *Journal of Child Language,* 1980, *7,* 413-472.

Read, C. Pre-school children's knowledge of English phonology. *Harvard Educational Review,* 1971, *41,* 1-34.

Rheingold, H., Gewirtz, J., & Ross, H. Social conditioning of vocalizations in the infant. *Journal of Comparative and Physiological Psychology,* 1959, *52,* 68-73.

Ritterman, S., & Freeman, N. Distinctive phonetic features as relevant and irrelevant stimulus dimensions in speech-sound discrimination learning. *Journal of Speech and Hearing Research,* 1974, *17,* 417-425.

Ross, G. Categorization in 1- to 2-year-olds. *Developmental Psychology,* 1980, *16,* 391-396.

Salus, P., & Salus, M. Developmental neurophysiology and phonological acquisition order. *Language,* 1974, *50,* 151-160.

Sander, E. When are speech sounds learned? *Journal of Speech and Hearing Disorders,* 1972, *37,* 55-63.

Sankoff, D. *Linguistic variation: Models and methods.* New York: Academic Press, 1978.

Schmauch, V., Panagos, J., & Klich, R. Syntax influences the accuracy of consonant production in language-disordered children. *Journal of Communication Disorders,* 1978, *11,* 315-323.

Schwartz, R. Assessment of speech sound disorders in children. In I. Meitus, & B. Weinberg (Eds.), *Diagnosis in speech-language pathology.* Baltimore: University Park Press, in press.

Schwartz, R., & Folger, M. Sensorimotor development and descriptions of child phonology: A preliminary view of phonological analysis for Stage I speech. *Papers and Reports on Child Language Development,* 1977, *13,* 8-15.

Schwartz, R., & Leonard, L. Do children pick and choose? An examination of phonological selection and avoidance in early lexical acquisition. *Journal of Child Language*, 1982, *9*, 319–336.

Schwartz, R., Leonard, L., Wilcox, M., & Folger, M. Again and again: Reduplication in child phonology. *Journal of Child Language*, 1980, *7*, 75–88.

Schwartz, R., & Prelock, P. Cognition and phonology. In J. Panagos (Ed.), Children's phonological disorders in language contexts. *Seminars in Speech, Language and Hearing*, 1982, *3*, New York: Thieme-Stratton.

Shibamoto, J., & Olmsted, D. Lexical and syllabic patterns in phonological acquisition. *Journal of Child Language*, 1978, *5*, 417–456.

Shriberg, L., & Kwiatkowski, J. *Natural process analysis*. New York: John Wiley, 1980.

Shriner, T., Halloway, M., & Daniloff, R. The relationship between articulatory deficits and syntax in speech defective children. *Journal of Speech and Hearing Research*, 1969, *12*, 319–325.

Shvachkin, N. The development of phonemic speech perception in early childhood. In C. Ferguson & D. Slobin (Eds.), *Studies of child language development*. New York: Holt, Rinehart & Winston, 1973.

Singh, S. *Distinctive features: Theory and validation*. Baltimore: University Park Press, 1976.

Smith, B. Temporal aspects of English speech production: A developmental perspective. *Journal of Phonetics*, 1978, *6*, 37–67.

Smith, N. *The acquisition of phonology: A case study*. London: Cambridge University Press, 1973.

Spring, D., & Dale, P. Discrimination of linguistic stress in early infancy. *Journal of Speech and Hearing Research*, 1977, *20*, 224–231.

Stampe, D. A dissertation on natural phonology. Unpublished doctoral dissertation, University of Chicago, 1973.

Stark, R. Stages of speech development in the first year of life. In G. Yeni-Komshian, J. Kavanaugh, & C. Ferguson, (Eds.), *Child phonology. Vol. I. Production*. New York: Academic Press, 1980.

Strange, W., & Broen, P. Perception and production of approximant consonants by 3-year-olds: A first study. In G. Yeni-Komshian, J. Kavanaugh, & C. Ferguson (Eds.), *Child phonology Vol. II. Perception*. New York: Academic Press, 1980.

Templin, M. Certain language skills in children: Their development and interrelationships. Institute of Child Welfare, Monograph 26, Minneapolis, University of Minnesota Press, 1957.

Tingley, B., & Allen, G. Development of speech timing control in children. *Child Development*, 1975, *46*, 186–194.

Toombs, M., Singh, S., & Hayden, M. Markedness of features in the articulatory substitutions of children. *Journal of Speech and Hearing Disorders*, 1981, *46*, 184–191.

Vihman, M. Phonology and the development of the lexicon: Evidence from children's errors. *Journal of Child Language*, 1981, *8*, 239–264.

Waterson, N. Child phonology: A prosodic view. *Journal of Linguistics*, 1971, *7*, 179–221.

Waterson, N. A tentative model of phonological representation. In T. Myers, J. Laver, & J. Anderson (Eds.), *The cognitive representation of speech*. Amsterdam: North-Holland, 1981.

Weiner, F. Systematic sound preference as a characteristic of phonological disability. *Journal of Speech and Hearing Disorders*, 1981, *46*, 281–286.

Weisberg, P. Social and nonsocial conditioning of infant vocalizations. *Child Development*, 1963, *34*, 377–388.

Weismer, G., Dinnsen, D., & Elbert, M. A study of the voicing distinction associated with omitted, word-final stops. *Journal of Speech and Hearing Disorders*, 1981, *46*, 320–328.

Wellman, B., Case, I., Mengurt, I., & Bradbury, D. Speech sounds of young children. *University of Iowa Studies in Child Welfare*, 1931, *5*.

Wepman, J. *Auditory discrimination test*. Chicago: University of Chicago Press, 1958.

Whitaker, J., Luper, H., & Pollio, H. General language deficits in children with articulation problems. *Language and Speech,* 1970, *13,* 231-239.

Williams, L., & Bush, M. The discrimination of voiced stop consonants by young infants with and without release bursts. *Journal of the Acoustical Society of America,* 1978, *63,* 1223-1225.

Winitz, H. *Articulatory acquisition and behavior.* New York: Appleton-Century-Crofts, 1969.

Zlatin, M., & Koenigsknecht, R. Development of the voicing contrast: A comparison of voice onset time in stop perception and production. *Journal of Speech and Hearing Research,* 1976, *19,* 93-111.

Zlatin Laufer, M., & Horii, Y. Fundamental frequency characteristics of infant non-distress vocalization during the first 24 weeks. *Journal of Child Language,* 1977, *4,* 171-184.

End Note

[1]Leonard, Newhoff, and Mesalam (1980) argued that this method leads to the uncertain assumption that this child would also produce *see* as [si] or[i] and *sun* as [tʌn]. Consequently, they would identify the phone classes as [t-d], [d-s-θ], [f], (b-p]. While this may be more accurate, it may be more difficult to compare with the adult system. The method employed should depend on the purpose of the analysis.

Frederick F. Weiner

A Phonologic Approach to Assessment and Treatment

Since the publication of *Phonological Disability in Children* (Ingram, 1976) the area of articulation disorders has taken a large turn in direction. The focus has broadened to include a phonologic thrust. With this new direction has come an interest in children with multiple misarticulations and unintelligible speech. Researchers and clinicians have viewed the patterns of sound production observed in these children as a separate aspect of language equal in importance to syntax, semantics, or pragmatics. Because of the orderliness of sound errors in these children, researchers have inferred that mentalistic rules must govern surface level sound production. In an attempt to determine the orderliness of sound errors, several evaluation procedures have been published. These include *Assessment of Phonological Processes* (Hodson, 1980), *Procedures for the Phonological Analysis of Children's Language* (Ingram, 1981), *Natural Process Analysis* (Shriberg & Kwiatkowski, 1980), and *Phonological Process Analysis* (Weiner, 1979).

Motivated by the publication of these procedures a great deal of work has been carried out in developing a better understanding of the theory behind a phonologic approach to misarticulation as well as suggestions for assessment and treatment of children who are unintelligible. This new work should certainly be considered as recent advances in the study of phonologic disability and will be summarized and discussed in this chapter. Specifically, the topics to follow will be: What is a Phonologic Process? Perceptual Testing for Phonologic Disorders, Systematic Sound Preference,

Phonologic Development for Unintelligible Speakers, and A Case for Using the Effects of Listener-Speaker Interactions to Facilitate the Treatment of Children with Phonologic Disability.

What is a Phonologic Process?

One of the most prominent characteristics of children with multiple misarticulations is the reduction of phonemic contrasts in comparison to the adult phonemic system. When the reduction in phonemic contrasts appears to be systematic, these patterns of errors have been called phonologic processes.

The term phonologic process, as used in analysis of misarticulation, comes from the theory of Natural Phonology (Donegan & Stampe, 1978). In the most recent version of this theory, it is assumed that the sound patterns of a language are governed by the constraints of the human speech capacity. These constraints include both the limitations of the human vocal tract and the perceptual system. Processes are mental substitutions which unconsciously adapt phonologic intentions to phonetic capacities.

By labeling a phonetic event a phonologic process we are saying that the speaker has subconsciously transformed a phonologic intention in a manner consistent with his phonetic capacity. In children, these phonologic intentions are based on what the child knows about the adult language. In this sense, the child is assumed to have an underlying phonologic representation fairly equivalent to the adult surface form. The phonologic process is a description of how the child subconsciously transforms underlying representations into surface level events. Because the child is in a more language-naive state than the adult, his or her phonetic output is highly subject to natural forces implicit in human vocalization and perception. As a consequence, many phonemic contrasts present in the adult language become obliterated. As children develop and come to know the language function of these phonemic contrasts, they begin to suppress the natural dynamics of vocalization in an attempt to establish these contrasts at the surface level. As a result, their surface level output becomes more like their internal representations.

Unfortunately, the mental events described by phonologic processes are not directly observable. They can only be inferred on the basis of phonetic output and perceptual responses. It is exactly for this reason that the usefulness of phonologic processes has been questioned. Being behaviorally oriented professionals, speech-language pathologists have felt uneasy about the description of events that are not directly observable. This uneasiness has led them to charge that "this kind of analysis appears no more than a relabeling of articulation errors, not a discovery of the operation of processes" (McReynolds & Elbert, 1981, p. 197).

At this time McReynolds and Elbert are correct in making such an assertion. To date there have been few published attempts to verify that phonologic processes are adaptations of internal representations to phonetic output. Furthermore, this concept has been overused by some investigators to the extent that all child misarticulations have been described as processes, whether justified or not. As a result, it is up to those who advocate the use of phonologic processes to justify their existence.

Criteria for the Occurrence of Phonologic Processes

In my view, the major substantiation of a phonologic process is showing that the child "knows" the adult phonemic contrast but does not use it. In this regard Dinnsen, Elbert, and Weismer (Note 1) have proposed three tests. The first is that the process must apply optionally. That is, if a child uses the correct form some of the time, we can infer that the adult form is known and an underlying representation exists. The second is that the adult contrast is expressed in an unconventional manner. An example would be when a child deletes the final consonant in *pig* and *pick*, but still maintains the contrast by lengthening the vowel in *pig*, but not in *pick*. The third test is that the process applies to a very limited class of segments. For example, if a process occurs for only the voiceless members of a class of sounds, the child is demonstrating knowledge of a voiced-voiceless distinction within that class. Assuming that these criteria are valid tests for establishment of processes, there are many examples in the literature and clinical reports of patterns of misarticulation that would qualify as phonologic processes.

As speech-language clinicians, we have all seen children who were inconsistent in their production of certain sounds or classes of sounds. Technically, these would qualify as phonologic processes. But, our assertion that phonologic processes exist would be strengthened if we could describe the conditions surrounding the inconsistency. For example, Dinnsen, Elbert, and Weismer (Note 1) described Jamie, a boy who deleted final consonants. His production of *dog* was /dɔ:/. But when he said the same word with the diminutive suffix added, his production was /dɔgI/. Here we can infer that the child had the underlying representation for /g/ but, because of the process of deletion of final consonants, did not use final /g/.

Another example comes from tests for assimilation. Ordinarily, a child who produces *dog* > /gɔg/ is assumed to assimilate the initial sound with the final /g/. This sound is described as a potential "culprit" which motivated the g/d substitution. To substantiate velar assimilation as a phonologic process, one should observe the child's other attempts to produce /d/ in words without final velar stops. If the child produces the /d/ sound correctly in words like *dish*, *do*, and *date* (words without the culprit /g/), then it might be assumed that the g/d substitution in dog > /gɔg/ was due to the phonologic process called velar assimilation.

A child in our clinic seemed to be using a process in words containing nasals. The following is a short corpus of his responses:

paint /neʔ/	sun /n:ʌʔ/
pig /pI/	soup /tʃup/
tent /nɛk/	swimming /nImI/
toothbrush /tutbʌs/	sweater /tawə\

In each case when the word contained a nasal, the first sound became a nasal. If the word did not have a nasal, then those same sounds were either produced correctly or were replaced by other nonnasal sounds. Here again is an example of a nasal assimilation that would qualify as a phonologic process because the child demonstrated that he had the underlying representation for many of the sounds that were replaced by /n/.

As an example of a child who demonstrated knowledge of an adult phonemic contrast without using that contrast as an adult would, the following short corpus is presented:

ski→/k⁼i/	swimming→/k⁼wImIŋ/
skate→/k⁼et/	sweater→/k⁼wevin/
sleeping→/tlpIn/	snake→/θneæ
sled→/tlek/	snowman→/ønomæ/

Even though this child does not produce these 4 cluster-types (/s/ + stop, /s/ + /l/, /s/ + /w/, and /s/ + nasal) as an adult would, he nevertheless has 4 different cluster-types. One interpretation of this finding could be that the child realizes that at least 4 different /s/ clusters occur in the adult language. From this realization it could be assumed that his underlying representation for the adult form is similar in many respects to that of the adult.

This final example shows the restricted use of a process:

five→/halv/	valentine→/bɑeldlhalm/
thin→/hIn/	this→/jIts/
soup→ /hup/	zipper→/dʒlpə/
shoe→ /hu/	

In this corpus the child replaces initial voiceless fricatives by /h/ yet other errors occur for initial voiced fricatives. This shows the restricted use of a process and verifies knowledge on the part of the child of a voiced-voiceless phonemic contrast among fricatives.

The above examples are presented to show how one can verify the presence of a process and to provide evidence that mentalistic phonological processes do occur. These examples are important because they demonstrate the role that language plays in sound production.

Perceptual Testing of Phonologic Disorders

In the previous section of this chapter, the point was made that many of a child's misarticulations may be classified as phonologic processes. Such classifications presume that surface speech productions are rule governed and based on an underlying phonemic system. One tool available to the speech-language pathologist to determine the distribution of phonemes in a child's phonologic system would be a description of his perceptual phonemic system. Unfortunately, the major perceptual tests and testing techniques will not provide valid information concerning phonemic perception. Instead, these tests only provide phonetic information. What follows are comments concerning methodological problems with popular perceptual tests and procedures to assess phonemic perception in children with phonologic disability.

By far, the most common form of discrimination testing used by speech clinicians is the same-different paradigm. The two published tests most representative of this paradigm are the *Auditory Discrimination Test* (Wepman, 1973) and a test commonly referred to as the *Templin Speech Sound Discrimination Test* (Templin, 1957). The *Auditory Discrimination Test* has pairs of words in which a single phoneme is contrastive, e.g., *pin - bin*. The *Templin Speech Sound Discrimination Test* has pairs of nonsense syllables. In both tests the child is instructed to say *same* if the paired items are identical, and *different* if the paired items are not identical.

Locke (1980a) presented a critical review of these tests. His review addressed many potential problems in interpretation of test results. First was the problem of the cognitive concept of same versus different. If a child being tested does not know the concept of same and different, incorrect responses may be more a function of this cognitive deficit than difficulty with perception.

Another problem arises when two sounds are allophones of the same phoneme for a child. If /f/ and /θ/ are allophones within a certain child's phonology, this child may respond to a pair of words like /fIn/-/θIn/ with a *same* response. This does not mean that the child does not perceive a difference between /f/ and /θ/. It merely means that the child did not consider the difference to be worth reporting. An analogy would be when an adult hears the words /hɑet⁻/ and /hɑetʰ/. These two words would most likely be reported as the same even though there is a phonetic difference between the two final /t/ sounds. In other words, the adult is capable of perceiving the difference between /t⁻/ and /tʰ/ but, similarly, does not consider this difference worth reporting. Interpretation, then, of the child's -*same* response to /fIn/-/θIn/ (using conventional testing) would be that the child cannot hear the difference between /f/ and /θ/ which may, in fact, be an erroneous conclusion.

Another factor is that some people feel that perception testing is useful as an explanation for faulty misarticulation (although this has not been clearly demonstrated empirically). Unfortunately, the items of most of the published discrimination tests have a poor correspondence with the most common misarticulations; i.e., those items which do relate to predictable misarticulations are only a small part of the test. This is further complicated by the two-alternative nature of these tests. This means that a child who is not correctly perceiving has a 50-50 chance of guessing some of these more difficult discriminations.

By far, the most powerful criticism offered by Locke (1980a) was that results of these tests do not help us answer the most important question, which is "whether the child detects a difference between the speech forms he is expected to acquire (that is, adult surface forms) and those already stored (that is, his internal representation)" (p.436). The same-different paradigm asks the child to make decisions concerning two surface forms spoken by the examiner. Locke argued that these decisions may not give us information about the child's phonemic system. For a child whose system held /f/ and /θ/ as allophones of the same phoneme, a /fIn/-/θIn/ item would require him to discriminate between his allophones. If this same child held /f/ and /θ/ as separate phonemes, then the discrimination would be between different phonemes. The problem is that we do not know the relationship between /f/ and /θ/ for the child. In fact, that is exactly the kind of information that our discrimination testing should give us.

On the basis of these criticisms, Locke (1980b) proposed a set of criteria for more efficient assessment of speech perception. These criteria are extremely useful and bear repeating here. The criteria are that the procedure must:

1. examine the child's perception of the replaced sound in relation to the replacing sound, that is, the target phoneme versus its substitution phoneme, or, as in the case of complete omission, silence;
2. observe the same phonemes in identical phoneme environments in production and perception;

3. permit a comparison of the child's performance of target and replacing sounds with his discrimination of target and perceptually similar control sounds;
4. be based on a comparison of an adult's surface form and the child's own internal representation;
5. present repeated opportunities for the child to reveal his perceptual decisions;
6. prevent nonperceptual errors from masquerading as perceptual errors;
7. require a response easily within a young child's conceptual capacities and repertoire of responses; and
8. allow a determination of the direction of misperception (p. 445).

On the basis of these criteria, Locke proposed a new form of discrimination testing called the Speech Production-Perception Task (SP-PT). To perform this test, the clinician first selects a production error such as /θʌm/ → /fʌm/. In this example /θ/ is considered the stimulus phoneme (SP) and /f/ is considered the replacement phoneme (RP). Next the clinician selects a control phoneme (CP). The CP is perceptually similar to the SP, such as /s/ for this example. The tester then selects a picture of *thumb* (the target word) and asks, "Is this /θʌm/? Is this /fʌm/? Is this /sʌm/?" The child is required to answer "Yes" or "No" to each of these questions. Each question is asked 6 times for a total of 18 responses and the order of presentation is randomized.

A child who had perception similar to adults would answer "Yes" to /θʌm/ and "No" to /fʌm/ and /sʌm/. This type of pattern of response would mean that the child's internal representation was the same as the adult's and, therefore, /f/ and /θ/ would be different phonemes in the child's external perceptual system. In the test administration, it is essential that the child answer "No" to the CPs (/sʌm/). Otherwise, the examiner cannot be certain that he is capable of performing to the conceptual requirements of the test. In other words, "No" responses to the CP items establish the validity of the child's responses. Once that is established, we can more readily believe what the child reports about SP and RP.

Some children tested by Locke showed a pattern of response wherein they said "Yes" to /θʌm/, "Yes" to /fʌm/, and "No" to /sʌm/. In this case, these children demonstrated that they were valid perceivers by responding "No" to /sʌm/. But, such children also responded as if /fʌm/ and /θʌm/ were appropriate descriptions of *thumb*. The conclusion to be drawn from this result is that /f/ and /θ/ are both allophones of /θ/ for these children because both, when produced by the adult, matched the children's internal representation for /θ/. In this instance, the children's misarticulation of f/θ was probably motivated by the fact that these two sounds were not contrasted in the children's perceptual phonology.

One other important point brought out by Locke (1980b) was that since different discrimination tests represent different levels of perception, we, as clinicians, should be able to use that information to our advantage in assessing our clients. Consider, for example, the child who answered "Yes" to /θʌm/, "Yes" to /fʌm/, and "No" to /sʌm/. On the basis of SP-PT testing, we know that /f/ and /θ/ are allophones of /θ/ and that the child did not discriminate between them. What we do not know, however, is if this child is capable of discriminating between them. To determine this we should follow up our testing with another form that has the potential to force a child to differentiate between allophones if he is capable. One such test protocol is referred to as an ABX procedure.

In an ABX procedure, the clinician could use two talking puppets, one for each hand. One puppet says "/θʌm/," the other says "/fʌm/," and the clinician asks, "Who said /θʌm/?" In this case, the child is forced to distinguish between his or her allophones. If the child were able to point to the appropriate puppet it would mean that although a distinction between /f/ and /θ/ was not made in the SP-PT test, the child was certainly capable of such a discrimination as was demonstrated by the ABX procedure. Failure to discriminate between /f/ and /θ/ in the ABX would suggest that the child's perceptual errors were not necessarily related to his or her phonemic system. Instead, he may have some form of gross perceptual deficit.

To further elucidate this point, an English-speaking adult with an intact language system can be similarly confronted with an SP-PT and ABX protocol to test perception of /t⁻/ and /tʰ/. For the SP-PT the adult would be shown a picture of a *baseball bat* and asked, "Is this /bæt⁻/?" and "Is this /bætʰ/?" Appropriate responses to both questions would be "Yes" because in English /t⁻/ and /tʰ/ are allophones of the same phoneme. Note that this procedure only tells us that /t⁻/ and /tʰ/ do not change the meaning of the word for the adult. That is, /t⁻/ and /tʰ/ have the same allophonic relationship for the adult as /f/ and /θ/ had for the child who accepted /θʌm/ and /fʌm/. We still do not know from this test whether the adult could distinguish between these allophones. For this, the ABX procedure is administered. In this procedure the examiner would say, "/bæt⁻/, /bætʰ/, which one was /bæt⁻/?" The adult would, no doubt, say that the first word presented was /bæt⁻/. Here the adult was asked to discriminate between the allophones /t⁻/ and /tʰ/ just as the child had been asked to distinguish between the allophones /f/ and /θ/. If the adult was not able to respond correctly in the ABX task we might assume the presence of some form of auditory deficit such as a peripheral hearing loss.

The importance of Locke's contribution was to remind us that there are at least two kinds of perception with which the clinician should be concerned. These types have been periodically referred to as phonetic and phonemic, or power and salience. Phonetic or power perception is most readily assessed when the child is required to make judgments about adult surface forms as in a same-different or ABX paradigm. A phonemic or salience decision is best assessed in a procedure where an internal representation must be compared with one presented by an adult, such as is required in SP-PT testing. In this respect, power decisions are nonlanguage perceptions, and salience decisions are language perceptions. Of course, children must have the ability to make power decisions. But perceptual testing designed to determine the motivation for misarticulation should be salience testing. In this regard, it is not only important for the child to be able to perceive the essential elements of sounds, but it is also important to ignore the nonessential elements. This is entirely different from power testing where children are required to distinguish minimal differences without regard to their function within the language.

Systematic Sound Preference

Whether the speech-language pathologist uses phonologic theory or relies on a more traditional philosophy during assessment, the clinician invariably looks for *patterns of misarticulation*. Sometimes, the patterns are present; other times, the speech-language pathologist describes misarticulation as being *inconsistent*.

Descriptions of inconsistent misarticulation can have at least two interpretations. The first is that the child really is inconsistent. The second is that the child is consistent but the conditions of consistency are not apparent to the clinician. For example, a child who substitutes n/f and p/f may be described as inconsistent. However, if we knew that the n/f substitution was limited to a specific phonetic context, and the p/f substitution was limited to another specific phonetic context, then the child's errors would be more predictable and, therefore, consistent.

Tests for phonologic processes described in the first section of this chapter were recommended when patterns of misarticulation were present. Consequently, before we can even test whether a phonologic process exists, the pattern of misarticulation must be described. To this end, the speech-language pathologist should be aware of some of the unique phonologic processes that potentially can occur in children.

In summarizing unique phonologic processes, Ingram (1976) noted that several children with phonologic disability overused nasalization in their speech. He described this excessive use of nasalization as nasal preference. Ingram also reported an occasional overuse of fricatives, which he similarly termed a fricative preference. Weiner (1981a), in assessing the speech of unintelligible children, found that many demonstrated sound preferences referred to by Ingram. The use of these sounds tended to be predictable. Weiner termed this phenomenon "systematic sound preference." At the same time, and quite independently, Edwards (Note 2) had made very similar observations about sound preference. She termed the phenomenon "favorite sounds" and, like Weiner, found that the occurrence of these sounds was systematic.

One characteristic of the sound preference phenomenon was that no specific favorite sound was seen to occur with any regularity across the children observed. The "choice" of the favorite sound did not seem to be related to sound difficulty, since many children used /k/, /tʃ/, or /θ/, usually acknowledged to be later developing and more difficult to produce. As stated above, the favorite sounds tended to occur systematically so that natural classes of sounds were regularly replaced. The most frequent natural class to be affected was fricatives. Occasionally, sound preference was limited to the voiceless members of a natural class with a further restriction that labials were not affected.

To demonstrate systematic sound preference the following corpus from a child seen in our speech and language clinic is presented:

short → /hɔr/	father → /hadə/
thumb → /hʌm/	this → /dI/
soup → /hup/	zipper → /bIpI/
fire → /faIr/	valentine → /bælɛʔaI/
sugar → /hʊdə/	vacuum → /baʔu/

The first 6 responses are to words beginning with voiceless fricatives. In each case, the voiceless fricative was replaced by /h/, the favorite sound. In the next four responses the words begin with voiced fricatives. For each of these words, the voiced fricative was replaced by a voiced stop. In this example, we see that the sound preference phenomenon affects a natural class of sounds (voiceless fricatives). In doing so, there is justification for considering this to be a phonologic process (see criteria for phonologic processes in the first section of this chapter). Being a phonologic process means that the child's underlying representation for voiceless fricatives is adapted in the above example to be expressed as /h/.

Why and how this happens is uncertain. One plausible explanation would be that for some reason /h/ is perceptually salient for this child. The form /hVC/ or /hVCV/ may be a perceptual structure into which words fall, in the tradition of Waterson (1971). Regardless of the reason, however, this phenomenon represents a neutralization of certain phonemic contrasts and is potentially important to the speech-language pathologists when determining whether a child's misarticulations are consistent or not.

Phonologic Development of Unintelligible Children

The preceding chapter by Richard Schwartz presents a theoretical perspective and discussion of recent issues concerning phonologic acquisition. The focus of his chapter was *normal* phonologic acquisition. The following section is included here because it presents some recent information about phonologic development in children with unintelligible speech. The reader should compare information concerning the normally developing child presented by Schwartz with characteristics of children who do not follow a normal developmental progression. Information concerning unintelligible children was gathered from a longitudinal investigation by Weiner and Wacker (1982).

In this investigation, children were administered the *Phonological Process Analysis* (Weiner, 1979) 3 times at 6-month intervals. The normally speaking children were 3 years of age at the first testing. This age group was selected because they were presumed to have normal developmental articulation errors. The unintelligible children were between 3 and 5 years of age. Results were analyzed in two ways. First, all speech productions were evaluated to determine whether there were patterns of misarticulation. Next, phonetic inventories were determined for each child. Phonetic inventory analysis determined which sounds were used by the children, regardless of target productions.

Results of the pattern analysis were predictable. That is, normally speaking children had too few errors for any patterns to appear. The errors present tended to be sound specific rather than to affect natural classes of sounds. Sound substitutions were generally within the same manner of production resulting in place errors as opposed to manner errors. Certain substitutions appeared over and over again. These were /ð/ → /d/, /θ/ → /f/, /s/ → /θ/, /ʃ/ → /s/, /r/ → /w/ and the replacement of liquids within clusters by /w/.

The unintelligible children, as expected, had many more misarticulations than the normally developing talkers. Substitution errors were patterned and predictable. If a child replaced a nasal by a homorganic stop in one situation, there was a tendency to do it to nasals in other words as well. The nature of substitution errors was also different. Whereas most of the substitution errors for normally developing speakers involved changes in place of articulation, the substitution errors for unintelligible talkers were replacements of one manner of production for another manner of production. In contrast to an f/θ substitution that might be present for an intelligible child, an unintelligible child would more likely replace /θ/ with /t/. Another difference involved the pervasiveness of errors. Normally developing children seemed to have errors for only fricatives and liquids. Unintelligible talkers, on the other hand, demonstrated errors across all manners of production.

In observing the development of phonology in these two groups over a 1-year period there were also other differences. Considering the number of words containing misarticulations in each of the 3 corpora collected from each child, there was greater improvement shown by the normally talking children. That is, they improved 40%, to only 10% for the unintelligible children. This means that sound errors in the children with phonologic disability were persistent, as was predicted by Ingram (1976).

There was also one other major difference in phonologic development between groups. This was the occurrence of *recidivism* among the intelligible children, which was not seen in the unintelligible talkers. Recidivism, as described by Weiner and Wacker (1982), was the correct production of a word at one developmental stage followed by incorrect production at another, later stage. Recidivism is not routinely reported in the literature because most studies of speech development have been cross-sectional. This study, however, was longitudinal, allowing investigators to observe articulation as it developed.

The second form of analysis, the phonetic inventory, yielded even more interesting results. From this analysis it was apparent that many more sounds were used by intelligible than by unintelligible children. Furthermore, sounds missing from the inventories of normally developing speakers seemed to be limited to the fricative-affricate manners, while unintelligible speakers had missing sounds across the whole phonetic spectrum. Another interesting finding was that unintelligible talkers tended to overuse certain sounds. Sometimes this was systematic, wherein an entire class was replaced by one phoneme (cf., Weiner, 1981). Other times, overuse was the result of a combination of phonologic processes. For example, a child who replaced fricatives by homorganic voiced stops would produce /s/, /θ/, /z/, /ð/, /ʃ/, and /ʒ/ as /d/. Therefore, in addition to attempts to use /d/, six fricatives in the child's corpus would appear as /d/, as well as clusters containing the fricative sounds just mentioned.

The greatest difference between groups in the phonetic inventory analysis appeared for clusters. Clusters were almost absent from the corpora of unintelligible children. At the beginning of the investigation, intelligible children used an average of 13.9 different word-initial clusters. Unintelligible children used an average of 4.5. By the end of the study, normally developing talkers used an average of 15.0 to only 5.67 for the unintelligible talkers. Therefore, one of the greatest discrepancies between groups, and a diagnostically significant result, was the frequency of cluster usage.

In summary, the unintelligible children had many patterns of errors. Most involved the replacement of one manner for another across all manners of production. Also, many sounds were completely missing from the phonetic inventories of these children. Sounds present tended to be overused resulting in stereotypic productions. Clusters were rare and slow to develop. And finally, the absolute number of errors seemed to persist over the course of the investigation.

A Case for Using Effects of Speaker-Listener Interactions to Facilitate the Treatment of Children with Phonologic Disability

As you will recall from the first section of this chapter, one of the major assumptions concerning a phonologic explanation for misarticulation is that the disorder is language-based rather than motoric. Given this assumption, the treatment method for unintelligible speech should parallel other methods of language remediation.

In this regard, there is a body of research which provides evidence that pragmatic factors present in the speaker-listener interaction can have a positive effect on communication including improved production of speech. This was demonstrated by Longhurst and Siegel (1973) where subjects were placed in a situation in which they were to provide listeners with instructions necessary to complete a task. The speaker and listener were separated from each other and the message listeners received was periodically distorted. When speakers observed that the listeners were confused, the speakers reduced speaking rates, became more elaborate in their instructions, and supplied more redundant information. Although there were no specific data showing improved articulation, the investigators concluded that the strategies the speakers selected seemed to contribute to improved communication.

This phenomenon was also demonstrated by Gallagher (1977), who intermittently asked the question, "What?" when gathering spontaneous speech samples from children. Results were that revision behaviors including linguistic elaborations, reductions, and sound substitutions occurred frequently. In addition, it was noted that 50% of the phonetic changes were interpreted as closer approximations to the adult model. Although the other 50% were not interpreted as positive changes, they were nevertheless changes. Thus, on the basis of listener responses, children in this investigation altered their phonetic output.

This effect has also been demonstrated in children with misarticulation. In a structured procedure Weiner and Ostrowski (1979) queried children about their misarticulations in three ways. If a child pronounced *fish* as /fIs/, he was asked one of the following 3 questions: (1) "Did you say fish?" (2) "Did you say /fIs/?" or (3) "Did you say /fIθ/?" In the first question, *fish* was produced correctly; in the second, *fish* was produced with the child's error; and in the third *fish* was produced incorrectly with a different error on the target sound than the child used. This procedure was repeated for a number of misarticulated words so that each query occurred an equal number of times for all subjects in the investigation. In response to the queries, children were trained to respond "Yes (or No), I said ____." The number of correct target sounds that occurred for each of the 3 types of queries were then compared to determine whether any or all of these query types had a positive effect on articulation. The results were that type 3 queries had the greatest effect in reducing misarticulation. In fact, a typical response to this type question was, "No!!! I said /fIsss/." The type 3 response was interpreted to convey the greatest amount of listener uncertainty because /fIθ/ was neither the target word nor the child's substitution for the target word. Here again, expressed misunderstanding resulted in changed articulation performance, but this time there was evidence that the change was in a positive direction.

In another investigation, Weiner and Ellis (Note 3) studied children's sound errors resulting in homonymy. An example of such a word pair is *bow* and *boat*, which would both be produced the same for children who delete final consonants. These children were then asked to produce their homonym pairs under 2 conditions. In the first, the words making up the homonym pairs were produced randomly. In the second, the words were presented as minimal pairs, side by side. Results were that children altered their productions of one or both members of the pairs in condition 2. Interpretation was that somehow the children sensed that there would be possible listener confusion in the paired condition and altered their productions to avoid such confusion.

In a discussion of the pragmatics of language, Greenfield and Smith (1976) wrote about the Principle of Informativeness, wherein the selection of elements for encoding by speakers are those perceived to resolve uncertainty. The above investigations provide examples of how this principle also exists at the phonologic level.

In clinical work, speech-language pathologists have also attempted to capitalize on the principle of informativeness. For a child with a w/l substitution, production of the words *white* and *light* would both normally be /waɪt/. If the clinician responded to the child's attempt to say *light* as though the child was saying *white,* the clinician would be sending a listener message similar to listener messages artificially constructed in the experiments described above. On the basis of this information, it would be predicted that the child would change the production of *light* so as to distinguish it from *white.*

This paradigm was used in a clinical investigation by Weiner (1981b). In this investigation, phonologic processes were treated using a minimal contrast paradigm. For the process stopping, word pairs such as *fin-pin, vase-base, zip-dip,* and *sea-tea* were selected. When stopping occurred, the 4 word pairs would be produced as 4 homonym pairs. Children were instructed to play a game where the object was for the clinician to pick up all the pictures of words beginning with fricatives. If the child's word started with a fricative, the clinician would pick it up. If the child pronounced the target sound as a stop, the clinician would pick up the wrong picture. Picking up the wrong picture was a sign of listener misunderstanding. Results of the experiment were that children were able to reduce the number of processes in their speech very rapidly. This was interpreted as support for listener response as a tool in the treatment of phonologic disability.

Of course, this is only one investigation supporting language training principles used to remediate misarticulation. Other investigations need to be conducted to verify effectiveness of some of the recently proposed articulation therapy methods. In fact, many of the methods currently used to treat misarticulation should be tested experimentally.

Conclusions

At this time, I would like to point out that over the past several years many new developments like phonologic theory have found their way into the area of speech-language pathology. Some of these new developments have not stood the test of time because they did not fully explain a particular disorder, nor did they provide useful clinical information. For clinicians to invest the time necessary to understand and use these new concepts, there must be some clinical gain.

In this chapter, I have tried to point out that description of misarticulation by phonologic analysis helps to explain articulation disorders as something more than a new label for an old pattern. But phonologic theory is not always easy to understand and apply. There are tests that must be employed to verify the existence of phonologic processes at both the productive and perceptual level. There are patterns of misarticulation that must be identified as potential phonologic processes. Some may be as unique as those described in the section on systematic sound preference. The point is that an adequate phonologic analysis can be difficult and time consuming. And, as with any new development, the ultimate test should not be the difficulty, but, rather, the clinical usefulness. That is, after having spent a great deal of time learning a new analysis technique, will clinicians be further ahead in treating their clients?

In this regard, I feel that the preliminary treatment data using speaker-listener interactions shows promise of being an effective therapeutic tool. Of course, phonologic theory applied to analysis and treatment of misarticulation is at a fairly early stage. A great deal more information is needed on both theoretical and clinical fronts. Therefore, I anxiously await the next round of "Recent Advances."

Reference Notes

1. Dinnsen, D., Elbert, M., & Weismer, G. On the characteristics of functional misarticulations. Paper presented to the Annual Convention of the American Speech-Language-Hearing Association, Atlanta, 1979.
2. Edwards, M.L. The use of "favorite sounds" by 14 children with phonological disorders. Paper presented at the Language Development Conference, Boston University, 1980.
3. Weiner, F., & Ellis, C. Tolerance for homonymy: A factor in children's misarticulations. Paper presented to the American Speech-Language-Hearing Association, Detroit, 1980.

References

Donegan, P., & Stampe, D. The study of natural phonology. In D. Dinnsen (Ed.), *Current approaches to phonological theory*. Bloomington: Indiana University Press, 1978.

Gallagher, T. Revision behaviors in the speech of normal children developing language. *Journal of Speech and Hearing Research*, 1977, *20*, 303-318.

Greenfield, P., & Smith, J. *Communication and the beginnings of language: The development of semantic structures in one-word speech and beyond*. New York: Academic Press, 1976.

Hodson, B. *The assessment of phonological processes*. Danville, Ill.: Interstate Printers and Publishers, 1980.

Ingram, D. *Phonological disability in children*. New York: American Elsevier Publishing, 1976.

Ingram, D. *Procedures for phonological analysis of children's language*. Baltimore, University Park Press, 1981.

Locke, J. The inference of speech perception in the phonologically disordered child. Part I: A rationale, some criteria, the conventional tests. *Journal of Speech and Hearing Disorders*, 1980, *45*, 431-444. (a)

Locke, J. The inference of speech perception in the phonologically disordered child. Part II: Some clinically novel procedures, their use, some findings. *Journal of Speech and Hearing Disorders*, 1980, *45*, 445-468. (b)

Longhurst, T., & Siegel, G. Effects of communication failure on speaker and listener behavior. *Journal of Speech and Hearing Research,* 1973, *16,* 128-140.

McReynolds, L., & Elbert, M. Criteria for phonological process analysis. *Journal of Speech and Hearing Disorders,* 1981, *46,* 197-204.

Shriberg, L., & Kwiatkowski, J. *Procedure for natural process analysis (NPA) of continuous speech samples: NPA application manual.* New York: John Wiley, 1980.

Templin, M.C. *Certain language skills in children.* Institute of Child Welfare, Monograph Series, No. 26. Minneapolis: University of Minnesota Press, 1957.

Waterson, N. Child phonology: A prosodic view. *Journal of Linguistics,* 1971, *7,* 179-221.

Weiner, F. *Phonological process analysis.* Baltimore: University Park Press, 1979.

Weiner, F. Systematic sound preference as a characteristic of phonological disability. *Journal of Speech and Hearing Disorders,* 1981, *46,* 281-286. (a)

Weiner, F. Treatment of phonological disability using the method of meaningful minimal contrast: Two case studies. *Journal of Speech and Hearing Disorders,* 1981, *46,* 97-103. (b)

Weiner, F., & Ostrowski, A. Effects of listener uncertainty on articulatory inconsistency. *Journal of Speech and Hearing Disorders,* 1979, *44,* 487-503.

Weiner, F., & Wacker, R. The development of phonology in unintelligible speakers. In N. Lass (Ed.), *Speech and language: Advance in Basic Research and Practice, Vol. 8.* New York: Academic Press, 1982.

Wepman, J.M. *Auditory discrimination test.* Chicago: Language Research Associates, 1973.

Elizabeth B. Cole and Marietta M. Paterson

Assessment and Treatment of Phonologic Disorders in the Hearing Impaired

In contemplating contributing yet another treatise on the topic of speech and hearing impairment, one gets a sense of both humility and frustration. The humility is from being in the company of clinicians, researchers, scholars, teachers, and parents who have struggled with the questions and the technology for literally centuries. (See, for example, the review in Ling, 1976, pp. 11-18). The frustration, on the other hand, is from the overwhelming feeling that it has all been said and done before—that there is very little new under the speech-for-the-deaf sun—and that still our overall results are dismal. Few would have been surprised by the statement in the 1979 American Speech-Language-Hearing Association's "Standards for Effective Oral Communication Programs" that "adequate oral communication frequently determines an individual's educational, social, and vocational success" (p. 1002). In view of that, we simply cannot be satisfied with speech intelligibility ratings of "barely intelligible," "not intelligible," and/or "would not speak" for 55.2% of the school-age hearing-impaired population (Jensema, Karchmer, & Trybus, 1978). True, the ratings are somewhat better for that proportion of the children with lesser degrees of hearing loss: 86.2% of those with losses of less than 70 dB were "very intelligible" or "intelligible." But only 54.8% of the children with losses ranging from 71-90 dB (at 500, 1000, 2000 Hz) were rated as "very intelligible" or "intelligible" and only 22.5% with losses greater than 90 dB were in that category.

In presenting speech workshops in the United States, Canada, and Australia, and in teaching graduate student teacher/clinicians, it has become apparent to both authors that the issues which are recurrently problematic regarding development of intelligibility can be divided into the following two broad areas:

Optimizing Input - guaranteeing that as much of the speech signal as possible is put within an accessible range for the child through optimum selection, fitting, and maintenance of amplification; and

Optimizing Instruction - teaching in ways that take into account information about learning, meaningful communication, oral language acquisition, acoustic phonetics, and articulatory phonetics; as well as teaching in ways that employ effective strategies for evoking and practicing motor speech skills, and for making the child's usage of good speech habits automatic in normal spontaneous oral language.

Both of these are areas which we believe require serious improvement in order for more hearing-impaired children to be achieving levels of maximum intelligibility. And, in both areas, there have been recent applications of innovative thought and research which merit widespread consideration and implementation.

Optimizing Input

Hearing Aids

That speech abilities are presently linked to the amount of auditory input available to the child seems undeniable. But reports showing a relationship between the amount of hearing loss and speech intelligibility, such as ones by Jensema, Karchmer, and Trybus (1978); Nickerson (1975); Smith (1975); and Subtelny, Whitehead, and Orlando (1980) tend to be misinterpreted by some professionals as indications of fixed and unchangeable causality. Can it be that the seriousness of the lack of audition (i.e., the simple fact of the hearing loss) makes intelligible speech a nearly unobtainable goal for the majority? Not so! comes the resounding answer from two directions:

1. from those who combine the selection and fitting of auditory prosthetic instruments with information about the acoustic properties of the spoken word; and
2. from competent users of a relatively recent program for teaching speech to hearing-impaired children, which has become popularly known as "The Ling Thing" (Ling, 1976).

When thinking about auditory input to the hearing-impaired child, one must think not only in terms of what the child's unaided thresholds are on the audiogram, but also (more so) in terms of what can become auditorily available to the child through appropriate amplification. It may be useful to employ the model of auditory learning suggested by Hirsh (1970) (detection, discrimination, identification, comprehension) in order to organize the issues surrounding this part of the problem. Detection is the necessary—but not sufficient—prerequisite for the other three abilities to be learned. Consequently, the first consideration is to provide sufficient gain in the child's amplification system to allow the child to detect all of the acoustic cues which he or she is capable of receiving. Recent processes for initial hearing aid selection (e.g., Berger, Hagberg, & Rane, 1977) have attempted to make the procedure a more precise and scientific process, and have consequently included information about speech spectrum characteristics in the calculations. As Byrne (1979), Libby (1980), and Yanick (1980) suggest, gain and output levels can be determined using prescriptive methods that are based on the speech spectrum. Then real ear measurements need to be used for optimizing the fitting by aid adjustments and/or by coupling modifications. In determining the appropriateness of the hearing aid selected and in making adjustments based on real ear (aided) responses, it is obviously critical to employ guidelines which take speech spectrum characteristics into account if the goal is to assure their maximum detectability. One such procedure is that suggested by Ling and Ling (1978). That is, in order for speech to be detected within a normal conversational distance of 2 meters or less, the child's aided responses need to fall within or above the range covered by a banana-shaped area on the audiogram, while maintaining relative proportions adequate for avoiding masking effects. This "speech banana" has approximately a 20 dB intensity range and extends from below 250 Hz through above 6000 Hz in order to account for all of the major acoustic cues in speech. At the present time, hearing aids do not routinely provide large amounts of gain at the upper end of that frequency range (6000 to 8000 Hz). However, there are now a number of aids providing significant amplification (peaks of 50 to 60 dB) at or above 5000 Hz (Rudmin, in press). With regard to amounts of gain possible, Rudmin (1982) found more than 80 models of ear level hearing aids whose (full-on) high frequency average gain was 60 dB or greater. Ling (1981b) offers the clinical observation that children with unaided thresholds down to the following levels can generally be provided gain sufficient to allow the children to detect the essential speech cues:

250	500	1000	2000	4000
85	100	115	115	95 dB

In other words, with a loss of 115 dB at 2000 Hz (for example), it is possible to provide enough real ear gain (65 to 75 dB) in order to expect the child to be evidencing aided responses at approximately 40 to 50 dB. If this were the case, the child could be expected to be able to detect (at a distance of 2 meters), the following acoustic cues which are centered around 2000 Hz ± ½ octave: the second formant of the front vowels, second transition place cues for most consonants, second and third transitions for liquids; turbulence of [ʃ]; [θ]; and [f]; and the third formant for some vowels (Ling, 1976).

In view of the present hearing aid technology, the 54.8% statistic for intelligibility among children with 71-90 dB losses is even more disturbing. Today, a 90 dB threshold at 4000 Hz represents a great deal of residual hearing *potentially* usable for speech cue detection, once optimally aided. However, it should be emphasized that hearing abilities within the speech banana are only potentially usable. That is, the ability to detect these elements auditorily will not automatically guarantee the use of that acoustic information, accessible as it is. A parallel could be drawn here to a normally hearing adult who is physically capable of detecting all of the essential speech sound contrasts in any language which is foreign to him. But the foreign language sounds like just so much verbal noise, unless, or until, the salient speech sound differences are brought to the adult's attention for communicative reasons, and/or through conscious effort on the part of a teacher. And even then, consciously knowing that the differences exist will not guarantee that henceforth the adult will immediately and automatically discriminate among them in listening to the native speaker's oral language. However, in order to even begin this auditory discrimination, identification, and comprehension process, the speech sounds initially must be accessible. Although often further compounded by a lack of normal clarity, the case is similar for a hearing-impaired child: detection is a necessary, but not sufficient, condition in order for auditory learning to occur.

Earmold Coupling Modifications

In addition to advances internal to the aid itself, another area of recent research and innovation is that of earmold coupling systems. (Gastmeier, 1981; Grave & Metzinger, 1981; Killion & Monser, 1980; Libby, 1980, 1981). Modifications can be made in the characteristics of venting, damper elements, and acoustic horns, and done either independently or simultaneously to produce controllable effects on the shape, bandwidth, and fidelity of the system. For example, using a fused mesh damper in the end of the earhook, a detrimental resonance peak at 1000 Hz can be smoothed (Gastmeier, 1981; Libby, 1980, 1981). Additionally, an increasing diameter in the earhook tubing-earmold tip sequence can be maintained producing an acoustic horn effect (Libby, 1980). The acoustic horn has been reported by Libby (1981) as typically producing improvement in sound field warble tone aided thresholds at 3000 to 4000 Hz of 5 to 15 dB (range = 0 to 24 dB). Similarly, Grave and Metzinger (1981) found an average of 13 dB improvement in functional gain at 4000 Hz using an undamped acoustic horn (range = 5 dB to +45 dB). It should be noted that the apparent increase in gain produced by modifications of the earmold coupling system is actually compensating for attenuation which normally occurs using standard earmold coupling procedures. This underlines once again the need to do real ear measurements and the lack of rationale for relying simply on hearing aid manufacturer's specifications in order to estimate amounts of gain being realized by the child. However, it also means that using personal hearing aids,[1] speech information (particularly consonantal) in the 2000 to 4000 Hz range may be more accessible for larger numbers of children who have some residual hearing in that range.

But what about the child who has only low frequency hearing (the frequently seen "corner" audiogram)? Even optimally aided, this child may not be capable of detecting the higher-frequency components of the speech signal. Fortunately, however, if he has aided responses between 30 to 45 dB even at only 250 Hz, he will still be able to detect the fundamental frequency of most female voices; some harmonics of male voices; the nasal murmur for [m, n, ŋ]; the first formant for some vowels; as well as cues for voicing, intonation, intensity, and duration. And, with instruction, these speech cues can make a major contribution toward making his voice sound "normal"—that is, without the hypernasal, monotone, arrhythmic qualities often cited as characterizing "deaf speech" (Nickerson, 1975; Smith, 1975; Subtelny et al., 1980).

Visual and Tactile Devices and Procedures

For the speech sounds with components which are auditorily undetectable, obviously sense modalities other than auditory (i.e., visual, tactile) will have to be employed for bringing the key elements of the sounds within range of the child's attention (Ling, 1976, p. 17, 45-65). Fortunately, spoken communication contains numerous contextual, lexical, semantic, and syntactic redundancies so that even normally hearing people are not utilizing all of the auditory information available to them in order to understand spoken messages (Fry, 1978, pp. 37-39). The underlying assumption seems to be that, using many of the visual and tactile devices, key element(s) can be brought to the child's attention, and then both recognition and production practiced to automaticity in selected linguistic contexts. Then, in normal conversational situations (without the device), the child's linguistic knowledge will allow use of some of those redundancies to comprehend messages and to produce sounds even when lacking acoustic cues. There are a number of workers in this area who have developed visual and tactile devices for recoding the speech signal in order to overcome hearing impairment which precludes auditory detection of the essential acoustic components. (See reviews in Boothroyd, 1975; Oller, Payne, & Gavin, 1980; Strong, 1975.)

When considering the use of visual and tactile devices or procedures for speech training with children, two cautions immediately arise. One concerns the choice of children with whom they are used. It should go without saying that it would be counterproductive to use a visual or tactile device with a child who could actually be detecting the targeted speech component(s) auditorily when optimally aided. (See Ling, 1976, pp. 22-65, for a discussion of the specific advantages of the ear in preference to either vision or taction for detecting speech patterns.)

The other caution particularly concerns those visual and tactile devices that are not portable, such as desk model vibratory devices. The problem with use of these devices is that tasks or abilities developed in using them may remain tied to that training situation and those devices. For example, although it has been possible to train severely-to-profoundly deaf adolescents to discriminate between word pairs based on tactile input alone (Oller et al., 1980), the sense of touch has yet to be successfully employed by itself for understanding speech in normal communication situations. As the Boothroyd (1975), Boothroyd, Archambault, Adams, and Storm (1975), and Strong (1975) results suggest, questions about carry-over from training on isolated parameters to real communication situations have yet to be fully answered.

One other speech recoding procedure should be mentioned at this juncture: the use of Cued Speech (Cornett, 1967). This is a visual system of gestures ("cues") which are used to reduce ambiguity among sounds that appear identical on the lips (e.g., there is a different hand position for signifying [d] versus [t] versus [n] since these three are visually synonymous). The gestures, performed by the speaker in conjunction with talking, are directly tied to the verbal message, and essentially provide a visible recoding of part of the phonetic information. Although use of Cued Speech has been adopted in a number of programs in North America and elsewhere since its introduction in 1967, there have been only three systematic studies of its effectiveness with hearing-impaired children. Results of all three studies have been generally favorable toward the use of cueing, specifically with profoundly hearing-impaired children. It has been shown, for example, that cueing can facilitate speech-reading of isolated sentences, phrases, and words (Clarke & Ling, 1976; Ling & Clarke, 1975). And the extensive study by Nicholls (Note 1) evidenced mean speech reception scores of over 95% for cues used with either lipreading or with lipreading and audition. (Note: "Speech reception" in the Nicholls study refers to prediction of the key word in sentence materials.) However, particularly in view of the need for continued research, the decision to use Cued Speech should be a carefully considered one to avoid some of the following pitfalls of its possible misuse.

As mentioned above, simply being capable of detecting speech features produced by a sender will not necessarily result in the automatic use of available hearing for discrimination and identification of the salient sound patterns, or for comprehension of the sender's message. The child's actual use of his or her auditory capabilities will depend on a variety of factors such as attention, motivation, and knowledge of the fact that verbal-auditory communications have meaning and value, as well as on training and experience with the acoustic elements whose differentiation is salient in the target language. Fortunately, Nicholls's (Note 1) results support the contention that use of cueing does not have a detrimental effect on the child's use of audition for speech reception (in fact, quite the reverse). But promoting the child's optimal use of whatever residual hearing exists will undoubtedly require continued attention and sustained effort on the part of the teacher.

A second possible problem is related to this statement by Cornett (1967):

> The teacher himself will have to spend many hours in practice before he becomes fluent enough to cue his speech . . . without so much preoccupation with the communication process as to impede spontaneity and flexibility of thought in the teaching process. (p. 11)

Along with possibly impeding "spontaneity and flexibility of thought," slow and belabored cueing can distort the normal rhythmic features and pitch variations of the spoken language it is accompanying. When these meaning-loaded components are distorted, several effects are likely:

1. the child may not learn that pitch and rhythm features have meaning and salience in spoken messages; and

2. since the distorted prosodic elements are those which can be auditorily detected by nearly all hearing-impaired children, then the very valuable information that the "corner" audiogram child can

listen to is not presented in a normal fashion. It would, consequently, not be surprising if that child's own speech were similarly arrhythmic and/or distorted in intonational contour.

Finally, having determined that fluency and continued attention to audition are necessary accompaniments to optimal usage of cueing with profoundly hearing-impaired children, the teacher needs to be fully aware that cueing is intended to be an adjunct to spoken language. While the studies cited above suggest that cueing helps the child's reception of oral messages, it should not be expected to simultaneously and automatically teach productive oral language, and/or productive speech skills (Cornett, 1975).

Cochlear Implants

The House Ear Institute (Los Angeles) began investigating the cochlear implant in 1960 with the goal of being able to restore hearing to the deaf by means of the implant (House, Bode, & Berliner, 1981). As of July 1981, a total of 178 persons had received single-electrode cochlear implants either at the Institute or through one of approximately 20 other co-investigators in the United States. Both objective and subjective responses have been generally quite positive in expressions of post-implant improvement (e.g., Campos, 1981; House, Bode, & Berliner, 1981; Luetje, 1981). Results of initial experimentation with multiple electrode implants have been similarly positive (Clark & Tong, 1981). For example, marked improvement in comprehension was obtained by two patients from means of 5% and 11% for a lipreading-alone condition, as compared to 32% and 38% comprehension for the condition when the implant was utilized in addition to lipreading (Martin, Tong, & Clark, 1981). At its present level of development, however, neither single nor multiple electrode implant restores hearing to the extent that it is possible to understand speech through its use alone, and continuing research is focused on developing improved ancillary devices for the processing of speech. What can be detected and used to advantage according to most reports are primarily voicing, nasality, intensity, and durational cues. That this voicing and prosodic information is beneficial is perhaps best attested to by the report that 152 of the 178 implant patients (associated with the House Institute co-investigation) are using the device on a regular basis (House, Bode, & Berliner, 1981). Obviously, selection of candidates for the implant is a crucial issue, and the cochlear implant is still considered an "investigational" procedure by the U.S. Food and Drug Administration (Luetje, 1981). Procedures and criteria for selection have consequently been carefully outlined by the researchers.

However, as Campos states,

> All possible non-invasive alternatives should be pursued with each candidate, prior to cochlear implantation. However, the cochlear implant. . . should continue to be available. . . as a viable means of communication when hearing aids are not helpful. (1981, p. 30)

It is possible that, with continued research, cochlear implants may become an increasingly viable part of the (re)habilitation procedure. It bears mentioning, however, that the rehabilitation problems presented by many post implant patients at the present time are largely different from those presented by the majority of hearing-impaired children who are learning language for the first time and who are doing that with the presence of some aidable residual hearing.

Summary

The foregoing discussion touches briefly on some of the present technological and procedural capabilities for optimizing the speech input to the child, whether auditorily, visually, or tactilely. Unfortunately, for a variety of reasons, capability is not necessarily accompanied by educational application and implementation.

Optimizing Instruction

The Problem

The problem is, basically, that in spite of all of the existing information and technology, more than half of our school-age hearing-impaired children are still rated as less than intelligible. Observations of characteristics of deaf speech by Hudgins and Numbers (1942) have been repeatedly and recently verified (see review in Ling, 1976; also, Nickerson, 1975; Smith, 1975; Subtelny et al., 1980). All authors mention such problems as inadequate breath control, excessive and inappropriate pauses, inappropriate pitch and intonation, hypernasality, excessive tenseness, inappropriate duration of both stressed and unstressed syllables, and omission or misarticulation of some phonemes.

Interestingly, there is not one characteristic of deaf speech mentioned by those authors that is not also mentioned by Ling (1976) as a remediable, or preferably, an avoidable problem. In what could be interpreted as an explanation for the continuing poor state of affairs, Ling wrote in 1976:

> Technological advances, emerging knowledge in speech science, and contributions from related areas are having little, or no impact on the speech patterns of many children. . . . It may be concluded that teachers do not have or are not using strategies which integrate current knowledge with compatible, traditional procedures. (pp. 17-18)

This assertion was essentially echoed by Hochberg, Levitt, and Osberger (1980) in a 3-year (U.S.) nationwide project whose long-term goal was to improve speech services to hearing-impaired children. Reasons cited for minimal progress in the area of speech-teaching included limited expectations for the children's speech and inadequate pre-service training in speech teaching. Although 80% of the classroom teachers felt speech-training was important, only 42% of the teachers spent as much as 6 to 20 minutes per day on speech development, and 30% spent between 1 and 15 minutes per day on speech maintenance. Approximately 37% and 45% of the teachers provided no speech development or maintenance (respectively) at all. In view of these numbers, one might wonder how it was ever possible at all for the 54.8% of the children with severe losses and 22.5% of the children with profound losses to achieve speech intelligibility ratings of "very intelligible" and "intelligible." Perhaps this is yet another case of children learning in spite of us, rather than because of us. Of course, some professionals are obtaining intelligibility scores for some hearing-impaired children that are not statistically different from the scores of their normally hearing peers (Ling, 1981a). This certainly lends credibility to the contention that the key to the solution lies in the child's education, and by extension, in the persons responsible for that education. And, in fact, teachers and speech specialists in the Hochberg et al. (1980) survey responded that 80-95% of them would benefit from continuing education in how to improve their competence in speech training. In order to begin to meet some of this need, Hochberg et al. instituted a pilot program of in-service training and a pilot pre-service workshop for faculty members of teacher-training programs. They note that "the magnitude of the problem is even more widespread and far-reaching than was initially supposed, and by and large, the professional personnel most directly involved in the provision of speech services. . . are unprepared to meet [the hearing-impaired children's] needs effectively" (p. 483).

Some Solutions

It would be an ambitious and futile project, indeed, to pretend to fully respond to the needs expressed by teachers and speech specialists by means of anything less than the Hochberg et al. (1980) programs mentioned above. As a partial and potentially very satisfying response, however, the authors would like to refer readers to the speech-teaching program and related ideas described in, for example, Ling (1976, 1978, 1979, 1981a, 1981b) and Ling and Ling (1978). This "Ling Thing," in the opinion of the authors, answers the need for a scientific and systematic program for teaching speech skills to school-age hearing-impaired children. Based on our own experience in using the program and in teaching others to use it, we have observed that there are a number of educational issues and techniques that are recurrently problematic for teachers and clinicians using the program. Space limitations require focusing on a selected few.

The essential concept in working on speech with hearing-impaired children is that the goal is intelligibility in spontaneous use of oral language (Ling, 1979). Somehow this goal often seems to become obscured. One source of the problem may be an over-emphasis on analytic teaching of specific speech segments. A "forest and trees" situation has apparently been created by teachers' desire for and comfort in using techniques primarily designed for simply evoking and rote-practicing speech sounds. Given time and skilled effort, this focus on the elements (albeit co-articulated) is likely to result in the child acquiring great facility in motor speech (articulation) skills. However, the expectation seems to be that intelligible, spontaneous, oral language will also automatically result from motor speech facility. And this is simply not the case. As Ling says, "Motor speech skills are essential but insufficient for the development of spoken communication" (1979, p. 217). A parallel could be drawn to a musician doing tone exercises and practicing memorized scales with the expectation that that would automatically enable him to play Mozart sonatas. Just as the ability to play a Mozart sonata requires a much greater knowledge of music, so does intelligible, spontaneous, oral language require a much greater knowledge of the conventions for communicating and encoding meaning in oral language. In fact, in terms of time allocation, the teacher's primary preoccupation needs to be with facilitating the growth of oral language in meaningful situations. Building speech intelligibility into such a program requires consistent overall expectations for maximum clarity, as well as planned occasions for both incidental and scheduled motor speech practice.

The next two sections of this chapter will offer concrete suggestions aimed at clarifying the intended focus on intelligibility in spontaneous oral language. The suggestions are intended to respond to two sources of misdirection regarding that goal: the overemphasis on speech element minutiae, and the neglect of prosody.

1. Organizing Learning/Teaching

The contention has been made that speech teaching has placed an overemphasis on the evocation and repetitious practice of coarticulated syllables. The question then arises as to how speech learning and teaching can be organized in order to include an appropriate emphasis on motor speech practice within the overall program. It should be noted that some parts of the following discussion could be classified as suggestions for the "transfer to phonology" of phonetic skills. However, the authors would prefer to avoid the exclusively "bottom-up" inference that may be inherent in the idea of phonologic transfer. Our approach is one that attempts to move quickly and recursively from whole to parts to whole (and so on), incorporating facets of "bottom-up" teaching into what is, fundamentally, a "top-down" view of oral language and speech development. Speech learning/teaching following this approach can be discussed in terms of incidental learning/teaching, and scheduled learning/teaching.

Incidental learning/teaching begins with the teacher's consistent expectation for maximum clarity of production of the speech aspects the child has mastered on a phonetic level. It is true that one of the most powerful motivations for children to use clear speech could be expected to be the fact that people understand them better when they speak clearly. However, listeners tend to fill in the gaps and mentally correct distortions from contextual and linguistic redundancy. That is, listeners familiar with the child may be able and willing to adjust their own speech perceptual mechanisms in such a way that they can understand the child even without hearing the level of speech clarity of which the child may be capable. However, unfamiliar listeners are much less likely to be able and willing to make the perceptual adjustments necessary for understanding the child, which has the effect of limiting the number of people with whom communication is possible. Consequently, in order to help the child speak as clearly as possible, as well as learn to automatically implement newly acquired skills, feedback-providing techniques can be consciously employed.

One such technique is positive reinforcement of the child's efforts toward overall clarity and/or of the clarity of specific speech aspects. This can be helpful since it indicates to the child what is being done correctly. Positive reinforcement is also likely to encourage the child's continued efforts, which can be especially important when intelligibility problems are multiple. Reinforcement can be verbal, accompanied or not by a smile, a pat, or a checkmark on the chalkboard.

Another technique for incidental learning/teaching is that of simply reminding the child to attend to speech clarity. This can be accomplished through adoption of a quizzical expression, for example, or by means of a verbal reminder about specific "tricky" words or sounds as they occur. Again, though, this kind of reminding is likely to be most useful for speech aspects that have been mastered on a motor speech level, and is preferably done in a gentle, good-humored fashion. Above all, it should be avoided if there is a chance that it could destroy a communicative event. Often the child's message or a conversational exchange will be judged more important than interrupting to practice a faulty /s/ or /r/. It is suggested that the reminding be accomplished unobtrusively and followed by immediate self-correction on the child's part. If this is not the case, then the teacher can make note of the specific difficulty and incorporate it into later scheduled practice.

The expectation for intelligibility and the techniques mentioned for skillful reinforcement and reminding are, perhaps, obvious to many readers. But these aspects are probably the most difficult ones to employ, as well as the most important ones in terms of actually realizing improvement in the child's intelligibility in spontaneous oral language. Naturally, the effort is likely to be most fruitful if it is a concerted one with all of the child's teachers and family involved to the greatest extent possible.

There is another kind of incidental speech learning/teaching which can occur at various times in the day. This is incidental phonetic practice of targets which a number of children have in common. One example of an activity for this kind of practice is the use of a "Speech Pocket." One could make a pocket out of construction paper and tape it to the back of the classroom door, then jot down a series of targets for the week on cards which fit in the pocket. For example, the group targets could be: (1) bama; (2) bibiBI; (3) fubufubu; (4) 1, 2, 3, 4, 5; (5)ʌs̪ la ʌs̪ la sla. Each time the class leaves the room, the children line up one by one and produce the target on the card chosen from the pocket as they file out of the room. For variety, the cards could have questions loaded with target sounds written on them, or simple games such as having everyone name a different animal, bird, fruit or state with the /m/ sound in it.

Scheduled learning/teaching can occur in a variety of ways. Ling (1976) recommends providing each child with several practice sessions of 2 to 3 minutes duration at spaced intervals during the day. On the other hand, some teachers have found that as they are becoming familiar with the system, one individual session of 8 to 10 minutes duration is more manageable. Organization of the activities during that individual session can follow a format such as that exemplified in Table 4-1.

Table 4-1
Sample of Individual Teaching Plan for Scheduled Practice

Name: _____   Date(s): _____

Target-Stage of Practice	Sense Modality		Techniques	Activities, Materials	Comments
1. /f/ - multiple reduplicated syllables, "legato," one breath fa fa fa fi fi fi fu fu fu	Vision Touch ↓	step 1.	Go from long ʌf and release into vowel ʌf‿a, slowly with control.	Move hand on table to show how long to hold /ʌf.../, when hand reaches pencil say /a/.	-Do again, same steps. -Attention to /fi, fu/. Loses frication when coarticulating.
	Audition	step 2.	Remove the crutch of /ʌ/- have child imitate vocalization of f‿a¹. Check for good coarticulation.		
		step 3.	Have child self-monitor, maintain, repeat 3 times for today with /a, i, u/		
2. ba/ma - a. auditory discrimination² b. multiple recursive syllables /ba‿ma ba‿ma ba‿ma/	Audition (free variation)	step 1.	Auditory discrimination - follow-up from last time, build confidence in ability to differentiate ba-ma	2 sets colored blocks	good ✓ -able to discriminate with confidence -able to do at normal rate

/bi‿mi/etc.
/bu‿mu/etc.

Then:
/bi‿ma/
/bu‿mi/

step 2.

Syllable practice.
Alternate each set 5 times.
Student will self-monitor.
Do once slowly; then try
normal rate.

-encourage more
correct produc-
tions in mean-
ingful contexts.

3. /p/ meaningful use
- in initial position
  only
- look for self
  correction
- consistent
  production

Audition
Vision
Touch

step 1.

Quickly review production
of /p/ with a range of
known vowels.

2 pens, 2 pandas,
2 pans, 2 pennies,
2 pears, 2 pigs.

-good practice,
-not fully
automatic at
meaningful
level

step 2.

Game round the table
a. Name objects.
   Q. What's that?
   A. It's a _____.

b. Take turns giving and
   following directions for
   placing objects in strange
   places.
   Pass me a/the _____
   Put a/the _____ in a/the _____.

- Trouble with
  /p/ after
  the word
  The -
  practice this
  context.

---

[1] The key is to hold the /f/ frication longer than necessary, and then release smoothly into the vowel.

[2] See Paterson, 1982.

Briefly, the lesson plan format specifies each of the following aspects:

- The stage of practice of each target. Particular targets could be at the stage, for example, of evocation; single, controlled production; multiple repetition (e.g., reduplicated syllables, alternated syllables, recursive or freely varied syllables); or meaningful use in selected words, phrases, expressions, or sentences.
- The appropriate sense modality to be used. This aspect requires knowledge of the child's aided audiogram, as well as some knowledge of acoustic phonetics. If the child has audition that will allow him to hear the salient acoustic elements of the target sound, then use of that auditory capability can be maximized. If, for example, the child has adequately aided hearing at 250 Hz and at 500 Hz, then the acoustic cues[2] distinguishing between /ba/ and /ma/ are available. Thus, the child can be expected to learn to auditorily discriminate between the two sounds. When the hearing loss precludes use of residual hearing, vision and touch will be helpful in evoking and practicing production of a number of sounds. Selective and combined use of sense modalities for speech teaching is described by Ling (1976) and Ling and Ling (1978); and the acoustic characteristics of English are detailed in a number of sources, including Fry (1976), Ling (1978), Minifie (1973), Pickett (1980).
- Techniques for evoking sounds for facilitating practice. Ling (1976) presents a large number of strategies for these purposes.
- Materials, reinforcers, activities. (Self-explanatory)
- The "comments" column is intended for any teacher comments during or after the session which will aid in planning further practice.

The intent of this section has been to describe the overall organization of an approach for speech learning/teaching, the goal of which is the child's use of maximum clarity in meaningful spontaneous productions. The motor speech practice sessions provide an increasing number of productive abilities which can subsequently begin to be required in spontaneous use. However, these scheduled sessions occur for, at most, a total of 15 to 20 minutes per day, and cannot be expected to automatically result in improved intelligibility in spontaneous oral language. Suggestions outlined above for incidental learning/teaching are intended to aid in that process.

2. Strategies for Development of Prosodic Elements

In addition to a need to redirect what appears to be an over-abundance of energy spent in coarticulated syllable practice, the authors perceive a concomitant need to direct more attention to the neglected area of prosody.

The prosodic components of speech in the Ling program are specified as vocalization, duration, intensity, and pitch. "Vocalization" can be interpreted to mean normal quality phonation, or use of an appropriately relaxed and oral voice. Use of normal voicing is important in order to avoid vocal strain, to make pitch and rhythmic changes, and to allow for the oral/nasal contrast. It is also aesthetically more pleasing for the listener. Automatic, controlled flexibility in use of the other three aspects (duration, intensity, and pitch) in speech allows the talker to implement stress, rhythm, and intonation conventions to mark constituent boundaries, as well as to express intent and emotion in ways which the listener will expect and understand. That the prosodic aspects are problem areas for hearing-impaired speakers has been repeatedly noted in the literature (Boone, 1966; Hudgins & Numbers, 1942; Ling, 1976; Nickerson, 1975; Martony, 1968; Smith, 1975; Subtelny et al., 1980). This is particularly distressing in view of the fact that voicing, duration, intensity, and pitch cues are generally available to adequately aided children, even those with · only minimal residual hearing (Ling, 1976). The problem seems to be grounded in a lack of information not only about the availability of the acoustic cues, but also about the mechanics of evoking and rehearsing these aspects in speech related ways, and about the necessity of continually and consciously employing and requiring normal variation in developing the segmental aspects.

The aspects of speech selected for separate discussion here include vocal quality, duration, nasality, intensity, and pitch. For each of the selected aspects, the following topics will be addressed: (a) typical problems; (b) physiologic causes; (c) aim of remediation; (d) auditory requirements; and (e) techniques for remediation. The first section to follow will outline techniques for evoking and practicing each aspect on a motor speech level. The final section will suggest activities for getting those practiced abilities to appear in the child's meaningful spoken language.

Vocal Quality and Duration

Typical problems

Hearing-impaired children judged as having an overall voice and breath control problem may evidence one or more of the following: harsh or strident voice quality, abnormal pitch variation, monotone voice, inability to control intensity differences, stop-start vocal production ("machine gun-like" speech), inability to maintain the voiced-voiceless distinction between consonants, talking on residual air, and nasal-sounding vocal production (Boone, 1966, pp. 636; Calvert & Silverman, 1975, pp. 183-190;

Ling, 1976, pp. 12–17; Monsen, 1976, p. 33, 1979, pp. 270–288; Mahashie, Note 2).

Physiologic causes

Hearing-impaired children are born with normal respiratory systems and the capacity for normal laryngeal/pharyngeal function. However, laryngeal abnormalities in the adduction and abduction of the vocal folds and in the production of subglottal pressure can be acquired over time (Pickett, 1980; Mahashie, Note 2). According to Ling (1976), reasons for such abnormality may be several: minimal practice in oral communication, inadequate exploitation of residual audition, a reliance on sensation of tactile vibration for monitoring of articulator placement, and poor voicing habits resulting from uninformed teaching strategies.

Aim of remediation

Remediation goals are to develop controlled vocalizations on well-supported oral breath, to promote correct use of subglottal pressure for controlled durational practice, to remediate improper vocal fold tension in vowel production, and to promote flexibility of tongue movement through coarticulation of vowels and some consonants.

Auditory requirements

Acoustic cues for the detection of the center fundamental frequency of the voice (F_0) for male, female, and child speakers range from approximately 100 to 265 Hertz (Pickett, 1980). As durational variation is one of several factors at least partially carried on the fundamental frequency, children with adequately aided residual audition extending only up to 500 Hz should be able to detect the presence or absence of voicing and subsequently be able to learn to judge durational differences (Ling, 1976, pp. 27–29; Pickett, 1980, pp. 46–47, 61).

Vocal quality work requires use of vowels. Consequently, it is relevant that with adequately aided residual hearing extending only up to 500 Hz, the first formants (F_1) of vowels are perceptible. Residual audition up to 1000 Hz renders F_1 of all vowels and the second formant (F_2) of the low and mid vowels audible. Residual audition up to 2500 Hz would render both formants of all vowels audible and discriminable (Ling, 1976, pp. 227–228; Ling & Ling, 1978, pp. 68–69).

Suggested techniques for remediation

Step 1. Produce a long, strong oral breathstream while holding the sound /a/. The child can feel the release of the teacher's breath with his or her own hand. Then the child could imitate the teacher, attempting to produce the same quality of breathstream while feeling the air flow across his or her own hand. Exaggerated breathiness can be encouraged at this stage with no danger to the child's speech production. Once the child develops flexibility and speed of vocalizations on the breathstream, the exaggerated breathiness will disappear.

Alternative techniques for step 1.

a. Whispering

If the child is unable to produce a breathy flow of air as per Step 1, then a more elemental strategy to evoke the oral breathstream may be required. One could have the child simply blow air from the mouth, making no attempt to voice the vowel /a/ and continue practice until the child is more comfortable with the feeling of the breath flow and is beginning to monitor the strength of the breath with his or her hand. In effect, the child is simply whispering the /h/ phoneme. The result of this is to eliminate vocal fold tension for the present and promote breathiness (Ling, 1976, pp. 204–220, 233). Then the child could make 3 to 5 productions in a row of the same "quality." There should be no harsh or sudden stopping at the end of a breath, but a relaxed cessation. Next, attempt to have the child softly voice /a/ as a syllable is initiated with /h/; the concentration should be on breath flow production. The goal is for the child to coordinate initiation of voicing (based on vocal fold tension) with release of breath (based on adequate subglottal pressure).

b. Panting

It is possible that, on demand, a child may be unable to produce any breathy flow of air at all, even through the whispering technique. To give the child an idea of the required response, it may be helpful to practice panting. The child could imitate short intakes and releases of air as a puppy would in panting and then monitor the resultant breath flow with his or her hand until the sensation of the air passing across the pharyngeal wall and the effect of diaphragmatic excursion feels comfortable. Then, the child could continue to produce multiple repetitions of the short panting but elongate the last breath. This would produce whispered /h/. Production could be stabilized by using the suggestions for whispering (Alternative technique "a").

Step 2. Next the child might produce a very long /a/ sound. The teacher should stop the child's vocalization of the vowel if the sound becomes nasal, harsh, or abnormal in pitch so that learning in error is not promoted. Point out the undesirable change so the child can learn to monitor the quality of his or her own vocalizations. Positively reinforce the child for improved production. Repeat this step until good quality, long duration production is stabilized.

Step 3. Here the child practices initiating, releasing, and re-initiating the vowel /a/, always with the same oral, breath-supported sound. It may be helpful for the teacher to use a hand cue to signal initiation and cessation of syllables and to indicate varying vowel durations. Other ideas for indicating changes in vowel duration include using different lengths of yarn or colored paper, having the child vocalize while tracing 12 inches of /a/ on a ruler, and having the child hold the sound for a given number of seconds.

Step 4. Next, one might move on to syllable practice, continuing to require a relaxed, oral sound, well supported by breath. The teacher could introduce a known consonant and have the child repeat the syllables so that phonation does not cease in-between (i.e., ba_ba_ba_ba). This type of practice is the remedial base for building coarticulation skill and can be likened to "legato" playing of a musical instrument. The object is to go smoothly from one sound to another with a minimal break in phonation. Having the child prolong the vowel prior to beginning the next syllable/consonant is a technique which can be beneficially used in early practice of all phonemes. Once brought to normal rate this technique has the potential of resulting in increased control and fluency of coarticulation.

Step 5. Next one might vary the length and speed of practice so that the child develops confidence and flexibility. "Legato" practice is facilitating at first, but now the child needs to add controlled "staccato" production of sounds to the repertoire. Staccato production occurs when phonation ceases after every syllable and the child must re-initiate with correct vocal-fold tension and subglottal pressure (i.e., ba-ba-ba-ba). The staccato productions shouuld be alternated with the legato (e.g., /ba-ba-ba_ba/ or /ba_ba_ba-ba-ba/) at varying rates of production. By the time the child's accuracy and ease of production have reached the Step 5 level, it is important to recursively integrate the suprasegmentals into the phonetic level practice. For example, as soon as the child has reached this stage of multiple repetitions, practice with stress change could be incorporated. Thus /ba-ba-ba/ becomes /BA-ba-ba/ or /ba-BA-ba/.

Step 6. At this stage of practice, voice and durational control can be generalized to practice of other vowels and diphthongs. Sets or combinations of vowels can be practiced to develop the flexibility in tongue control needed for accuracy, speed, and economical coarticulation in connected speech. That is, once the first 3 vowels /a/, /i/, /u/ have been stabilized in multiple repeated consonant-vowel syllables, combinations of these vowels can be encouraged in free variation with each other. It may be especially helpful to begin this varied vowel practice with one of the high front vowels gliding into one of the back vowels (e.g., /i‿u/). This type of articulatory contrast will produce the greatest amount of obvious tongue movement. It also will highlight the transitions in second formants for the child with adequate hearing. The goal is to obviate the "neutral quality" typical in many hearing-impaired persons' speech (Rothman, 1976, p. 129). Other helpful combinations include: /aI/, /au/, /Ia/, /Iu/. Those combined with /I/ promote the production of the /j/ semivowel which can thus be taught just after the diphthongs in the First Step vowels. (See Ling's [1976] "Phonetic Level Evaluation" form.) For both diphthongs and the /j/ semivowel, the child might initially prolong the first element of the combination until given a hand cue to continue onto the second element (e.g., /a‿i/ or /aI‿ja/).

Step 7. All subsequently acquired phonemes should be practiced with good voice quality and control of duration as described above.

Nasality

NOTE: Nasality is not a prosodic feature. However, production of nasal-sounding voice is inextricably linked with voice and breath production. Furthermore, it merits separate treatment since it is one of the most commonly cited characteristics of "deaf speech."

Typical problems

The child with hypernasality exhibits speech that is excessively nasal, neutral, or central-sounding rather than oral, clear, forward-sounding.

Physiologic causes

As is well known to speech-language pathologists and audiologists, production of oral or nasal sounds is controlled by the movement of the velum in closing or opening the velopharyngeal port. Hearing-impaired children at birth have the capacity for the development of normal functioning of the velopharynx. However, they often seem to acquire problems making appropriate oral/nasal contrasts. Abnormalities in the opening/closing action of the velum can be acquired through insufficient use of the auditory modality to monitor production of oral sounds, inadequate teaching of the oral/nasal contrast in motor speech production resulting in practiced error on the part of the child, and overall insufficient oral stimulation and practice. (For a more complete discussion of nasality, the reader is directed to Ling, 1976, pp. 249-251.)

Aim of remediation

Remediation goals are to improve auditory awareness of the difference between oral and nasal production of sounds, to develop the oral/nasal contrast in motor speech production, and to remediate faulty velopharyngeal function through practice of facilitative sets of syllables.

Auditory requirements

Children with adequately aided residual audition only up to 500 Hz can detect and discriminate nasality, since the nasal murmur or steady state band of energy which identifies the nasal sounds falls at or below 300 Hz (Ling, 1976, pp. 262-263).

Techniques for remediation

Step 1. The teacher could begin by establishing the ability to auditorily discriminate a nasal from an oral sound. The /ba/ versus /ma/ sounds are suggested initially, since they represent one of the most typical auditory and articulatory confusions. One can simply use two sets of colored blocks and have the child select the color which represents either the /ba/ or the /ma/ as the teacher says one or the other. At first it may be helpful for the teacher to slightly exaggerate the length of the nasal in the syllable [ma] or the plosive burst in the syllable [ba] in order that the child focuses on the salient acoustic properties of the two sounds. After the child has consistently discriminated auditorily between the two syllables, the roles then can be reversed so that the child is producing the /ma/ and /ba/ syllables. More ideas for this and other types of auditory discrimination work are described by Paterson (1982).

Step 2. Reteach phonemes which have already been acquired but which are produced with excessive nasality. Use the steps outlined for remediation of vocal quality and duration to help promote oral sounds.

Step 3. Sets of syllables with adjacent nasal and oral consonants can be practiced in order to facilitate rapid and smooth opening and closing of the velum. All consonant manners of production can be contrasted with all nasal sounds. Initially, however, the voiceless fricatives are especially useful because of their very strong breathstream, which reminds the child of oral production and seems to promote it. The following are examples of various facilitative combinations of syllables:

Condition 1: (a) /m, n, or ŋ/ versus /f, ʃ, θ/, and later /s/
            e.g., /ʌmʃa ʌmʃa ʌmʃa ʌmʃi/
            /ʌnfa ʌnfi ʌnfu/

(b) /m, n, or ŋ/ versus any other oral consonant
with free variation.

e.g., /ʌmba ʌmba ʌmbɒ ʌmbi/
/aInda ʌnda aInda/

and groups of/ omwa; ʌnga; amlav; Imtu/, etc.

Condition 2:   any oral consonant versus /m, n, or ŋ/ with free
variation: e.g., groups of /olna, Iʃma; æbmi;
ɔfno; Isnav/, etc.

Intensity

Typical problems

Intensity problems may be evident from the child's difficulty in producing intensity extremes: that is, a controlled shout versus a whisper. But it may be even more damaging to conversational fluency and intelligibility if the child does not use the stress patterns and vowel lengthenings required in spoken language. Since English is a stress-timed language, a hearing-impaired child's failure to employ expected rhythmic stress patterns in sentences can make it difficult for a listener to detect boundaries among thought groups within a sentence. In addition, the use of stress indicates a meaning difference between a number of word pairs, such as the following:

The désert/dessért is hot.

Physiologic causes

Intensity control is linked to the amount and control of subglottal pressure and is coordinated with vocal fold tension (Ling, 1976; Pickett, 1980, p.87). Syllables receiving strongest stress in a phrase receive both an increase in vocal fold tension and in subglottal pressure (Pickett, 1980, p. 88). This is the reason that hearing-impaired children with poor voice quality and inadequate breath control often exhibit concomitant problems with both intensity and pitch. However, the hearing-impaired child has the physiologic capacity to produce conventional intensity and stress contrasts. With adequate training, the ability can be realized.

Aim of remediation

Remediation goals are to provide children with the ability to monitor and produce vocalizations varying in intensity over a comfortable range and to produce controlled and flexible intensity contrasts (in combination with durational aspects) for sentence stress.

Auditory requirements

Acoustic cues for the detection and discrimination of intensity differences should be available to adequately aided children with residual hearing up to 500 Hz (Ling, 1976, p. 27-29).

Techniques for remediation

Step 1. The teacher could begin by initiating teaching with the voice and breath work described under "Vocal Quality" above. Once the child has reached the stage of practice of repetition of multiple reduplicated syllables, the teaching of intensity changes could begin.

Step 2. In order to evoke use of loud voice, our experience has shown it useful to send the child to the other side of the room and speak audibly. Thus, the use of a loud voice performance is logical and meaningful.

Step 3. Intensity steps: Once the child is used to practicing a loud voice from across the room, one can work on decreasing volume in a controlled manner by having the child come toward you in stages. The routine is that the child will start off talking in a very loud voice away from the listener and by the time 5 giant steps have been taken the child should be next to the listener talking in a whisper. Five steps are suggested to coordinate with 5 levels of vocal intensity (very loud, loud, normal, soft, whisper). By reversing the procedure, the child practices going from a whisper to a shout by going away from the listener. Any amount of variety is possible once the child indicates good control. Steps can be jumped so that the child goes straight from normal voice to whisper, or shout to normal voice level. Teachers can invent many individual and group games for this kind of exercise. At this gross level we recommend first working with consonant-vowel combinations, which are the easiest for the child (e.g., ba), and always insisting on the oral supported sound as explained under "Vocal Quality."

Pitch

Typical problems

Difficulties with pitch evidence themselves in monotonous voice quality, incorrect voice register, uncontrolled pitch changes, confusion of pitch for intensity changes, and/or poor use of intonational contours in language.

Physiologic causes

Usually pitch problems are related to too little vocal fold tension, which is realized in a low, monotone voice with little or no sentence intonation. However, occasionally, a child evidences too much vocal fold tension, which results in an abnormally high-pitched voice. In addition to vocal fold tension, insufficient control of subglottal pressure may also be a factor in pitch problems. As mentioned above, differences in subglottal pressure and vocal fold tension also produce intensity contrasts. Consequently, pitch problems and intensity problems are often linked.

Aim of remediation

Remediation goals are to establish controlled and flexible production of pitch contrasts leading to normal intonational contours in running speech.

Auditory requirements

Acoustic cues for the establishment of pitch control necessary for intonation changes are available to children even with residual hearing only up to 500 Hz (Ling, 1976, p. 190).

Techniques for remediation

Step 1. A reasonable starting place would be to initiate breath and voice work as described under "Vocal Quality" above. (Usually pitch would be the last suprasegmental aspect to be specifically remediated.)

Step 2. Once controlled voice and breath production have been accomplished, one can simply ask the child to imitate the teacher's varied pitch production. If this is unsuccessful, hand cues to indicate high, medium, and low pitch might be used. If additional strategies are necessary, Steps 3 and 4 suggested below could be helpful.

Step 3. Lowering pitch:

  a. Yawning relaxes the child and lowers the larynx. As this occurs the only possible type of sound to emerge is an oral one. If the child is instructed to think of a low sound at the same time, it is likely to emerge. The child could do this several times while extending the length of vocalization on /a/ and this might be repeated until the child has developed control. Then the child could vocalize and change pitch on the oral stream of air (think of waves of sound) e.g., /a∿∿a/.
  b. Requesting the child to lower the head to the chest while vocalizing may result in a lowering of the larynx and a change in pitch. The child should listen to the change and feel the movement of the larynx

so that what is happening can be understood. This should be repeated until the child can change pitch without the artificial head movement.

   c. The child could begin this activity by continuously voicing /a/ while the teacher walks toward him. Any pitch level would be acceptable to begin with. The longer the child has to hold this sound on one breath, the more effort it will take for him to hold an abnormal pitch placement. Gradually a drop in pitch will usually be noticed as the child releases the faulty placement and allows a more natural, easier placement to occur. The child should be made aware that the lower, more natural voice is the desired one.

Step 4. Raising pitch:

   a. This activity could begin by having the child prepare to vocalize, but wait in anticipation of a hand signal to begin. This procedure should have the effect of causing vocal fold adduction in preparation for the emission of a high sound. In essence, one tricks the child into producing the amount of tension required at vocal fold level for a high-pitched sound.

   b. The child is then given a mental picture of higher pitch by touching the top of the head gently as the spot to aim for when vocalizing.

   c. The vocal folds could then be artificially tensed by having the child push with his or her arms against the table or try to pull upwards while holding firmly to the sides of the chair. When voicing is initiated, the sound produced should be high in pitch.

Step 5. As soon as the child is able to consistently produce pitch change at the gross level with a single vowel, practice with vowel transitions can begin. One could practice gliding downwards and upwards in pitch in a continuous manner. Support this on one breath, i.e.,

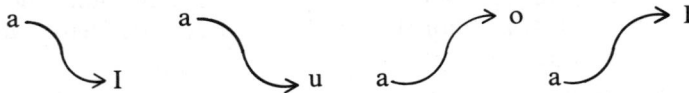

This step is only possible if the child has been progressing well through the vocal quality remediation section.

   The preceding section has offered techniques for the remediation and practice of the prosodic elements of speech at the motor speech level. It has also been suggested that work on these minute aspects of motor speech—though necessary to the remediation process—will not automatically result in the child's overall improvement in speech flexibility nor in improved intelligibility to the listener. In order to effect change, elements practiced at the motor speech level must rapidly be used in meaningful situations. The next logical step for a child at this level of remediation is to create and allow for opportunities for meaningful usage of prosodic features in both scheduled and incidental ways.

Scheduled Practice of Prosodic Elements in Limited Meaningful Contexts

NOTE: As the child is applying the newly acquired prosodic skills to meaningful language, it is important to use linguistic structures and content which are already familiar. (This is an extension of a principle for language learning/teaching cited in Kretschmer & Kretschmer, 1978, p. 257.)

1. Targets:

Parameters of speech production selected for treatment are vocal quality and breath control integrated with stress, intonation, and rhythm.

Requirements:

— Articulation ability at the multiple alternating syllable stage;
— Prior understanding of the linguistic structures involved.

Sample Activities:

a. Children could practice the following common sentences which combine all of the aforementioned elements. It seems useful for the teacher to think of linking each syllable to the next in order to be reminded of how coarticulation might occur. Vowels may be lengthened at first to facilitate movement and joining without destroying intonation and stress.

$$\text{I have} \begin{cases} a \\ the \end{cases} \underline{\hspace{2cm}}. = [\text{aɪ hæ ya} \underline{\hspace{2cm}}]$$

$$\text{Do you have} \begin{cases} a \\ the \end{cases} \underline{\hspace{2cm}}? = [\text{du ju hæ ya} \underline{\hspace{2cm}}?]$$

Games can be devised to allow for rapid multi-practice of these variations which are naturally implied (*He has; Do they have?; I don't have; She does,* etc.). Activities should emphasize the conversational/interactional constraints inherent in the sentences and not become a series of rote repetitions of the same sentence. The objective is to allow for scheduled practice and helpful encouragement in using the correct intonational patterns and stress markers, but only to impel growth. Once the child facilitates production through one or two repetitions of a game, responsibility for some aspect of the practice in incidental conversation would be appropriate.

b. Another activity could involve several children and the teacher having one or more objects to toss around, as in the "Hot Potato" game. Whoever is holding the object could say the key sentence or a variation: "Now, I have the ____." That child then passes it on to the next player and says, "Mary, it's yours" or "Catch it, Mary!" "You have it now!", etc.

2. Target: Nasality

Requirements:
— Establishment of the nasal/oral contrast in specific phoneme discrimination;
— Articulation at the multiple syllable level;
— Prior understanding of the linguistic structures involved.
a. Once the child has learned to recognize nasality in a controlled discrimination set, discrimination between oral and nasal sounding production of coarticulated speech in phrases and sentences is appropriate. This highlights again the fact that a difference can be discerned and allows the teacher to begin to pass responsibility on to the child for monitoring of vocal production.

e.g. Oral, Clear,   Nasal, Neutral
      Forward sounding   sounding

      _____   _____

      May I go out.   May I go out.

The teacher provides both stimuli; the child then simply marks or indicates which was heard. The role reversal technique works well in this instance, with the child attempting to give only the desirable oral production.
b. The following linguistic context can be used for meaningful practice of /d/ versus /n/ after it has been established at the motor speech level.

e.g. Do you need some | ____?
                 a, the |

      Yes, I do! Yes, I
             do need a | ____.
                   the |

      No, I don't!
      No, I don't need a | ____.
                     the |

Games can be devised which emphasize the interactional/conversational use of those structures. For example, a small group or an individual could prepare a recipe with the teacher. Nonsense or inappropriate objects, utensils, or ingredients could be offered which would create an element of fun, surprise, and spontaneity, as the preparation continued.

c. A game of 20 questions could be played using the same linguistic patterns, while the child or children attempt to guess "how" a task can be completed.

> e.g. Answer: "to build a house." Questions: Do you need some wood? Do you need paint? Do you need many people?

d. Selected phrases from social routines may be chosen for special attention in scheduled practice prior to incidental reminding. Once the nasal/oral contrast has been established, such common phrases as "Hello! Thank you! Good-bye!" should no longer be accepted when produced with nasal-sounding voice.

3. Targets:

Stress (intensity) change in conversation, monitoring of appropriate stress patterns versus monotone or incorrect stress/timing; integrating stress variations with duration and intonation.

Requirements:

— Parameters of speech production selected for treatment are previous establishment of the ability to change intensity production at motor speech level;
— Prior knowledge of the linguistic structures involved.

Sample activities:

a. Through the use of audition and some play-like situations, one could attempt to have the child imitate the production of the modeled loudness of voice. For example, with a young child one can put a doll to bed and say "ssh, ssh" in a whispered voice and then play at waking the doll up by shouting "Boo!" Or games could be arranged so that the children must call out the name of another person very loudly or very softly in order for them to turn around or follow an instruction.

b. Almost all hearing-impaired children shout on the playground. It may be necessary to utilize playground games to practice vocal variety in stress and then remove the work to indoors. The game of "Stop and Go" can be played outside with children taking turns as callers. "Simon Says" is another game that facilitates rapid practice of stress and grosser intensity changes in sentences.

4. Targets:

Parameters of vocal production pinpointed for treatment are intonation (pitch) change in conversation, self-monitoring of intonation pattern versus monotone speaking, and integrating intonational variation with stress and duration.

Requirements:
— Ability to vary pitch grossly at the motor speech level of production;
— Prior understanding of the linguistic structures involved.

Sample activities:
a. Selected phrases from social routines could be chosen for specific, scheduled practice prior to incidental practice. Monotone production should be avoided with attention to correct stress, duration, and overall intonation pattern being most important. Misarticulations could be ignored for the present until flexibility and greater automatic production of prosodic elements is achieved. Some sample phrases are: "Thank you"/"Pardon me!"/"I'm sorry!"/"Excuse me!"

b. Younger children especially enjoy acting out fairy stories, which lend themselves naturally to wide intonational contour variation. This affords children the opportunity to listen closely for intonational change and also to practice production. For example, "Goldilocks" provides the three varied voices of Papa Bear (low voice), Mama Bear (medium voice), and Baby Bear (high voice). Thus, flexibility in use of a consistent specific pitch level is incorporated with the overall intonational contour of the lines of spoken dialogue.

c. Games can be created that specifically encourage practice of the rising intonation patterns associated with Yes/No questions,

    e.g., "Are you big?" "Is this something yellow?"

Twenty questions is an obvious game for this type of scheduled practice.

d. Each child can be given the task of finding pictures that convey the intent of common expressions of emotion.

e.g., "She's mad/sad/happy/crying."
"You're crazy"/"Don't touch"/"Look out!"
"That's so funny" "Uh – oh" . . .
A quick flashcard game could then be played with the children offering in turn an expression chosen to describe the picture from those currently selected for scheduled practice.

5. Targets:
Speech production parameters selected for treatment are duration variation of syllabic groups in sentences, integration of duration with stress and intonation, continued auditory awareness of durational differences.

Requirements:
— The ability to alternate multiple syllables on one breath;
— The ability to whisper;
— Prior understanding of the specific linguistic structures involved.

Sample activities:
Young, hearing-impaired infants (like their hearing counterparts) can learn durational differences through play by associating certain sounds with a wide range of selected toys. For example: a frog or other jumping animal becomes associated with "hop, hop, hop". An airplane flying can be associated with a long vowel variation a⌒I; short duration can be emphasized in expressive phrases—"He's mad! Stop him! Make him go! No! No!" Similar sorts of strategies can be adapted for work with older children.

Incidental Practice of Prosodic Features
The sample ideas and activities outlined above are intended to show how carry-over of aspects of prosody from scheduled to incidental practice can be achieved. Fundamental to all of these activities is the fact that the teacher must create an environment of high expectations for speech.
The expectations for the child include taking responsibility for:
— Beginning to incorporate into the daily routine the aspects of prosody covered in scheduled practice;
— Using better voice quality and intonational contours in all utterances.
Teacher responsibility then includes:
1. Positive reinforcement for oral-sounding speech. A brief reminder to "begin your talking on your breath" is often sufficient to produce

oral sound. Similarly, the phrase "make your sounds more forward" can help jog the child's memory.

2. Organizing learning/teaching to best facilitate change.
   — Establishing an environment in which children are allowed and encouraged to talk a great deal.
   — Correcting selectively. That is, while establishing improved vocal quality and prosodic skills, many misarticulations probably should be ignored in order to give the child a change to recuperate some of the flexibility in voice use which was not fostered adequately earlier.
   — Keeping in mind that the overall aim is for the child to use spoken language with maximum ease and intelligibility.

Summary

In a recent survey of the school-age hearing-impaired population in the United States, more than half of the children received unacceptable intelligibility ratings (Jensema, Karchmer, & Trybus, 1978). In order for more children to achieve maximum clarity of speech in spontaneous oral conversation, two broad areas require serious improvement: input and instruction. Applications of recent research and innovative thought in each area have been presented in light of the contributions they may make toward achieving the goal of intelligibility. Systematic empirical study of these and other treatment techniques is now needed in order for future advances to be made.

End Notes

[1] A discussion of auditory training systems presently in use (hardwire systems, portable desk trainers, and loop systems, radio frequency direct systems, infared light systems) is outside the scope of this paper. Probably the greatest advantage of these systems is improvement in signal-to-noise ratio, which can be essential in many communication situations both in and out of the classroom. For more information, the reader is directed to (Børrild, 1978; Libby, 1973; Ling, 1978; Ross, 1977; Staab & O'Gara, 1974).

[2] The voiced plosive burst characteristic of the /b/ contrasts greatly with the 200 to 300 Hz nasal murmur of the /m/.

Reference Notes

1. Nicholls, G. Cued speech and the reception of spoken language. Unpublished Master's thesis, McGill University, 1979.

2. Mahashie, J. J. Deaf speakers' laryngeal behavior. Unpublished doctoral dissertation, Syracuse University, 1980.

References

American Speech-Language-Hearing Association. Standards for effective oral communication programs. *ASHA,* 1979, *21,* 198–1002.

Berger, K. W., Hagberg, E. N., & Rane, R. L. *Description of hearing aids: Rationale, procedures and results.* Kent, O: Herald Publishing House, 1977.

Boone, D. Modification of the voices of deaf children. *The Volta Review,* 1966, *68,* 686–692.

Boothroyd, A. Technology and deafness. *The Volta Review,* 1975, *77,* 27–34.

Boothroyd, A., Archambault, P., Adams, R. E., & Storm, R. D. Use of a computer-based system for speech training aids for deaf persons. *The Volta Review,* 1975, *77,* 178–193.

Børrild, K. Classroom acoustics. In M. Ross & T. G. Giolas (Eds.), *Auditory management of hearing-impaired children.* Baltimore: University Park Press, 1978.

Byrne, D. Hearing aid selection: An analysis and point of view. *Archives Otolaryngologica,* 1979, *105,* 519–525.

Calvert, D. R., & Silverman, S. R. *Speech and deafness.* Washington, D. C.: A. G. Bell Association for the Deaf, 1975.

Campos, C. T. Co-investigator experience with the cochlear implant: A report from the Denver Ear Institute. *Hearing Instruments,* 1981, *32,* 26–30.

Clark, G. M., & Tong, Y. C. Multiple-electrode cochlear implant for profound or total hearing loss: A review. *Medical Journal of Australia,* 1981, *1,* 428–429.

Clarke, B. R., & Ling, D. The effects of cued speech: A follow-up study. *The Volta Review,* 1976, *78,* 23–24.

Cornett, R. O. Cued speech. *American Annals of the Deaf,* 1967, *112,* 3–13.

Cornett, R. O. Cued speech and oralism: An analysis. *Audiology and Hearing Education,* 1975, *1,* 26–33.

Fry, D. B. *Acoustic phonetics. A course of basic readings.* Cambridge: Cambridge University Press, 1976.

Fry, D. B. The role and primacy of the auditory channel in speech and language development. In M. Ross & T. G. Giolas (Eds.), *Auditory management of hearing-impaired children.* Baltimore: University Park Press, 1978.

Gastmeier, W. J. The acoustically damped earhook. *Hearing Instruments,* 1981, *32,* 14–15.

Grave, J., & Metzinger, M. The effects of stepped diameter coupling systems on hearing-impaired children. *Hearing Instruments,* 1981, *32,* 27, 66.

Hirsh, I. J. Auditory training. In H. Davis & S. Silverman (Eds.), *Hearing and deafness.* New York: Holt, Rinehart and Winston, 1970.

Hochberg, I., Levitt, H., & Osberger, M. J. Improving speech services to hearing-impaired children. *ASHA,* 1980, *2,* 280–284.

House, W. F., Bode, D. L., & Berliner, K. I. The cochlear implant: Performance of deaf patients. *Hearing Instruments,* 1981, *32,* 13–18.

Hudgins, C. V., & Numbers, C. V. An investigation of intelligibility of speech of the deaf. *General Psychology Monograph,* 1942, *25,* 289–292.

Jensema, C. J., Karchmer, M. A., & Trybus, R. J. The rated speech intelligibility of hearing-impaired children: Basic relationships and a detailed analysis. Office of Demographic Studies, Gallaudet College, Washington, D. C., 1978.

Killion, M. C., & Monser, E. L. CORFIG. In G. A. Studebaker & I. Hochberg (Eds.), *Acoustical factors affecting hearing aid performance.* Baltimore: University Park Press, 1980.

Kretschmer, R. R., & Kretschmer, L. W. *Language development and intervention with the hearing impaired.* Baltimore: University Park Press, 1978.

Libby, E. R., The achievement of optimal amplification for the hearing-impaired child. *The Hearing Dealer,* July, 1973. (reprint).

Libby, E. R. Smooth wideband hearing aid responses: The new frontier. *Hearing Instruments,* 1980, *31,* 12–13, 15, 18, 43.

Libby E. R. Achieving a transparent, smooth, wideband hearing aid response. *Hearing Instruments,* 1981, *32,* 9–12.

Ling, D. *Speech and the hearing-impaired child: Theory and practice.* Washington, D. C.: A. G. Bell Association for the Deaf, 1976.

Ling, D. Auditory coding and recoding: An analysis of auditory training procedures for young children. In M. Ross & T. G. Giolas (Eds.), *Auditory management of hearing-impaired children.* Baltimore: University Park Press, 1978, 181–218.

Ling, D. Principles underlying the development of speech communication skills among hearing-impaired children. *The Volta Review,* 1979, *81,* 211–223.

Ling, D. Early speech development. In S. Gerber & G. Mencher (Eds.), *Early management of hearing loss.* New York: Grune & Stratton, 1981. (a)

Ling, D. Keep your hearing-impaired child within earshot. *Newsounds,* 1981, *6,* 5–6. (b)

Ling, D. & Clarke, B. R. Cued speech: An evaluative study. *American Annals of the Deaf,* 1975, *120,* 480–488.

Ling, D., & Ling, A. H. *Aural habilitation: The foundations of verbal learning in hearing-impaired children.* Washington, D. C.: A. G. Bell Association for the Deaf, 1978.

Luetje, C. M. Single-electrode cochlear implant: Practicality in clinical otologic practice. *Hearing Instruments,* 1981, *39,* 20–23.

Martin, L. F., Tong, Y. C., & Clark, G. M. A multiple-channel cochlear implant: Evaluation using speech tracking. *Archives of Otolaryngology,* 1981, *107,* 157–159.

Martony, J. On the correction of the voice pitch level for severely hard of hearing subjects. *American Annals of the Deaf,* 1968, *119,* 195–202.

Minifie, F. Speech acoustics. In F. Minifie, T. J. Hixon, & F. Williams (Eds.), *Normal aspects of speech, hearing and language.* Englewood Cliffs, N.J.: Prentice-Hall, 1973.

Monsen, R. B. The production of English stop consonants in the speech of deaf children. *Journal of Phonetics,* 1976, *4,* 29–41.

Monsen, R. B. Acoustic qualities of phonation in deaf children. *Journal of Speech and Hearing Research,* 1979, *22,* 270–288.

Nickerson, R.S. Characteristics of the speech of deaf persons. *The Volta Review,* 1975, *77,* 342–362.

Oller, K. D., Payne, S. L., & Gavin, W. J. Tactual speech perception by minimally trained deaf subjects. *Journal of Speech and Hearing Research,* 1980, *23,* 757–768.

Paterson, M. M. Integration of auditory training with speech and spoken language development. In D. G. Sims, G. Walter, & R. Whitehead (Eds.), *Communication training for the severely hearing impaired.* Baltimore: Waverly Press, 1982.

Pickett, J. M. *The sounds of speech communication.* Baltimore: University Park Press, 1980.

Ross, M. Classroom amplification. In W. Hodgson & P. Skinner (Eds.), *Hearing aid assessment and use in audiologic habilitation.*Baltimore: Williams & Wilkins, 1977.

Rothman, H. B. A spectrographic investigation of consonant-vowel transitions in the speech of deaf adults. *Journal of Phonetics,* 1976, *4,* 129–136.

Rudmin, F. R. Letters to the editor: Comment on "Judgments of hearing aid processed music." *Ear and Hearing,* 1982, *3,* 238–239.

Rudmin, F. R. The why and how of hearing /s/. *The Volta Review.* (in press)

Smith, C. R. Residual hearing and speech production in deaf children. *Journal of Speech and Hearing Research,* 1975, *18,* 795–811.

Staab, W. J., & O'Gara, E. J. Auditory training systems for the hearing-impaired: A discussion of types, advantages, and uses. *Hearing Instruments,* September, 1974. (reprint)

Strong, W. J. Speech aids for the profoundly/severely hearing impaired: Requirements, overview, projections. *The Volta Review,* 1975, *77,* 536–556.

Subtelny, J. D., Whitehead, R. L., & Orlando, N. A. Description and evaluation of an instructional program to improve speech and voice diagnosis of the hearing-impaired. *The Volta Review,* 1980, *82,* 85–95.

Yanick, P. Speech processing and hearing rehabilitation. *Hearing Instruments,* 1980, *31,* 24, 26–27.

Dennis M. Ruscello

Motor Learning as a Model for Articulation Instruction

Introduction

Individuals who exhibit articulatory production errors comprise a large segment of speech-language clinicians' caseloads (Weston & Leonard, 1976). In the typical assessment/intervention program, a client's specific production errors are identified, and then a treatment is administered for the purpose of modifying the pattern of misarticulation. There are a number of available treatments that appear to reflect either different theoretical positions (Bernthal & Bankson, 1981) or service delivery models (Costello & Onstine, 1976). Regardless of the clinician's orientation, the productive component of the treatment strategies is directed toward target sound establishment in a variety of training units. The training units can include levels that range from isolated sound practice to spontaneous conversational speech.

If one simply focuses on the training units employed, it appears that two main generalizations become apparent (Ruscello, Note 1). First, the treatment plan proceeds from less complex to more complex units of production training. The initial training level will depend on the client's competence with the target sound, since successful completion of a particular unit facilitates the introduction of more advanced tasks. Second, early treatment sessions involve discrete production such as isolated sound or word practice, while later sessions incorporate usage in continuous discourse. The aforementioned characterization is closely allied with concepts presented in the theoretical constructs of motor skill learning (Ellis, 1972). That is, skilled movements are composed of a series of finely controlled responses which are organized in various sequences. Initially a person practices a motor skill in limited contexts until correct execution of the movement is achieved. As the person continues practice, the movement is carried out in combination with others. Conscious control of the skilled movement eventually shifts to enactment in an automatic, effortless manner.

Salient features in the discussion of motor skill learning include stages of response development and the role of practice in such development. The purpose of this chapter is to present a viewpoint that articulatory training can be conceptualized as a skilled motor learning phenomenon. Literature to be discussed will include the purposes for which practice is used in developing different aspects of motor behavior and the theoretical positions that have been proposed in motor skill learning. In addition, articulatory studies that have investigated various skill learning variables will be reviewed. Finally, clinical implications of theory and research will be presented.

Purposes of Motor Practice

Shelton (1963) presented a position paper that discussed the different purposes of motor practice. Depending on the interests of the learner, practice can be utilized to: increase strength, develop endurance, increase range of motion, or acquire various motor skills. Each of these different purposes requires practice; however, practice techniques will vary as a function of the goal. For example, procedures employed to build strength might include the use of resistance placed against a muscle or muscle group. A person interested in developing strength would carry out practice trials against the resistance. Additional resistance would gradually be introduced as the individual increased strength capabilities.

In contrast to the strength building example, the formation of a motor skill requires the execution of a series of coordinated muscular movements. Initially, the act is novel to a learner; consequently, practice is necessary for the development of the motor skill. The act of throwing a ball involves both arm and general body movement in synchrony. A thrower attempts to achieve some type of target through coordinated movement. The learner who tries to perfect the skilled act practices it under various response conditions. These two examples suggest that practice is an important requisite in both areas; however, the end or terminal behavior dictates the type of practice that is appropriate.

While disciplines such as physical therapy might use motor practice techniques in any of the ways mentioned, the speech-language pathologist is generally involved in skill building (Shelton, Hahn, & Morris, 1968; Shelton, Morris, & McWilliams, 1973).[1] That is, articulatory training may be explained as a process within a framework of motor skill building. In this framework it is necessary to distinguish between a motor pattern and motor skills. Godfrey and Kephart (1969) have stated that a motor pattern consists of a series of skilled motor acts. The acts are performed for the accomplishment of some specific overall purpose. Motor skills, on the other hand, are movements or groups of movements which are components of an overall motor pattern.

In adapting the two-level hierarchy of Godfrey and Kephart to articulatory production, the motor pattern would be analogous to coordinated sequences of movements of the articulators during speech production. The formation of the individual speech sounds would be the skills or subroutines in the overall speech production pattern. The use of this characterization is somewhat of an oversimplification and is not intended to present articulatory production as simply a pattern composed of discrete skilled movements. The author recognizes that production is a dynamic process (Daniloff & Hammarberg, 1973) that defies individual sound segmentation on either acoustic or physiologic bases (Curtis, 1970).

Netsell (1982) has indicated that speech motor production is not a function of stored movement routines or muscle contraction patterns, but a flexible internalized plan that allows for adaptation. The internalized plan of reference is formed through the analysis of afferent information that is available during speech production. In this way modifications may be enacted to insure that motor production goals are realized.

Motor skills have been divided into open and closed categories (Poulton, 1957). In closed skill development an individual learns a movement which is appropriate for a particular goal. Open skill development also involves patterned movement formation; however, the movement is such that it must be executed under varying environmental conditions (Gentile, 1972). Learners must adjust their skilled responses so that they might respond appropriately in different situational contexts. The teaching of articulatory movements would appear more like an open skilled task, since the target behavior must ultimately be used across a variety of phonetic contexts in a number of different speaking environments.

Johnson (1972) has described skilled learning as "the ability to execute a pattern of behavioral elements in proper relation to a certain environment" (p. 10). When evaluating motor skill development, researchers study one or more of the following variables: speed, accuracy, form, and adaptability. Each variable shows some degree of change when a learner develops and eventually perfects a particular skill.

Speed refers to the time in which a skilled movement task is completed. As one perfects a skill, speed will increase to some asymptote which, of course, is dependent on the skill being developed in training. In addition to reduction in execution time, the accurate enactment of a skill also improves through practice. Accurate response is suggestive of stabilization since error rate is minimized. As previously mentioned, motor skill learning involves the proper execution of a movement that is composed of certain behavioral elements. Form refers to the correct sequencing of the behavioral elements to achieve the desired movement. Finally, use of a motor skill across a variety of conditions and situations indicates that the learner has achieved a degree of adaptability. The skill has, in fact, become a part of the learner's repertoire of skilled movements.

In summary, it was stated that there are a number of different purposes for engaging in various motor practice techniques. One purpose which appears relevant to the work of the speech-language pathologist is skill building. Motor skills are coordinated movements organized within a motor pattern. The motor pattern is an organizational hierarchy of a group of related motor skills. It was proposed that speech sounds are skilled movements and the movements are part of the overall motor pattern of speech production. When an individual develops a particular skill through practice, there are measurable components that change as a function of skill refinement.

Theories of Skill Learning

The study of motor skills had undergone a very gradual evolution until the advent of World War II (Schmidt, 1975a). At that time individuals were required to learn complex skills necessary for military occupations, so research efforts in the area were intensified. Following the war, research activities continued and investigators collected data to test various hypotheses. The hypotheses, however, were tied into general learning theory; they did not deal with the question of motor skills exclusively. It was not until the 1960s that theories particular to motor skill were formally introduced. Emergence of theoretical explanations appears related to an increased need for understanding the complexities of motor skill training across many disciplines. Investigators from the fields of industrial engineering, psychology, physical education, special education, and sports medicine were, and are currently, involved in motor skills research and application.

The diversity among disciplines is evident in the various theories that have been formulated.

Fitts (1962) has proposed that a learner passes through certain phases of development when perfecting a skill. The phases indentified by Fitts are cognition, fixation, and automation. Although distinct labels are employed, Fitts has indicated that there is overlap among the stages, and the passage between them is a continuous, rather than a discrete, type of progression.

As Fitts describes it, the cognitive stage is one of mental analysis because the learner is attempting to master the task at hand. The requirements of the task must be determined, and strategies to perform the skill correctly must be formed. During early practice trials the learner continually makes motor adjustments based on the cognitive analysis of previous performance. The adjustments are mediated via internal verbalization and based on the demands of the particular skill.

Following the period of conceptual scrutiny, practice is aimed at fixating the skilled behavior pattern. Continued practice results in enactment at a very low error rate. Gradually, fixation gives way to automation, wherein the execution time required for the skill declines. The motor skill is produced effortlessly and without conscious control under a variety of situations and conditions; it has been automated for inclusion into one's repertoire of skilled motor behavior.

A more physiologic approach in explaining the patterning of skilled movement was proposed by Palliard (1960) through his acquisition-automatization model. In his phase progression, the initial effort or acquisition stage constitutes practice guided via conscious mental control. There is a general tension or stiffness in the musculature that is evident when observing the succession of voluntary movements. The tension gradually dissipates when the person perfects the pattern through practice. Palliard suggested that repetition of the skilled act creates new feedback circuits. For example, early visual reliance might be replaced by other sensory modalities like kinesthetic feedback. The transfer among feedback mechanisms occurs because the movement becomes more automatic to the learner. In addition, voluntary control becomes diminished following automatization; its role becomes delegated to starting and terminating the motor behavior. The desired act is carried out largely on an unconscious basis.

A more recent hypothesis explains skill learning in terms of a problem that necessitates some form of solution (Adams, 1971). During the early period of skill formation a learner executes a movement, but knowledge of results is heavily relied upon. The feedback information is obtained through the learner's own assessment of the performance and that provided by an external source such as an observer. Modifications leading toward correct execution are coded verbally for future trials and the movement pattern is stored in what Adams calls a perceptual trace. The trace is feedback dependent and is frequently modified until the movement pattern becomes stabilized. Since verbal coding strategies are so vital initially, the author refers to this inceptive stage as the Verbal-Motor Stage.

The former stage is gradually replaced by the Motor Stage. The learner has finally altered the perceptual trace so that error is negligible; the process is achieved through practice. Feedback or knowledge of results is no longer vital, since the perceptual trace is stored in a motor memory trace. The learner may recall the movement pattern which is coded into the perceptual trace and stored in a motor memory trace at will. Adams indicates that the perceptual trace is an error dependent or closed loop mechanism, while the memory trace is an open loop phenomenon.

Schmidt (1975b) has presented a theoretical position of skill learning that emphasizes the creation of motor schema. A schema is an internalized rule that allows the application of a particular skilled movement across a variety of contexts. At first a learner tries to form a particular movement pattern through practice; the unsteady movement is eventually transformed into a coordinated, effortless performance. According to Schmidt, when the learner forms the movement pattern, related information is stored was well. The information includes: the existing environmental conditions, the requirements of the motor program, the sensory feedback received following enactment of the skilled pattern, and the outcome of the response. Repetition of the movement results in the abstraction of information regarding the four informational variables and thus a schema is formed.

The novel feature of Schmidt's proposal is his provision of extended use under differing response conditions. A person who perfects a skill with training must generally use it in circumstances that do not clearly parallel practice conditions. For example, a basketball player may learn a shot with practice; however, actual game conditions force him to shoot differently each time. A successful shooter in Schmidt's proposal would have formed a general schema that enables him to carry out the movement without any problem under a variety of circumstances.

Finally, Shelton and McReynolds (1979) reviewed a conceptualization of perceptual-motor performance which was based on the work of Marteniuk (1976). Marteniuk's proposal emphasizes the utilization of information processing by the learner. The central nervous system extracts information that is subject to evaluation, prior to and during a movement sequence. The less familiar the learner is with the movement pattern, the more information there is to consider and, presumably, the slower the patterned-movement time. After the movement pattern is stabilized, the informational load is reduced because the learner need not be concerned with numerous alternatives.

Information processing skills are superimposed on the components of Marteniuk's performance model. The components of perception, decision making, and enactment interplay with incoming information which is available to the learner. Relevant data are perceived and then organized for analysis so that decisions may be made. The importance of perception in initiating the chain of events assumes that perceptually dependent mechanisms of selective attention, short term memory, and long term memory are adequate for task purposes.

According to Marteniuk, following evaluation of the perceptual information, a decision is made concerning a plan of action. As the learner becomes more familiar with the movement task, the decision-making process occurs on an unconscious level. Processing time is then devoted to the actual movement and not to a decision concerning the requirements of the movement. The learner ultimately forms a motor program through continued practice. The motor program operates in an open loop mode and is tied into a general motor schema. The schema is a closed loop process that enables an individual to produce various forms of motor behavior. The hierarchial relation of schema and motor programs permits adaptive regulation of actions requiring skilled motor behavior.

In summary, the theoretical discussions of skill learning use somewhat differing terminology, but they do seem to exhibit a very decided interrelatedness. The authors of these conceptualizations appear to be dealing with skilled learning in much the same way. The salient features among theories center on the variables of: practice, stages of motor skill development, cognitive analysis, and feedback processes.

The use of practice for development, improvement, and subsequent refinement of a particular motor skill is a universal notion. As the learner practices a particular motor skill, modifications from internal or external sources are received and processed for the purpose of establishing performance at a high level of accuracy. Moreover, performance on a motor skill is monitored through observation of practice trials. It is clear that regardless of the hypotheses, practice is the key variable thought necessary for mastery of skilled motor behavior.

Another common feature, stages of motor skill development, is explicitly described by Fitts (1962), Palliard (1960), and Adams (1971) and implicitly mentioned by Schmidt (1975b) and Marteniuk (1976). With the former group, specific stages of skill development through which the learner proceeds are posited. For example, Palliard states that early in skilled learning there is a sluggishness in execution because the learner is acquiring the movement. Following acquisition, further practice strengthens the movement so that it can be used correctly in a variety of contexts. When accurate, effortless use is achieved, automatization has taken place. Schmidt and Marteniuk do not outline distinct stages, but instead discuss the progression of changes which correlate with the learner's competence in performing the movement. Marteniuk suggests that enactment time lessens with proficiency because a correct motor program has been formulated.

In addition, there is a universal provision for some type of cognitive analysis, expecially during the preliminary phase of movement formation. It appears to be a requisite since each theorist states that a prospective learner must evaluate his performance mentally and then incorporate necessary adjustments. Once stabilization has occurred, attention toward mentalistic planning types of activities is minimized. According to Adams (1971), a learner cognitively searches for a solution to the motor problem at hand. Schmidt (1975b) presented the position that correct performance is predicated upon the mental analysis of data during the outset of practice.

The mentalistic notions discussed above appear tied into feedback processes that also figure prominently among theorists. That is, early in the development of a skill, feedback is thought to be of great importance. Incoming sensory information is hypothesized to be employed in guiding movement until it is executed in consistently accurate fashion. When error responses diminish, feedback may be minimized (Adams, 1971; Schmidt, 1975b) or altered in some fashion (Marteniuk, 1976; Palliard, 1960).

Finally, although not a point of similarity, it is interesting to see how the mechanism of general skill developmment has been handled among the various theories. Fitts (1962) and Palliard (1960) did not address the issue; however, Adams (1971) hinted at such a proposal with his introdution of a motor trace. The motor trace is a storage mechanism or collector of motor skills within the learner's repertoire. Schmidt (1975b) further modified the storage idea with his notion of a schema—a generalized motor program for a given class of movement. In Marteniuk's (1976) thinking, a schema is also important for storing general motor routines that can be applied when needed. The generality or inherent flexibility of schema is thought necessary since it would be prohibitive to store a very large number of motor programs. It is obvious that the theorists have progressed from suggested explanations of skill learning to ways in which general motor skills might be organized for utilization.

Each theory has a certain amount of credibility, since various components of each have been submitted to empirical test and supportive data have been obtained (e.g., Carson & Wiegand, 1979); however, the establishment of one theoretical explanation over the others has not occurred. Many of the constructs incorporated into the theories are somewhat difficult to evaluate empirically. Execution of responses can certainly be observed and evaluated, but determination of stages within response development is problematic from a measurement standpoint. For example, Fitts discussed stages of response development but suggested that the skill development process was continuous rather than a series of discrete stages. Similarly, cognitive scrutiny and the role of feedback mechanisms in the establishment of motor skills pose similar measurement problems. Rather than emphasize the above limitations, it should be noted that theory development has greatly expanded and empirical evaluation is continuing (Kelso & Norman, 1978).

Utilization of Skill Development in Articulatory Training

Up to this point, it has been suggested that concepts from motor skill learning be applied to the treatment of articulatory disorders. A direct analogy was suggested between speech production and the motor pattern-motor skills hierarchy that has been discussed. Moreover, a review of motor skill theories indicated a number of parallels between them and certain processes that occur in clinical training. For example, the sluggishness alluded to in early skill acquisition appears to have an articulatory correlate, since some clients initially prolong an articulatory position they are learning. Ruscello and Shelton (1979) conducted an articulatory treatment study that introduced a planning feature prior to the execution of individual practice trials. In their discussion the authors reported the "two subjects indicated they were thinking about what they should do." The observation cited is compatible with the mentalistic analysis outlined in the different motor skill theories. The similarities also have great appeal on an intuitive basis.

Kent and Lybolt (1982) have also proposed that concepts from motor skill learning be used as a basis for treating persons with articulatory disorders. The authors suggest that speakers form motor schema which are codings of intended speech movement targets. The schema are generalized motor routines that allow for flexibility in the achievement of a movement target. That is, a particular target could be realized through various movements that are incorporated into the schema. Since there is so much variability in speech production from factors such as phonetic context, schema could account very nicely for the diversity.

It must be emphasized that the incorporation of motor skill concepts in articulatory training is not meant to imply a direct isomorphic relationship. There is an inherent distortion that one should be aware of when choosing to implement such a model: the model has been adapted from another discipline. Such adaptation, however, is not unusual since training models in speech-language pathology have traditionally been taken from other fields (Schultz, 1972). Schultz summarized his position on models in the following way:

> In summary, then, any rational therapy strategy has an underlying model which provides direction to and constraints on the clinician in his planning and execution. This shaping of therapy occurs even though the clinician may be unaware of the model he is using. The profession should initiate systematic exploration and public discussion of the various theories of therapy and their resultant models upon which clincial interactions are based. (p. 121)

The introduction of a motor skill model in articulation training is not a novel approach since others have also presented training models based on different theoretical underpinnings. (Readers are referred to an excellent discussion of different therapy models that was prepared by Shelton and McReynolds [1979]). It is the position here that the teaching of phonetic production skills may be conceptualized as a motor learning phenomenon. The motor skill model provides an organizational structure and a set of guiding principles applicable to the treatment of persons with articulatory disorders. In line with this conceptualization, articulatory errors are modified through practice in either of two ways. Movements may be taught in place of other movements, or movements may be taught where they were formerly absent. The orientation toward articulatory errors is a reflection of the physiologic nature of motor skill learning; the characterization appears compatible with both the traditional classifications of articulatory errors and the different forms of articulatory pattern analysis (Bernthal & Bankson, 1981).[2]

Studies Employing Motor Skill Model

A number of different theoretical models were described in the previous section of the paper; however, studies to be reviewed below have generally operated under the acquisition-automatization model proposed by Palliard (1960). Nevertheless, issues dealt with are relevant, regardless of the specific model one might use. This section is not meant to be exhaustive but, rather, a selective review of studies pertaining to motor skill learning in articulation.

Measurement of Articulation

In two separate investigations, Shelton and his associates (Elbert, Shelton, & Arndt, 1967; Shelton, Elbert, & Arndt, 1967) developed an articulation assessment procedure from which evolved a methodology for sensitive measurement of articulatory change during articulation instruction. Subjects in both investigations were given lessons based on motor skill-learning principles. Before, during (at beginning or end of every session), and following training, subjects were administered imitative protocols which the authors designated Sound Production Tasks (SPTs). The tasks sampled individually the target phonemes of interest in contexts of isolation, syllables, word pairs, and sentences. The target phonemes occurring in word pairs and sentences were arranged in specific sound environments patterned after the work of McDonald (1964a; 1964b). Subjects in both studies demonstrated statistically significant changes in their SPT scores. Subjects had relatively few correct responses prior to initiation of treatment, but progressed during therapy. In the Shelton, Elbert, and Arndt (1967) study, subjects maintained their SPT production capabilities even after therapy had been terminated for approximately 5 months.

Shelton and his colleagues concluded that SPTs were reliable assessment devices which were sensitive to a subject's change in target sound production. Changes in SPT scores illustrated improvement with training. The authors suggested that the SPT procedure furnished information on the acquisition stage of skill learning but not on automatization. Consequently, Shelton, Elbert and Arndt (1967) stated the following:

> We are currently studying the relationship between task scores and a measure of more spontaneous articulation usage. Measurement of articulation acquisition and of automatization may be expected to contribute to solution of the "carry-over" problem. This solution will probably involve recognition of satisfactory acquisition followed by use of methods to encourage and reinforce correct usage in a variety of speaking situations. (p. 585)

In this statement, Shelton et al. emphasized the need for comparison measures of a target sound production that would be more sensitive to automatization. The inclusion of such a procedure would aid in determining whether a person had transferred target sound production to more spontaneous or conversational-like conditions. Depending on one's theoretical underpinnings, the correct use of a formerly misarticulated sound in novel contexts has been labeled carry-over, generalization, or transfer of training (Mowrer, 1971). In line with a motor skill orientation, generalization is synonymous with the term adaptability.

The final report (Wright, Shelton, & Arndt, 1969) in the series of measurement studies done in Shelton's laboratory introduced more spontaneous measures of articulation production. Talking tasks (TTs) and reading tasks (RTs) were employed in conjunction with SPTs. A TT consisted of 30 samples of the target sound recorded while the subject described various pictures. For RTs, subjects read aloud until 30 tokens of the target sound had been produced. All subjects received treatment based on a motor skills learning model. The findings indicated that subjects showed positive change in TTs and RTs, just as they did with the SPTs; however, the magnitude of the measured change differed among the tasks. SPTs exhibited the greatest improvement followed by the RTs and TTs. The investigators felt that the performance on the sampling tasks suggested subjects had acquired correct articulation of the target sounds; however, automatic usage was not complete. These findings illustrate that differential information concerning acquisition and automatization might be examined by monitoring practice through progressive levels of training material (Ruscello, 1975) and periodic sampling on nontraining types of tasks such as SPTs, TTs, and RTs.

The early treatment studies of Shelton and his colleagues dealt primarily with the methodological consideration of measuring change with treatment based on motor learning principles. Following the development of appropriate measurement tools, additional treatment studies were undertaken so that a number of treatment related issues could be examined.

Acquisition

Chisum, Shelton, Arndt, and Elbert (1969) conducted an articulatory treatment study with subjects who had palatal closure deficits. The authors indicated that their treatment was based on motor skill-learning principles. Training was initiated, when necessary, at the isolated sound level and progressed through nonsense syllables, words, sentences, and conversation. During individual training trials, subjects were instructed to observe and listen while the clinician produced the target item. Following presentation of the target item, the subject attempted to imitate it. The production was evaluated by the clinician and the appropriate feedback given to the subject. Correct responses were verified with verbal affirmation. Incorrect responses were identified. The clinician also furnished placement information thought to be pertinent in assisting the subjects to achieve correct production of the target sound.

The results showed a statistically significant difference between word articulation test scores administered before and after training. Despite the positive treatment change, correlations between articulation difference scores and numbers of practice responses did not demonstrate a significant relationship. In discussing the lack of relationship between articulation change and practice responses, Chisum et al. wrote: "The importance of practice and reinforcement to motor learning is so well established that other factors must be found to account for the relatively low correlations obtained in this study (p. 62)."

They discussed a number of possible reasons including the following:

Another possible explanation for the low correlations involves the relationship between rate of learning and number of practice responses. For instance, one individual may require 100 practice responses to change an incorrect response to a correct one, whereas another individual may require 200 practice responses to accomplish the same task. The relationship between rate of learning and treatment activities should be studied in future investigations. (p. 63).

The latter explanation seems most plausible in explaining the fact that degree of change on the criterion measure did not correspond with the number of responses that subjects produced in therapy. Individuals require different amounts of practice to attain a specified level of proficiency, and clinicians should be cognizant of this fact. Practice is not synonomous simply with repetition but must be specific to the individual's learning requirements.

One of the more frequent features of the motor skill-learning theories is the emphasis on mentalistic analysis, particulary during the early stages of skill development. Consequently, Ruscello and Shelton (1979) evaluated a treatment that incorporated mental planning and self-assessment features during response acquisition. The authors reasoned that initial practice units should be carried out differently from later practice activities. Utilizing the acquisition-automatization distinction proposed by Palliard (1960), practiced units were dichotomized. Isolated sound, nonsense syllables, and word practice were considered acquisition level activities, and sentences and conversation were automatization. Drill with acquisition level units was done under the conditions of mentalistic focus and self-assessment. That is, subjects in one training group (Group I) were instructed to consider articulatory movements mentally before producing them and then assess their productions. A second group (Group II) also received articulation instruction, but the treatment did not contain mentalistic or self-assessment components. The insertion of the mental focus and self-assessment was prompted by the cognitive participation alluded to by Palliard (1960) and others (Adams, 1971; Schmidt, 1975b). Initially, the experimenter described the movements of the target sound and then presented the actual practice item. The subject was told to "think" about the movement before enactment. Following production, subjects evaluated their responses. The experimenter verified the subjects' assessments or provided other feedback, whichever was necessary. When subjects progressed to sentences and conversation, the mental focus and self-assessment components were withdrawn.

The results indicated a statistically significant advantage for Group I on SPT and TT measures, which were obtained periodically during the instructional period when the planning and self-assessment features were in effect. Group I also required significantly fewer trials in order to complete the acquisition phase of the study. The data suggest that the planning aspect of the experimental treatment was the differentiating feature between the 2 groups because subjects' self-assessments were not generally accurate. They typically identified their correct responses but consistently erred on responses that were misarticulated. Although the authors indicated that the results supported the planning concept, they cautioned against extensive generalization until further study resolved certain experimental issues. In addition, the statistical superiority of Group I was not maintained during sentence and conversational training. It appears that the initial treatment effect which was found did not enhance the performance of Group I subjects during later stages of treatment.

Automatization Treatments

Instead of the usual progression from acquisition to automatization, Johnson, Shelton, Ruscello, and Arndt (1979) evaluated a treatment that was intended to involve simultaneous acquisition-automatization techniques. The investigation was prompted by Diedrich's (1971) observation that some children demonstrated changes in conversational probes even though they had only received instruction directed toward acquisition. In the Johnson et al. investigation a total of 34 preschool subjects were assigned randomly to 1 of 2 treatment groups. Each group practiced similar materials via lessons provided by the experimenters. The difference between groups was that one also had their parents conduct home practice. The home activities, which were carried out in individual practice periods, were introduced when the children demonstrated the ability to articulate correctly their target sound in practice words. At that time, training activities were carried out in both the clinic and home. Prior to beginning home practice, parents received individual instruction on discriminating between correct and incorrect target productions. During the home practice periods, parents monitored the productions of their children. They verbally rewarded correct target phoneme productions and had their children repeat incorrect productions correctly. The number of target sounds evaluated by the parents was gradually increased from 10 to 30 productions each day. Home training advancement was contingent upon the performance of the children during the experimenter-based lessons. Periodic sampling of imitative and conversational skills revealed that both groups improved significantly with training, but there was no statistical difference between the 2 treatment groups. The results indicate that the combined treatment did not result in a decided advantage for those subjects who received it. Since the subjects who also practiced with their parents received even more treatment than the other group, yet showed no superiority in articulation performance, the inclusion of this method of simultaneous acquisition-automatization training is questionable.

Bankson and Byrne (1972) approached automatization through the use of a timed response task. That is, the experimenters speculated that gradual reductions in the time necessary to complete a block of training trials might facilitate automatization. Experimental subjects consisted of five elementary school subjects who had previously acquired correct production of their target sounds but were inconsistent in conversation. For automatization training purposes, subjects read word lists aloud. Each list contained 60 words; lists were read 25 times per day for 10 consecutive days. Reading times were taken with a stopwatch and were gradually required to be decreased as subjects read lists without misarticulating the target sound. Initially, subjects needed approximately 60 seconds to read a list, but with practice and differential reinforcement for decreasing times, times were reduced to a range of 17 to 33 seconds. Conversational probes were obtained in the children's homes, in the clinic, and by an unfamiliar observer on the final day of practice. Despite the fact that accuracy was maintained with increments in speed, performance errors on the conversational probes indicated automatization was not complete. The authors concluded the following:

> The approach we used, based on the concept that articulation is a learned set of motor events, stressed the motor skill. We wanted production of the phoneme to be correct, effortless, and automatic both at the drill level and in spontaneous speech in all of the three settings—at home with a parent, at school with the clinician, and in a new setting with a stranger. In a total of five hours of individual therapy time with each child, a great deal was accomplished, but additional carryover is needed for all of them. Further refinement of this procedure seems warranted. (p. 167).

Shelton, Johnson, and Arndt (1972) evaluated the merits of using exclusive parent participation to produce automatization in the use of formerly misarticulated speech sounds. Before treatment, the 8 school children who served as subjects demonstrated imitative control of their target sounds, but erred inconsistently in conversation. TTs and RTs were measured before treatment, during treatment, and 4 months following the final lesson. The treatment was administered after the parents had received appropriate instruction concerning the identification of correct and incorrect sound productions. The parent-child lessons were carried out daily for a period of 5 weeks. During the first week, parents conducted word drills and monitored target sound productions in conversation. The remaining 4 weeks were devoted to daily conversational monitoring. Parents provided appropriate verbal feedback for correct responses and had the children repeat their errors. Children earned performance points which could be exchanged for small prizes. Statistical analysis showed no significant differences for pre- and post-treatment SPT measures, which was expected since subjects were required to have imitative control of their target sounds prior to treatment and, therefore, produced relatively high pretreatment SPT scores. There were, however, significant differences between pre- and posttreatment TT and RT measures. Comparison of the immediate posttreatment measures with data collected approximately 4 months later showed no significant difference, indicating that the observed treatment change was maintained.

A similar study investigated the development of automatization through parent training activities with preschool children (Shelton, Johnson, Willis, & Arndt, 1975). The 10 children who received the treatment practiced with an experimenter before the parent intervention plan was begun. When the subjects produced a group of training words correctly, practice shifted to the home. The parent program was basically the same as that described in the previous investigation (Shelton, Johnson, & Arndt, 1972). Statistically significant differences were found for pre- and posttreatment comparisons of both imitative and spontaneous measures of articulation. The magnitude of change, however, was greater for the imitative measure (SPT) than the spontaneous measure (TT).

The studies in this particular section have incorporated more spontaneous sampling measures as indices to automatization of target phones. TTs and RTs have been used and gains documented, but the degree of change has been somewhat limited. Overall findings indicate that average posttreatment TT scores are substantially lower than the imitative SPTs scores (Johnson et al., 1979). These data suggest that the teaching strategies were effective in facilitating acquisition when evaluated via SPTs, but limited in the development of automatization as demonstrated in TT scores. Since the goal of articulation training for most individuals is automatic use of target sounds, more effective treatments are still in need of development.

Automatization Measures

The following investigations are not treatment reports but have operated within a motor skill model. Manning and his associates have used auditory masking procedures to estimate the level of automatization achieved by children who had been enrolled in articulatory remediation. The underlying assumption is that reliance on auditory feedback is minimized when target productions are produced on an automatic basis. Manning, Keappock, and Stick (1976) gave the McDonald Deep Test (1964a) to a group of elementary school children who were receiving articulation lessons. Subjects were first given the test under normal test conditions and then in the presence of auditory masking, if they had received a test score of 90% or better on the initial administration. The masking stimulus was 86dB SPL of white noise presented binaurally through head sets. Approximately 4 months after the initial testing, the McDonald test was given again without masking. Subject performance under normal test conditions and masking were compared with results obtained at the end of the 4-month period. Data indicate that performance on the masking condition was more accurate in predicting target sound stability following 4 months with no treatment. While articulation test scores without masking might prove to be an acceptable dismissal criterion for some cases, the masking technique appeared more stringent, thus resulting in a more accurate dismissal procedure.

Manning, Wittstruck, Loyd, and Campbell (1977) categorized a group of misarticulating children into 2 subgroups based on posttreatment McDonald Deep Test scores. Those subjects who scored 80% or higher were placed in the high-acquisition group while those scoring below 80% were placed in a low-acquisition group. After categorization, subjects underwent further McDonald Deep testing with 85dB SPL of competing speech presented binaurally. The children in the low-acquisition group exhibited performance decrements under the masking condition that were significantly greater than those observed for the high-acquisition group. It appears that auditory masking exhibits more disrupting influence for children who have not achieved a high level of sound acquisition/automatization as measured with the McDonald Deep Test.

Summary

To summarize, a number of investigations that have operated within a skill-learning model have been reviewed. Initially, methodological studies were used to develop measurement tools which could substantiate treatment effects. Implementation of the measurement tools across investigations suggest that treatments have been successful in altering patterns of mis-articulation. The generalization of target sounds to untaught items has generally been greater on measurement tasks similar to acquisition-type training levels (syllables and words) rather than to more spontaneous or automatic levels. Johnson et al. (1979) stated:

> We have come to consider 33% correct in posttreatment talking tasks (TTs) as a rough comparison point to be surpassed in future articulation research involving subjects who initially make five or fewer correct responses on a sound production task. This presents a challenge to identify or develop a treatment that will better improve conversational speech in a relatively short period of time. (p. 346)

Finally, the response of subjects who were at various levels of response development showed variations in production when responding under auditory masking conditions implying that responses on such a measure might be indicative of one's level of mastery or automatization of an articulatory motor skill.

Treatment Implications

The implications of motor-learning theory and investigative research will be discussed in reference to a number of instructional variables that have been covered in the previous sections. Literature from both skill learning and articulation treatment research will be cited where it appears pertinent.

Practice

The key ingredient in the typical skill-learning paradigm, and also a primary feature in articulation treatment, is practice. An individual is taught to produce a target sound correctly and then it is practiced in various phonetic contexts. An individual executes a particular skill in practice until it has been formed. Jones (1969) has indicated that learning is achieved through various combinations of practice. Practice is intertwined with all aspects of a training program and can be discussed in terms of the scheduling of practice, establishment of performance criteria, and differential practice methods.

In the parlance of motor learning, the issue of scheduling practice is one of distributed versus massed practice (Irion, 1969). Distributed practice consists of periodic responding across some specified time interval. For example, one could practice a particular motor skill a total of 15 times per training session for 5 consecutive days. In a massed practice plan, the motor skill is practiced equally frequently but during a single training session. An example would be a situation wherein the person practices a motor skill during a training session for 75 repetitions once a week. A correspondence in articulatory training would be the clinician's use of either block or intermittent scheduling for clients (Bernthal & Bankson, 1981). The block plan would be analogous to distributed practice, since remediation activities are carried out for short periods over a specific time span. The speech-language pathologist might see a child for 15 minute sessions, 4 times per week, so that opportunities for practice are distributed over a span of 4 sessions. Intermittent scheduling is similar to the massed form of practice; the client responds more frequently over a limited period of time. A child may be seen twice a week for 30 minute articulatory training sessions. Consequently, opportunities for practice must be massed into the allotted time rather than being distributed over a number of sessions.

Bernthal and Bankson (1981) summarized the scheduling data and indicated that block scheduling was slightly superior to intermittent scheduling in terms of dismissal rate. Motor-learning research has supported the employment of distributed practice (Catalano, 1978) in the teaching of motor skills. The agreement from both areas of research suggests that a block schedule would be more amenable to effecting change in articulatory training. However, there is a qualification that needs to be made concerning the issue. Research in motor learning indicates that the difference between massed and distributed practice is one of actual performance, not learning (Dunham, 1976). That is, subjects engaging in massed practice will often show decrements in practice trial performance which have been attributed to factors such as motivation and fatigue. However, comparison between massed and distributed practice groups does not reveal significant differences on adaptability or transfer of training tasks (Schmidt, 1975a).

In consideration of the above factors, we would recommend distributed practice, since this form of responding is more resistant to performance decrements. However, the feasibility of such scheduling is not always a viable option for many speech-language pathologists. Cognizant of the limitation, we would suggest that clinicians utilizing massed practice examine the response records of their clients to determine if performance reductions occur. For example, a client may practice the target sound in word size units during a particular training session. When reviewing the client's practice trials, there might be a drop in response accuracy toward the end of the session. The pattern would be suggestive of a performance drop described earlier. Verification of the performance reduction could be studied through the inclusion of some type of adaptability or transfer of training measure. One would predict stability or improvement in transfer despite transient fluctuations in session performance. If there was also a corresponding decrement in transfer rather than the pattern formerly described, the clinician would need to examine the teaching strategy utilized so that possible modifications might be made.

A common feature of skill-learning research and application is the establishment of performance criteria (Schmidt, 1975b). Similarly, articulatory training procedures that are guided by other theoretical frameworks also incorporate some type of performance criteria in their lesson materials (Costello, 1977; Gerber, 1977). A client must accomplish a training goal under certain conditions that have been set by the clinician. After the conditions have been met, the client is given some different type of practice material. Examples of performance criteria presented by Costello (1977) include: accuracy percentages across a group of trials (e.g., 90% accuracy in a block of 30 training trials); a set number of consecutively correct trials (e.g., 7 correct trials in succession); or some form of time designation (90% accuracy in a 5-minute segment of conversation).

From a skill-learning viewpoint, performance criteria are used because of the tremendous heterogeneity among subjects concerning the amount of practice needed. To illustrate, Ruscello and Shelton (1979) compared 2 groups of children who were receiving different training procedures, but practicing the same materials. The authors set a response achievement criterion of 80% for a block of 10 training trials in each of the levels of isolation, syllables, words, and sentence imitation. The number of responses necessary for individual subjects in either group to reach the imitative sentence condition ranged from 372 to 912 responses. Some subjects required a very limited number of practice trials at each level, while others needed a substantially higher amount of practice across the training levels. The figures reflect individual learning rates that may also be observed in clinical work. In order to allow for individual learning rate differences, one should include response achievement criteria in a training plan.

The final topic in this section concerns differential practice methods that would be suggested from skill learning theory. The various theories that were summarized describe stages of response development. It seems plausible, therefore, that different practice techniques might be beneficial at one stage but discarded eventually in favor of different procedures for subsequent stages. Practice would not simply be sheer repetition, but instead, pursuit of the most economic resolution in the most efficient manner (Bernstein, 1967). Cross (1967) stated that certain practice techniques might be helpful at one stage, but totally inappropriate at some other level of training.

The previously discussed investigation conducted by Ruscello and Shelton (1979) is an example of a treatment plan that incorporated differential practice methods. During the acquisition stage of training, subjects were requested to "think" about the impending movement of their target sound prior to producing it. Following production of the target sound, they judged the accuracy of the sound and received appropriate feedback information from the experimenter. The mentalistic and self-assessment features were eliminated from training when subjects reached sentence and conversational practice levels. By structuring therapy in this way, an effort was made to develop practice methods consistent with Palliard's acquisition-automatization distinction (Palliard, 1960).

The acquisition treatment appeared to influence positively the subjects' misarticulations, and, in particular, the mental participation activity was thought responsible. Nevertheless, there are a number of issues which must be resolved before the treatment is clinically feasible. Mentalistic participation is an abstract concept that must be inferred since it can not be observed or measured directly. Schmidt (1975a) indicated that the mental practice notion has received attention in the skill learning literature, and data suggest that the procedure is of benefit. He believes that mentalistic participation facilitates the formation of execution strategies and other verbal rehearsal features. In addition, the learner probably reviews performance from prior trials so that appropriate adjustments might be implemented in future practice trials (Gallagher & Thomas, 1980). As task familiarity increases, mental participation is of less importance to the learner; it appears to have no effect on performance after the skill has been acquired (Marteniuk, 1976).

Another example of differential practice which might be introduced clinically is the speed drill technique evaluated by Bankson and Byrne (1972). Drill times were gradually reduced while subjects maintained high response accuracy rates. The method was not completely successful; nevertheless, subjects did improve with treatment. Rate drills might enhance the stability of a target response following acquisition, thus assisting with the establishment of effortless, automatic use (Poulton, 1972).

Feedback and Knowledge of Results

The motor learning literature distinguishes between feedback and knowledge of results (Adams, 1971). Feedback is information that learners obtain from evaluation of their own performance. The learner has acccess to various types of incoming sensory information which function as feedback sources. The incoming information is analyzed internally so that appropriate alterations may be made by the learners. In contrast to feedback, knowledge of results is performance data furnished by an external source. Generally, the speech-language teacher or clinician will evaluate individual responses and provide the learner with information that presumably is useful for future practice. Knowledge of results can be qualitative in nature; for example, a response could be judged either correct or incorrect. Conversely, the experimenter might employ some form of quantitative information which would furnish an accurate index to degree of error. For example, a learner might execute a movement task for the purpose of achieving some specific target. Practice attempts which are not successful in reaching the target could be measured and the off target distances relayed to the learner for future consideration.

Knowledge of results has been systematically studied and a number of generalizations have emerged. Foremost is the fact that knowledge of results is a primary component in facilitating accurate skilled performance, (Newell & Kennedy, 1978). Moreover, the frequency of knowledge of results is directly related to the learning of a motor skill (Bilodeau, 1969). That is, the more frequent the knowledge of results, the better the opportunity for learning to occur. Another generalization is the consistent finding that delays in the dispensation of knowledge of results do not impede, but may aid, in learning (Adams, 1971). Although this might seem to be somewhat in conflict with operant learning principles which emphasize the immediacy of reinforcement following a response (e.g., Costello, 1977), the former statement holds true only when the delay period does not exceed the time between the response that received knowledge of results and the succeeding reponse. It should also be emphasized that delays are in the range of seconds, and there are no intervening activities within the delay period. Presumably, the delay period is an interval wherein response information is stored and later compared with the knowledge of results information that follows. When the learner has firmly established the motor skill, knowledge of results may be withdrawn without adversely affecting performance. According to Schmidt (1975a) feedback takes over when knowledge of results is no longer necessary, and occasional performance problems are identified by an error-detecting mechanism which the learner has constructed internally.

Although the concepts of knowledge of results and feedback have not garnered much attention in articulatory training, the idea of response information or reinforcement has usually been a part of speech treatment discussions (Bernthal & Bankson, 1981; McReynolds, 1970; Van Riper, 1963). The misarticulating client produces a treatment item, then receives information concerning adequacy of the production. Application of the motor skill concepts to articulatory training would be somewhat similar to current practices (Costello, 1977; Gerber, 1977); however, there would be certain procedural differences. The similarity between current practices and the concept of knowledge of results is that the observer evaluates a response and furnishes information to the learner. The proposed differences involve use of delays in providing knowledge of results and frequency of dispensation of knowledge of results. In the typical articulatory treatment, knowledge of results delays in the range of 3 to 15 seconds would be suggested. Delays in excess of the suggested time period have not proven to be effective (Irwin, Nickles, & Hulit, 1973) and such excessive delays would greatly limit opportunities for practice within sessions. In addition, knowledge of results should be given continously, since establishment of a motor skill is dependent on such initial information to the learner. Once acquisition has been accomplished, knowledge of results might be completely eliminated instead of shifting to some intermittent schedule, as utilized in other learning conceptualizations (Sloane & MacAulay, 1968). It should be noted that the above statements require empirical validation since they have not been studied with articulatory-disordered children.

One of the primary goals of any teaching strategy is that the learner eventually spontaneously uses the taught behaviors in novel encounters. If this did not occur, the speech clinician would be faced with the insurmountable task of teaching a target sound in a seemingly endless number of phonetic contexts and environmental situations. In both motor skills (Carson & Wiegand, 1979) and articulatory research (Elbert, Shelton, & Arndt, 1967), tasks that provide indices to novel usage have been administered before treatment, during treatment, and following the conclusion of treatment. Motor skills investigators obtain information on the adaptability of persons with a motor skill (Johnson, 1972), while proponents of learning theory collect information concerning generalization (Costello & Bosler, 1976). In other descriptions, the term carry-over is employed when discussing this phenomenon (Mowrer, 1971). Shelton, Elbert, and Arndt (1967) advocated the inclusion of adaptability measures, since the measures appear sensitive to changes obtained through training. Diedrich and Bangert (1980) stated that periodic use of adaptability measures supplant the traditional procedures of simply administering an articulation test prior to and following treatment.

In this chapter's earlier reviews of some of the other training implications, concepts from skill learning and other disciplines were presented relative to their similarities and differences; however, such a discussion approach appears unnecessary here. Adaptability and generalization are constructs considered relatively homogeneous by the writer.[3] The classic work of Shelton and his associates (Elbert, Shelton, & Arndt, 1967; Shelton, Elbert, & Arndt, 1967; Wright, Shelton, & Arndt, 1969) has had a great influence in articulatory research and training with their development of SPTs and TTs. Their treatment procedures were carried out under the guise of motor learning theory, and the measures were used to evaluate treatment effects.

If clinicians do not wish to use the standard measures that have been recommended, they can create their own adaptability tasks. However, this writer suggests that the self-made measures reflect Shelton's format. That is, adaptability assessment should incorporate provision for a contrived task and a spontaneous task. The contrived task should contain items that span the usual acquisition regimen and include the target sound in isolation, syllables, words, and phrases. Items used for training purposes should not be presented in the contrived task. The spontaneous task should entail some form of conversational usage by the client and the more natural, the better. Recall that Bankson and Byrne (1972) evaluated spontaneous utilization of target sounds in their clients' homes, in the clinic, and in the presence of an observer unfamiliar to the clients. The clinician should also be sure that an adequate number of tokens have been collected for each task. Bernthal and Bankson (1981) present an excellent account of methods which may be utilized in tabulating adaptability data. In addition, they present very detailed procedures concerning ways in which the clinician may document changes in articulatory behavior.

The sampling format presented above is suggested for two specific reasons: (1) the method is clinically feasible for practicing clinicians; and (2) the tasks provide an estimate of adaptability along the acquisition-automatization continuum. The typical response pattern that has emerged from the employ of SPTs (contrived task) and TTs (spontaneous task) is one that this author refers to as a shadow effect. Generally, the SPTs show an earlier and more rapid departure from pretraining levels than the TTs. The superiority of the SPTs is maintained with the TTs continuing to shadow the short utterance, imitative measurements. Treatment sutdies incorporating these measures (Johnson et al., 1979; Ruscello, 1977) have usually been shorter in duration than actual training intervention and as a consequence have not furnished precise guidelines regarding the measures and terminal performance. However, Diedrich and Bangert (1980) carried out a long-term investigation of /r/ and /s/ misarticulating children who received training from public school speech clinicians. SPTs and TTs were given to the children throughout training and Diedrich and Bangert's recommendations are as follows:

> We believe that children who achieve 75% correct or better on the target phonemes /r/ or /s/ in conversation for two successive probes (one week apart) should be dismissed from therapy. A follow-up probe should be made at four weeks. If the child is still above 75%, but not at 95%, continue with eight-week interval probes. Stop follow-up probes when child is at 95% or better. Reinstate child in therapy if follow-up probes fall below 75% correct. (p. 233).

The masking technique reported by Manning and his group (Manning et al., 1976, 1977) is a somewhat different form of adaptability testing that appears to differentiate between those who have or have not achieved automatic use of their target sounds. The technique does have appeal and could probably be implemented without much difficulty by school speech-language pathologists. It might be particularly helpful in deciding which clients should receive supplementary articulation instruction in the summer months when school is not in session.

The position of this chapter has been that the teaching of articulatory movements could be likened to the teaching of other motor skills. Therefore, theoretical constructs from the discipline of motor learning served as a framework for organizing treatment research and making predictions concerning treatment outcomes. The studies reviewed suggest positive changes have occurred in the production capabilities of experimental subjects when their instruction has been derived from these motor learning constructs, thus adding credence to motor learning theory. We are, however, far from validating a particular motor learning theory; and for that matter, so is the field of motor learning. The constructs applied herein to treatment are more similar to, than different from, constructs from other theoretical proposals because each is directed to one specific end: learning correct articulations. Future studies must explore treatment variables that may result in more efficient teaching strategies. Efficiency in this context is reduced practice time with increased adaptability.

End Notes

[1] Speech-language pathologists have, in certain instances, formulated treatments which focus on one of the other purposes of therapeutic exercise. Interested readers are referred to a paper by Ruscello (1982) for a more detailed discussion.

[2] The physiologic slant is similar to the position of McDonald (1964b), who discussed the overlapping, ballistic movements of the speech articulators.

[3] Generalization in articulatory research has been examined in numerous ways (Costello & Bosler, 1976); however, studies undertaken within a motor learning framework have not explored novel target use in such depth. Consistent with the current discussion, the analogy between adaptability and generalization is limited to that level which Costello and Bosler refer to as intratherapy generalization.

Reference Note

1. Ruscello, D.M. The use of a mental practice feature during the initial stages of phone learning. Unpublished doctoral dissertation, University of Arizona, 1977.

References

Adams, J.A. A closed-loop theory of motor learning. *Journal of Motor Behavior,* 1971, *3,* 111-145.

Bankson. N.W., & Byrne, M.C. The effect of a timed correct sound production task on carryover. *Journal of Speech and Hearing Research,* 1972, *15,* 160-168.

Bernstein, N. *The coordination and regulation of movement.* Englewood Cliffs, N.J.: Prentice-Hall, 1967.

Bernthal, J.E., & Bankson, N.W. *Articulation disorders.* Englewood Cliffs, N.J.: Prentice-Hall, 1981.

Bilodeau, I. McD. Information feedback. In E.A. Bilodeau (Ed.), *Principles of skill acquisition.* New York: Academic Press, 1969.

Carson, L.M., & Wiegand, R.L. Motor schema formation and retention in young children: A test of Schmidt's Schema Theory. *Journal of Motor Behavior,* 1979, *11,* 247-251.

Catalano, J.F. The effect of rest following massed practice of continuous and discrete motor tasks. *Journal of Motor Behavior,* 1978, *10,* 63-67.

Chisum, L. Shelton, R.L., Arndt, W.B., & Elbert, M. The relationship between remedial speech instruction activities and articulation change. *Cleft Palate Journal,* 1969, *6,* 57-64.

Costello, J.M. Programmed instruction. *Journal of Speech and Hearing Disorders,* 1977, *42,* 3-28.

Costello, J., & Bosler, C. Generalization and articulation instruction. *Journal of Speech and Hearing Disorders,* 1976, *41,* 359-373.

Costello, J., & Onstine, J. The modification of multiple articulation errors based on distinctive feature theory. *Journal of Speech and Hearing Disorders,* 1976, *41,* 199-215.

Cross, K.D. Role of practice in perceptual-motor learning. *American Journal of Physical Medicine,* 1967, *46,* 487-510.

Curtis, J.F. Segmenting the stream of speech. In J. Griffith and J.E. Miner (Eds.), *The first Lincolnland conference on dialectology.* Tuscaloosa: University of Alabama Press, 1970.

Daniloff, R.G., & Hammarberg, R.E. On defining coarticulation. *Journal of Phonetics,* 1973, *1,* 239-248.

Diedrich, W.M. Procedures for counting and charting a target phoneme. *Language, Speech, and Hearing Services in Schools,* 1971, 18-32.

Diedrich, W.M., & Bangert, J. *Articulation learning.* Houston, Texas: College-Hill, 1980.

Dunham, P. Distribution of practice as a factor affecting learning and/or performance. *Journal of Motor Behavior,* 1976, *8,* 305-307.

Elbert, M., Shelton, R.L., & Arndt, W.B. A task for evaluation of articulation change: I. Development of methodology. *Journal of Speech and Hearing Research,* 1967, *10,* 281-288.

Ellis, H.C. *Fundamentals of human learning and cognition.* Dubuque, Ia.: W.M.C. Brown, 1972.

Fitts, P. Factors in complex skill training. In R. Glaser (Ed.), *Training research and education.* New York: Wiley, 1962.

Gallagher, J.D., & Thomas, J.R. Effects of varying post-KR intervals upon childrens' motor performance. *Journal of Motor Behavior,* 1980, *12,* 41-46.

Gentile, A.M. A working model of skill acquisition with application to teaching. *Quest,* 1972, *17,* 3-23.

Gerber, A. Programming for articulation modification. *Journal of Speech and Hearing Disorders,* 1977, *42,* 29-43.

Godfrey, B.B., & Kephart, N.C. *Movement patterns and motor education.* New York: Appleton-Century-Crofts, 1969.

Irion, A.L. Historical introduction. In E.A. Bilodeau (Ed.), *Principles of skill acquisition.* New York: Academic Press, 1969.

Irwin, R.B., Nickles, A., & Hulit, L.M. Effects of varying latencies in the stimulus-response paradigm of speech therapy. *Perceptual and Motor Skills,* 1973, *37,* 707-713.

Johnson, A.F., Shelton, R.L., Ruscello, D.M., & Arndt, W.B. A comparison of two articulation treatments: Acquisition and acquisition-automatization. *Human Communication,* 1979, *4,* 337-348.

Johnson, H.W. Skill = speed x accuracy x form x adaptability. In R.N. Singer (Ed.), *Readings in motor learning.* Philadelphia: Lea & Febiger, 1972.

Jones, M.B. Differential processes in acquisition. In E.A. Bilodau, (Ed.), *Principles of skill acquisition.* New York: Academic Press, 1969.

Kelso, J.A.S., & Norman, P.E. Motor schema formation in children. *Developmental Psychology,* 1978, *14,* 153-156.

Kent, R.D., & Lybolt, J.T. Techniques of therapy based on motor learning theory. In W.H. Perkins (Ed.), *Current therapy of communication disorders: General principles of therapy.* New York: Thieme-Stratton, 1982.

Manning, W.H., Keappock, N.E., & Stick, S.L. The use of auditory masking to estimate automatization of correct articulatory production. *Journal of Speech and Hearing Disorders,* 1976, *41,* 143-149.

Manning, W.H., Wittstruck, M.L., Loyd, R.R., & Campbell, T.F. Automatization of correct production at two levels of articulatory acquisition. *Journal of Speech and Hearing Disorders,* 1977, *42,* 358-363.

Marteniuk, R.G., *Information processing in motor skills.* New York: Holt, 1976.

McDonald, E.T. *A Deep Test of Articulation.* Pittsburgh: Stanwix House Publications, 1964. (a)

McDonald, E.T. *Articulation testing and treatment: A sensory-motor approach.* Pittsburgh: Stanwix House, 1964. (b)

McReynolds, L.V. Contingencies and consequences in speech therapy. *Journal of Speech and Hearing Disorders,* 1970, *35,* 12-24.

Mower, D.E. Transfer of training in articulation therapy. *Journal of Speech and Hearing Disorders,* 1971, *36,* 427-446.

Netsell, R. Speech motor control: Theoretical issues with clinical impact. In W. Berry (Ed.), *Clinical dysarthria.* San Diego: College-Hill, 1982.

Newell, K.M., & Kennedy, J.A. Knowledge of results and children's motor learning. *Developmental Psychology,* 1978, *14,* 531-536.

Palliard, J. The patterning of skilled movements. In J. Field (Ed.), *Handbook of physiology (Vol. III, Section I) Neurophysiology.* Baltimore: Waverly, 1960.

Poulton, E.C. On prediction in skilled movements. *Psychological Bulletin,* 1957, *54,* 467-473.

Poulton, E.C. Skilled performance. In R.N. Singer (Ed.), *The psychomotor domain: Movement behavior.* Philadelphia: Lea & Febiger, 1972.

Ruscello, D.M. The importance of word position in articulation therapy. *Language, Speech, and Hearing Services in Schools,* 1975, *6,* 190-196.

Ruscello, D.M. A selected review of palatal training procedures. *Cleft Palate Journal,* 1982, *3,* 181-193.

Ruscello, D.M. & Shelton, R.L. Planning and self-assessment in articulatory training. *Journal of Speech and Hearing Disorders,* 1979, *44, 504-512.*

Schmidt, R.A. *Motor Skills.* New York: Harper & Row, 1975. (a)

Schmidt, R.A. A schema theory of discrete motor skill learning. *Psychological Review,* 1975, *82,* 225-260. (b)

Schultz, M.C. The bases of speech pathology and audiology: What are appropriate models. *Journal of Speech and Hearing Disorders,* 1972, *37,* 118-122.

Shelton, R.L. Therapeutic exercise and speech pathology. *Asha.* 1963, *5,* 855-859.

Shelton, R.L., Elbert, M., & Arndt, W.B. A task for evaluation of articulation change: II. Comparison of task scores during baseline and lesson series testing. *Journal of Speech and Hearing Research,*1967, *10,* 578-586.

Shelton, R.L., Hahn, E., & Morris, H. Diagnosis and therapy. In D.C. Spriestersbach & D. Sherman (Eds.), *Cleft palate and communication.* New York: Academic Press, 1968.

Shelton, R.L., Johnson, A.F., & Arndt, W.B. Monitoring and reinforcement by parents as a means of automating articulatory responses. *Perceptual and Motor Skills,* 1972, *35,* 759-767.

Shelton, R.L., Johnson, A.F., Willis, V., & Arndt, W.B. Monitoring and reinforcement by parents as a means of automating articulatory responses: II. Study of preschool children. *Perceptual and Motor Skills,* 1975, *40,* 599-610.

Shelton, R.L., & McReynolds, L.V. Functional articulation disorders: Preliminaries to treatment. In N.J. Lass (Ed.), *Speech and language: Advances in basic research and practice* (Vol. II). New York: Academic Press, 1979.

Shelton, R.L., Morris, H., & McWilliams, B.J. Nonsurgical management of cleft palate speech problems. In Report from the Committee. *Speech, language, and psychosocial aspects of cleft lip and cleft palate: The state of the art:* ASHA Reports number 9. Washington, D.C.: American Speech and Hearing Association, 1973.

Sloane, H.N. & MacAulay, B.D. Teaching and environmental control of verbal behavior. In H.N. Sloane & B.D. MacAulay (Eds.), *Operant procedures in remedial speech and language training.* New York: Houghton Mifflin, 1968.

Van Riper, C. *Speech correction: Principles and methods* (4th ed.). Englewood Cliffs, N.J.: Prentice-Hall, 1963.

Weston, A.J., & Leonard, L.B. *Articulation disorders: Methods of evaluation and therapy.* Lincoln, Neb.: Cliff Notes, 1976.

Wright, V., Shelton, R.L., & Arndt, W.B. A task for evaluation of articulation change: III. Imitative task scores compared with scores for more spontaneous tasks. *Journal of Speech and Hearing Research,* 1969, *12,* 875-884.

Mata B. Jaffe

Neurological Impairment of Speech Production: Assessment and Treatment

Introduction

Among the neurogenic disorders of communication in children are motor speech disorders: dysarthria and developmental apraxia of speech. Unfortunately, the situation is more complex than that simple statement. These two disorders may coexist and may also accompany a language disorder. Furthermore, some clinicians and researchers feel that there is insufficient evidence to justify the diagnosis of apraxia of speech of a developmental nature. The concept of developmental apraxia of speech is surrounded by controversy, and this chapter will address that controversy.

According to Nicolosi, Harryman, and Kresheck (1978), the term "dysarthria" refers to a collection of motor speech disorders. The impairment originates in the central or peripheral nervous system. Respiration, phonation, resonance, prosody, articulation, chewing and swallowing, and movements of the jaw and tongue may all be affected. The diagnosis of dysarthria excludes apraxia, functional articulation disorders and central language disorders.

Apraxia of speech is defined by Nicolosi et al. (1978) as a nonlinguistic sensorimotor articulation disorder. It is characterized by impairment of the ability to program the positions of the musculature used for speaking and to sequence the movements for producing phonemes. "Dyspraxia" is the term sometimes used to label a less severe form of apraxia. In developmental apraxia of speech (DAS), a congenital condition is assumed. However, as intimated above, even the definition of DAS is somewhat controversial.

These are the two motor speech disorders in children that we will examine: dysarthria and developmental apraxia of speech.

Dysarthria

In the past 10 to 15 years, the role of the speech-language pathologist has changed substantially in relation to neurologically impaired infants and children. These clinicians are working with younger and more severely involved children in an expanded capacity. Some even work with infants in neonatal intensive care units. This shift is due to changes in legislation, earlier identification of neurologically compromised infants or infants at risk for neurologic impairment, evidence from normal infant research concerning the neonate's capacity to learn, and recognition of the efficacy of early identification and intervention with neurologically impaired children and their families.

The Handicapped Children's Early Education Act of 1968 led to establishment of early intervention programs for cerebral palsied and developmentally disabled infants. Some infant stimulation programs use a transdisciplinary approach whereby each team member must have the basic skills needed for total therapeutic interaction with the child and parents. In addition to responsibilities for the development of speech and language, then, the therapist must help the mother in all types of activities that include proper feeding, handling, positioning, and facilitation of gross and fine motor skills. In such settings, the trend has been for therapists to work with very young children (beginning as young as a few months of age) and to demonstrate a wider range of skills than has been the tradition in our field.

Another important legislative act was the Education of All Handicapped Children's Act, PL 94-142, which mandated special education programming for students to 21 years of age regardless of the severity of their handicap. Passage of this law in 1975 made speech and language therapy available to individuals who previously were considered too involved, mentally and/or physically, to benefit from such services. Many of these youngsters were nonverbal, with poor potential for developing serviceable speech. Their needs were part of the incentive for recent advances in nonvocal communication systems and aids and in evaluation and treatment procedures for the feeding and prespeech behaviors which occur during the developmental period that precedes the first word. It is this author's observation and conviction that the clinician who works with younger and/or more severely handicapped children requires knowledge and skills in assessment and treatment in the area of prespeech and feeding.

However, many colleagues, especially university instructors, remain unconvinced that it is the speech-language pathologist's role to feed children or do other nonlanguage-oriented activities. Thus, universities seldom include specific training of this kind in their programs. Their graduates, ill prepared in the areas of prespeech, feeding, and early oral motor development, take jobs in rehabilitation centers, hospitals, and infant-toddler programs where they are expected to have expertise in all that pertains to the oral area.

Augmenting university training programs are training courses in Neuro-Developmental Treatment. This training is particularly useful for clinicians who treat neurologically impaired infants and young children. Such courses are offered in this country and around the world. Guided by the work of Berta Bobath (1967, 1971a, 1971b), Karel Bobath, (1966, 1971), and both together (Bobath & Bobath, 1972), instructors in neuro-developmental treatment (NDT) teach sophisticated assessment and therapy procedures through articles, books, courses, workshops, and conference presentations. Long waiting lists for the basic 8 week NDT course offered to physical, occupational, and speech-language therapists affirm the need for this kind of continuing education. The relatively few speech-language pathologists with NDT training regularly receive letters from programs across the country soliciting their application for jobs that specify an NDT background.

One reason that university programs do not address feeding and oral motor development, assessment, and treatment in more detail is perhaps that the relationship between these early oral motor behaviors and subsequent speech and language development has not been established empirically.

Research in the area of prespeech and feeding with neurologically impaired children is difficult, but not impossible. Morris (1982a) has conducted 2 pilot studies of early feeding and vocal development. The first utilized a screening questionnaire that a paraprofessional or a professional could administer to parents of high risk infants. Questionnaires on 30 infants who failed a prespeech screening and had an abnormal diagnosis at 12 and 24 months were compared with approximately 460 infants with a normal diagnosis at 12 and 24 months. The study attempted to find a cluster of clearly defined problems or prognosticators that would identify children with handicapping conditions associated with a high incidence of speech production problems. There were difficulties inherent in the data collection and analysis. Different diagnostic tools and different criteria for normalcy were used, and there was no consistent follow-up evaluation by a speech-language pathologist. However, the results of this pilot study showed that no single prespeech item or discrete cluster of items clearly separated normal children and children with developmental disabilities.

In a retrospective study, Morris (1982a) sent another set of questionnaires to therapists and parents of infants from 4 to 24 months of age who were in active programs of prespeech and feeding therapy. Diagnostic labels of the 150 infants included cerebral palsy, developmental delay, mental retardation, and chromosomal abnormalities. Preliminary data are currently available on the prenatal history, the children's early feeding history, and the parents' concerns and attempts at finding help. One conclusion was that parents typically identified a feeding problem and looked to the medical community for help, but intervention was regularly postponed. It seemed that pediatricians did not know how to help the parent and infant, probably due to lack of information and lack of standardized tests for identifying infants who should be referred for further evaluation. Parents' reports of feeding problems in their infants were in agreement at least 80% of the time with therapists' descriptions. Recently, a new *Pre-Speech Screening Questionnaire* has been developed to provide a tightly structured study in 2 high-risk-infant follow-up programs. This questionnaire will be available for distribution when field testing with groups of children without unusual birth histories and groups of children at risk has been completed.

Morris (1982a) also conducted a longitudinal study. She observed and filmed the feeding of 6 normally developing infants between birth and 36 months. The infants were studied monthly during the first year, quarterly during the second year, and, finally, at 3 years of age. Morris describes the components of oral movement and their significance in later development of feeding and speech movements, and the parallel relationships between movements and processes described as necessary for both speech production and feeding skills. Major components in the development of both early speech production and feeding skills are the increase in the number and variety of oral movements and positions, differentiation of movements, and more complex coordination ability. Morris suggests that a factor such as gross and/or fine motor development may be involved in the motor skills for both speech and feeding, and thus be responsible for the parallel development of both functions.

Love, Hagerman, and Taimi (1980) examined the relationship between nonspeech oral motor behaviors (biting, sucking, swallowing, and chewing, and 9 infantile oral reflexes) and speech performance in 60 children and young adults with cerebral palsy. They reported a trend, although not completely systematic, for subjects with adequate feeding skills to have better speech. Results generally supported the value of treatment to improve feeding in cerebral palsy, if only to make eating easier and faster and to stimulate gross movement of the oral musculature.

Years ago, in the orientation of Harold Westlake (1951) and Martin Palmer (1947), programs began in which feeding was used as a means of improving oral motor functioning for speech. Then, our profession rejected the concept of the interrelationship of oral movements for speech and for eating. However, clinicians today have been using the feeding process as part of their treatment programs with the working hypothesis that it may improve sensorimotor patterns for better speech and communicative interactions, as well as the child's feeding skills. If we are to meet the challenge of assessing and treating neurologically impaired infants and very young children, we must gather research data to verify the activities that we hypothesize as being clinically appropriate. Morris (1982a) suggests that the group of children with severe gastrointestinal problems, but intact nervous systems, who have not been fed by mouth may offer the opportunity to explore the interrelationship issues.

The following sections will discuss assessment and treatment. The most recent advances in the area of dysarthria in children are in prespeech behaviors.

Assessment

Representing a significant contribution for evaluating speech disorders in neurologically impaired children is the Pre-Speech Assessment Scale (PSAS), a rating scale for the measurement of prespeech behaviors from birth through 2 years (Morris, 1982b). Standardized tools to measure articulation and other speech and language parameters of the older, verbal child have been available, but none were capable of evaluating the prespeech development of the child with sensorimotor impairment. The PSAS can be used with a wide variety of children with delayed or disordered development, including children with cerebral palsy, apraxia of speech, mental retardation, sensory-integrative dysfunction, and other developmental disabilities. Any child functioning below the 2-year level in prespeech development can be appropriately tested.

The PSAS systematically examines feeding, respiration-phonation, and sound play—sensorimotor skills considered to be important for the later development of the more complex act of speech production. The clinician is encouraged to make extensive clinical observations of overall postural tone and movement, head and trunk control, response to sensory stimulation, and response to specific treatment techniques.

Both gross motor and prespeech behaviors of the neurologically impaired child can be divided into abnormal movement patterns, primitive movement patterns, and higher developmental movement patterns. The PSAS provides a way of simultaneously observing and scoring behaviors within the normal developmental ranges of 1 to 24 months on an equal interval scale, and pathological or abnormal behaviors on an ordinal scale. A double-scaling system takes into account the normal/abnormal contrast for prespeech development by measuring the child's performance in each area against specific behavioral descriptions in a section on normal development and a section on abnormal development. The PSAS attempts to place the child's behavior in a specific performance area according to a developmental age range while acknowledging that performance may still be somewhat different qualitatively from that of a normal infant at that age.

The scores are transferred to a graph which allows the therapist to compare the child's levels and problems within each area, to compare developmental abilities across categories, to assign or revise treatment goals and priorities, and to note progress or lack of progress from one evaluation period to the next.

Scoring protocols for the PSAS were based on the above-referenced longitudinal study of 6 normal infants who were filmed from birth to 36 months, and on the scored profiles of approximately 800 developmentally disabled children. Over 200 therapists who have undergone training in the use of the PSAS have provided extensive clinical input into its development and into its content, format, and organization. Studies of interexaminer reliability for behavioral observations and for scoring have indicated that therapists trained in a 4-day workshop can use the PSAS with a clinically acceptable level of reliability.

In addition to its use as an evaluation tool, the PSAS can be recommended because it provides probably the most definitive and complete information on normal sequential development and abnormal deviations of the precursors of speech available in one volume.

Another recent assessment tool was developed by Mysak (1980), who has long been interested in cerebral palsy and dysarthria. Central to Mysak's approach is the concept of neuroevolution of speech viewed as "the progressive integration and elaboration of lower sensorimotor integration centers by higher ones until the ultimate integration of integration centers results in bipedal standing, walking, and talking behavior" (Mysak, 1980, p. 19). He traces this evolution phylogenetically and ontogenetically. Mysak's (1980) *Neurophysiological Speech Index* (NSI) is a clinical tool for evaluating the development of a child relative to a "neurophysiological speaking age". It includes behaviors that children normally achieve by 18 to 24+ months of age. The NSI has ratings based on expected reflexes in infants and ratings based on the presence of persisting infantile reflexes in older infants and children. It is a composite of the Basic Movements

Index and the Skilled Movements Index. The author suggests using the *Neurophysiological Speech Index* primarily as a guide for planning therapy and judging progress and, secondarily, as an index of the child's neurophysiological speech age.

In this author's opinion, Mysak's recent work continues to be difficult reading, hampered by use of idiosyncratic terminology such as "face talk." Furthermore, the NSI lacks standardization, validity, and reliability information. Developmental milestones are based on normative data which are not referenced. Speech-language pathologists would probably find the *Neurophysiological Speech Index* difficult to use.

Treatment

Treatment of dysarthria in children is not researched in the most recent literature. However, corresponding to the interest in prespeech and feeding assessment and the development of assessment tools is an interest in early intervention and in the principles and strategies for treating prespeech and feeding problems of the young and/or severely neurologically impaired child. Much of the current sensorimotor programming for neurologically impaired children is based on the writings of Mueller (1972, 1975) and based on the NDT approach. A review of recent writings on treatment, emphasizing feeding, follows.

Perske, Clifton, McLean, and Stein (1977) have collected contributions by "knowledgeable persons" about their programs and handicapped persons at mealtimes. While this is not a how-to-do-it handbook, it does attempt to increase the sensitivities and skills of those who feed seriously handicapped persons. The editors point to a movement toward making mealtimes as important for handicapped persons as for the rest of us. Contrasting in style, Gallender (1979) presents the anatomic and physiologic aspects of eating handicaps and relates and illustrates specific techniques and instructional materials on particular eating handicaps.

Campbell (1982) developed a problem-oriented approach to make the therapist, teacher, or parent "the expert" in identifying problems and creating solutions to help the child with feeding difficulties acquire basic feeding skills. The material is divided into 3 major parts. The first section introduces approaches to feeding problems and general methods for handling specific concerns. Five major feeding problems are presented in the second section in a flow chart format so the reader can identify the child's specific difficulties, develop appropriate goals, select possible solutions, and evaluate their effectiveness. The last section includes some common techniques for the management of the feeding problems identified.

Morris (1977) developed a manual primarily for use with young children with mild to severe degrees of neurologic impairment with or without mental retardation. It is designed to instruct teachers, therapists, and parents how to help children develop better control for eating. Program guidelines, many illustrated with photographs, are suggested according to the probable causes of the child's feeding difficulties. Morris points out that often the solution to the problem of feeding depends on physically handling and positioning the cerebral palsied child to decrease spasticity or involuntary movements of the total body as well as the mouth, face, and throat. She also emphasizes the critical importance of involving the parents or parent substitutes as active participants in the treatment program. They must understand the goals, underlying rationales, and the steps in the program, and learn the specific procedures. Further, the therapist must understand the family situation and routine and the difficulty parents and child may have in changing their ways of feeding.

Davis (1978) describes prespeech development in normal and atypical children. Early intervention is advocated with the major goal of establishing muscle tone and neuromuscular patterns–which are as normal as possible–in respiration and feeding, as a foundation for achieving more normal speech development. Davis describes intervention and specific activities.

Unfortunately, there are many excellent clinicians, especially those trained in neuro-developmental treatment, who have the most to offer in the area of prespeech treatment and who present workshops and courses of exceptional quality, but who have not published their work. Morris (1982a), however, has written about prespeech and speech therapy with neurologically impaired children, emphasizing early intervention and a physiologic and neurologic orientation toward treatment. Morris considers the following as important concepts:

1. Abnormal postural tone and movement patterns interfere with speech (and feeding) patterns. Abnormal tone reduces the options for normal movement and normal sensory feedback.
2. Hypersensitivity and hyposensitivity to sensory stimulation can reduce the opportunities for learning.
3. Motor learning is predominantly motor-sensory-motor learning. There is a need to prevent the establishment of abnormal patterns and to provide a spontaneous option for the child to feel and sense a different, more normal way of moving.
4. Early automatic patterns of oral movement provide a model for similar movements to be incorporated later into speech production.
5. Treatment is an ongoing process and way of life to be incorporated throughout the day.

With these assumptions, Morris offers the following basic goals for a communication skills program for children with neurologic deficits:
1. normalization of the child's postural tone through inhibition of abnormal and strong postural reflexes;
2. simultaneous stimulation and facilitation of normal postural reactions and automatic responses;
3. feedback to the child's system of correct tone and performance; and
4. constant awareness of the communication dynamics between the child and others in the environment.

In the assessment section of this chapter Mysak's assessment procedure, the *Neurophysiological Speech Index,* was discussed. Mysak (1980) chooses the term "neurospeech therapy" to designate his treatment approach to emphasize the overall neurologic focus in speech therapy with the cerebral palsied child. His theory is based on "the progressive and successive integration of lower sensorimotor integration centers by higher centers and, finally, the integration of the right hemisphere by the left hemisphere" (p.184). He, too, advocates beginning therapy with children below 1 year of age, during the prespeech period, because the plasticity of the infant brain could prevent fixation of abnormal movement patterns, deformities, and contractures.

Mysak considers the stimulation of basic listening movements, speech postures, hand movements, and basic speech movements to be fundamental to neurospeech therapy. He describes preparatory physical maneuvers to enrich sensorimotor experiences, to induce relaxation, to normalize tone, posture, and movement, and to facilitate integration and elaboration of reflexes. His suggestions for normalizing facial and oral area sensitivity and facilitation of drinking and eating movements are similar to those suggested by aforementioned authors (Campbell (1982); Davis (1978); Gallender (1979); Morris (1977, 1982a); Mueller (1972, 1975).)

Mysak facilitates speech postures through various postures of the body, head, and parts of the oral mechanism, and through isolation of body parts and movements. He combines these with appropriately timed speech sound stimulation. He suggests neuro-facilitation techniques, such as resisted movement manuevers or reversed movement maneuvers, to counteract limitations in direction and range of articulatory movement. To increase sensory awareness, he recommends exercises such as increased pressure for bilabial sounds, longer contacts for stop and continuant sounds, and elongated vowel sounds. Symbolic facial and hand gestural communications are viewed as facilitators of speech and enhancers of communication.

Treatment programs for young children with dysarthria can successfully include simultaneous goals and treatment to improve prespeech, feeding, phonation-respiration, and language functions. Successful treatment of the child with central nervous system dysfunction requires an integrated approach. The therapy will be effective if the therapist does not rely on specific techniques but observes thoughtfully, reevaluates continually, and modifies treatment according to the responses of the child.

In summary, our profession is faced with the reality of assessing and treating younger and more severely involved children with neurologic impairment. The recent trend, clinically if not academically, is to approach this challenge by working in transdisciplinary and interdisciplinary teams toward common goals for the child and family. Such an integrated approach generally includes the area of prespeech and feeding as well as the more traditional speech-language assessment and therapy for dysarthria. To be effective, the therapist needs to understand and treat the child's entire system, not just the mechanisms directly involved in speech. There are many unanswered questions about the efficacy of this kind of treatment. Though difficult, research in this area is sorely needed.

Developmental Apraxia of Speech

Known by a variety of labels such as "developmental motor aphasia", "articulatory apraxia or dyspraxia", and "childhood verbal apraxia", a motor programming disorder in children was first described by Hadden in 1891. Currently the most common term is developmental apraxia of speech (DAS). This speech disorder is characterized by impaired ability to program, combine, and sequence the elements of speech. It is considered to be a neurologic, sensorimotor speech disorder and is differentiated from dysarthria and functional articulation disorders in children (Nicolosi et al., 1978). The apraxic child demonstrates impairment, in varying degrees, in the ability to position the articulators consistently to produce speech and sound combinations.

There is confusion in the literature as to the behaviors that are important for the diagnosis of DAS. Thus, the practicing clinician often does not feel confident in labeling a given child's speech pattern as developmental apraxia of speech. Table 6-1 illustrates the wide range of characteristics that have been suggested to be part of DAS. Some of the problem is due to assumptions based on the adult literature on verbal apraxia, even though the differences between children and adults are great enough that perhaps the terminology should not be the same. Rosenbek (Note 1) pointed out differences in apraxia of speech between adults and children and suggested reasons for these differences.

Apraxia is defined by a symptom cluster—another source of confusion. Not *all* symptoms must be present; no *one* characteristic or symptom *must*

TABLE 6-1
Reported characteristics of developmental apraxia of speech

CHARACTERISTICS	AUTHORS
Early History	
History of feeding problems; noninformative crying; little distinguishable vocal play, babbling, imitation, or self-imitation during infancy	Aram & Glasson, Note 2 Eisenson, 1966
Family History	
Strong family history of speech, language, and learning disorders	Aram & Glasson, Note 2 Morley, 1972 Saleeby, Hadjian, Martinkosky, & Swift, Note 3
Neurological Findings	
High incidence of "soft" neurological findings; generalized dyspraxia	Crary, Note 4 Eisenson, 1966 McClumpha & Logue, Note 5 Yoss & Darley, 1974a
Nonspeech Findings	
Deficits in oral perception	Loevner, Note 6 Prichard, Tekieli, & Kozup, 1979
Oral nonverbal apraxia co-occuring	Aram & Glasson, Note 2 Chappell, 1973 Eisenson, 1966 Rosenbek & Wertz, 1972 Yoss & Darley, 1974a
Poor self monitoring	Edwards, 1973 Fawcus, 1971 Morley, 1972 Morley & Fox, 1969 Yoss & Darley, 1974a
Gross motor incoordination	Aram & Glasson, Note 2
Speech	
Markedly reduced repertoire of phonemes	Aram & Glasson, Note 2 Chappell, 1973 Edwards, 1973 Fawcus, 1971 Morley, 1972
Extraordinarily poor imitative skills for articulation	Chappell, 1973 McClumpha & Logue, Note 5 Rosenbek, Hansen, Baughman, & Lemme, 1974

TABLE 6-1 (cont.)
Reported characteristics of developmental apraxia of speech

CHARACTERISTICS	AUTHORS
Speech (cont.)	
Significant problems in phonetic synthesis for speech	McClumpha & Logue, Note 5
Highly inconsistent errors	Nicolosi et al., 1978
	Rosenbek & Wertz, 1972
Misarticulations that are grossly inconsistent at the imitative level and generally consistent (primarily simplifications) in spontaneous speech	McClumpha & Logue, Note 5
	Rosenbek, Note 1
Delayed and deviant speech development	Aram & Glasson, Note 2
	Rosenbek & Wertz, 1972
Prominent phonemic errors: omissions (errors are more often omissions than substitutions of sounds and syllables), distortions, additions, repetitions, prolongations	Rosenbek & Wertz, 1972
Frequent methathetic errors, sequential sound production difficulties	Aram & Glasson, Note 2
	Edwards, 1973
	Morley, 1972
	Rosenbek & Wertz, 1972
Misarticulations of vowels as well as consonants	Rosenbek & Wertz, 1972
Adequate repetitions of sounds in isolation; connected speech more unintelligible than would be expected on the basis of single word articulation tests results	Rosenbek & Wertz, 1972
Errors varying with the complexity of articulatory adjustment; most frequent errors on fricatives, affricates, and consonant clusters	Crary, Note 4
	Rosenbek & Wertz, 1972
Groping trial-and-error behavior manifested as sound prolongations, repetitions, or silent posturing which may precede or interrupt imitative utterances	Rosenbek & Wertz, 1972
Oral diadochokinetic rates, especially for /pʌ tʌ kʌ/, slower than normal and often incorrectly sequenced	Aram & Glasson, Note 2
	Crary, Note 4
	Yoss & Darley, 1974a
More voicing errors than by children with functional articulation disorder	Yoss & Darley, 1974a
2- and 3-feature errors, prolongations and repetitions of sounds and syllables, additions, and distortions present in repetition speech tasks	Yoss & Darley, 1974a

CHARACTERISTICS	AUTHORS
Speech (cont.)	
Distortions, 1- place feature errors, additions, and omissions in spontaneous speech	Yoss & Darley, 1974a
Prosodic disturbances, such as slower rate and equalized stress	Edwards, 1973 Glasson, Note 7 Rosenbek & Wertz, 1972 Yoss & Darley, 1974a
Difficulty sequencing sounds and larger speech units, with the complexity and length of the utterance governing the degree of verbal apraxia evidenced; greater difficulty on polysyllabic words	Aram & Glasson, Note 2 Chappell, 1973 Edwards, 1973 Eisenson, 1966 Glasson, Note 7 Morley, 1972 Rosenbek & Wertz, 1972 Yoss & Darley, 1974a
Oral-nasal resonance confusions	Glasson, Note 7 Yoss & Darley, 1974a
More omission errors than in functional articulation disorder	Smartt, LaLance, Gray, and Hibbett, 1976
Breakdown in the spatial and temporal coordination of speech	Crary, Note 4; Note 8 Glasson, Note 7
Language	
Receptive abilities inordinately superior to expressive abilities	Aram & Glasson, Note 2 Rosenbek & Wertz, 1972 McClumpha & Logue, Note 5
Pervasive expressive language disorder	Aram & Glasson, Note 2 Ekelman, Note 9 Ekelman & Aram, 1983 Rosenbek, Note 1
Co-occurrence with aphasia, dysarthria, specific learning disability	Aram & Glasson, Note 2 Rosenbek & Wertz, 1972 Yoss & Darley, 1974a
Disordered basic language processes	Aram & Glasson, Note 2 Ekelman, Note 9 Ekelman & Aram, 1983 Loevner, Note 6 Rosenbek, Note 1
Prognosis	
Very slow in improving speech; typically poor response to "traditional" speech therapy	Chappell, 1973 Court & Harris, 1965 Daly, Cantrell, Cantrell & Aman, 1972 Fawcus, 1971 Rosenbek et al., 1974

be present; and the typically reported symptoms are not *exclusive* to developmental apraxia of speech. Compounding the problem is the observation that children change over time. For example, one client was diagnosed as apraxic at 3 years of age when he was essentially nonverbal. Without knowing his history, it is doubtful that a speech pathologist first meeting this child when he was 5½ years old would consider the label "developmental apraxia of speech". By this time he displayed a mild to moderate expressive language disorder and misarticulations characterized by a frontal lisp, distorted /l/ and /r/, and productions such as "whipskers" for whiskers and "ephalant" for elephant.

It is also extremely difficult to conduct research on a disorder for which identification of subjects is a problem. Many clinicians feel that this is a heterogeneous, rather than homogeneous population. Logue (Note 10) believes that single subject research is the most promising way to study DAS. In research to date, subjects represent a wide range of age, IQ, severity of communication disorder, concomitant disabilities, and organic signs. While there are children for whom neurologists have designated a neurologic basis for their speech disorder, it is currently debated whether the children under discussion actually have neurologic disorders. There is a small body of literature about developmental apraxia of speech: probably the major works have yet to be written.

American journal articles describing apraxic children began to appear in the 1970s with Rosenbek and Wertz in 1972, then Yoss and Darley (1974a), and Rosenbek et al., in 1974. Presentations at national, regional, and state conventions addressing verbal apraxia in children have been particularly popular in the last 10 years. There is a strong clinical interest in the disorder, even though a relatively small percentage of children receive this diagnostic label. Clinicians have found the diagnosis of developmental apraxia of speech useful for a number of children whose speech is particularly resistant to change, and many clinicians diagnose apraxia by first eliminating all else. Now it appears that the pendulum has swung again with writers who are challenging the existence of developmental apraxia of speech as a clinical entity. There are those who believe that we have embraced the area of apraxia without proper evidence—either empirical or clinical.

Behavioral Descriptions of the Symptomatology of Developmental Apraxia of Speech

Various authors have described the behavioral characteristics of apraxia. As indicated above, Table 6-1 lists these characteristics and includes earlier as well as recent authors. Perusal of this table may provide insight for the reader regarding the problems that arise in pinpointing the defining characteristics of this disorder.

A recent critical review of the literature written about developmental apraxia of speech by Guyette and Diedrich (1981) has spurred the controversy, which is likely to continue. In their survey of over 100 publications on adult and childhood apraxia and on principles of diagnosis, they conclude that there are as yet no convincing empirical bases to support assumptions regarding the existence of a readily differentiated DAS clinical population. Regarding nonspeech symptoms sometimes reported to characterize DAS (neurological "soft" signs; poor oral motor and diadochokinetic skills; the presence of concurrent language, sensory and/or intellectual deficits; positive family histories for speech disorders; the imbalanced distribution of the disorder between males and females; and the wide range of prognoses that have been claimed for DAS), Guyette and Diedrich illustrate the myriad of contradictory findings reported in that literature, leaving none of those characteristics to be reliable indicators of DAS. Further, they draw the same conclusions when they report the literature's findings on the speech symptoms various writers have attributed to DAS children. They discuss supposed symptoms such as articulatory inconsistency; inability to imitate; the display of particular articulatory error patterns related to sound omissions, vowel productions, or errors on consonant clusters, fricatives, and affricates; increasing errors with increasing lengths of utterances; and problems of prosody (including the classic groping behaviors of adult apraxia), sequencing, voicing, and oral-nasal differentiation. They suggest that most of these reported speech symptoms have been based on clinical impressions, and the few that have been studied empirically either have been shown not to occur in the speech of supposed DAS subjects or not to differentiate that speech from the speech of children with functional disorders of articulation.

Further, Guyette and Diedrich suggest that it is no wonder the literature is so diverse and inconclusive where the behavioral description of DAS children is concerned, considering the ways in which subjects have been selected for the studies that have produced these inconsistent findings. It is exceedingly circular to select subjects on the basis of behavioral characteristics that the study itself is designed to discover. So, their observation that subjects have been selected on the basis of defective oral movement skills (Smartt et al., 1976; Yoss & Darley, 1974a), or because someone has previously diagnosed them as apraxic by some unknown criteria (Prichard, Tekieli, & Kozup, 1979; Rosenbek & Wertz, 1972), or because they've made insignificant progress in therapy (Ferry, Hall & Hicks, 1975; Prichard et al., 1979; Aram and Glasson, Note 2), would almost necessarily produce a highly heterogeneous population. And that is, in fact, what has been shown in comparative reviews of the literature.

Guyette and Diedrich (1981; in press) make one further observation regarding the ways in which DAS children have been studied in the literature. They point out the absence of treatment studies demonstrating such children to be positively affected by certain treatments and not by others. In fact, treatment research in general is quite sparse with this population, so one has to wonder about the value of providing a diagnostic label from which no specific treatment has yet evolved.

More doubt regarding the likelihood of reliably identifying subgroups of DAS children is raised in an empirical study conducted by Williams, Ingham, and Rosenthal (1981). This study was, in fact, a direct replication of the Yoss and Darley (1974a) study that was essentially the first experimental attempt to determine whether a group of misarticulating children could be realistically described as DAS and shown to be different from other misarticulating children. In both studies essentially the same battery of speech and nonspeech tasks was given to 30 children with moderately to severely defective articulation but normal intelligence, hearing, and language development, and no apparent primary organic etiology. In both studies the same battery was also administered to an age- and sex-matched control group.

While Yoss and Darley found several characteristics that appeared to distinguish between children with apparently functional misarticulations and those whom they suggest could be called DAS children (separated arbitrarily on the basis of their isolated volitional oral movement—IVOM—scores), the findings of Williams et al. were at variance with almost every Yoss and Darley conclusion. Whereas Yoss and Darley's 2 groups of misarticulating subjects were significantly different on nonspeech IVOM scores, SVOM (sequenced volitional oral movements), and neurologic findings, in the Williams et al. study the 2 groups of misarticulators differed only on the variable used to divide the groups originally—IVOM scores. The 3 measures mentioned above might be assumed to be hallmarks of DAS, but they were not differentiating for the Williams et al. subjects. By conducting a discriminant function analysis on 14 speech variables, both studies pinpointed 6 variables that significantly discriminated the 2 speech disordered groups on the basis of the repeated speech tasks in the test battery, but only 2 variables overlapped: the sum of 2-feature errors and the sum of addition errors. Yoss and Darley's groups were differentiated primarily by neurologic findings which were uninfluential variables for the Williams et al. subjects. For spontaneous speech tasks, Yoss and Darley's analysis pinpointed 5 variables that could reliably separate the 2 groups of speech disordered subjects, with neurologic findings leading the way once again; but the Williams et al. analysis found no variables that could reliably separate the 2 groups of subjects. Essentially the only variable upon which the 2 studies agreed was a finding that diadochokinetic rates for the production of /kʌ/ were significantly slower for the potentially DAS group of subjects. Although Williams et al. appropriately suggest differences between the 2 studies that might account for differences in their findings (severity differences between the 2 potential DAS groups, differences in referral sources and, therefore, in the likelihood of the presence of neurologic "soft" signs, etc.), one is again left wondering whether it is currently possible to unambiguously differentiate DAS children from other misarticulating children.

Apparently there are those who believe it is, because work continues in relation to this disorder. Recent investigations which hold promise for a better understanding of this disorder are by Crary (Note 4; Note 8), Comeau & Crary (Note 12), and Towne and Crary (Note 13). They suggest a neurolinguistic perspective, and take the position that DAS usually encompasses both phonology and syntax. They state that the underlying deficit in phonologic development is limitation in the control of the spatial and temporal properties of articulation. Glasson's (Note 7) spectrographic analysis also suggested temporal coordination difficulties in DAS. The studies by Crary and his colleagues describe phonologic process profiles and investigate phonologic influence on syntactic performance. The authors suggest that the expansion of syntactic skills may depend on a certain level of proficiency in production of closed-syllable shapes. These studies, in general, support the studies by Aram and Glasson (Note 2), Ekelman (Note 9), Ekelman & Aram (1983) and Loevner (Note 6), as well as observations by many clinicians, that language processes may also be disordered in DAS.

Clearly, most investigators who are interested in DAS do not doubt its existence, but do feel a need for further delineation and exploration. It is anticipated that the many questions surrounding differential diagnosis will be addressed over the next few years. Some clinicans suggest that the advantages of making such a diagnosis are that it can provide a rationale for intensifying therapy, may prevent mismanagement, may direct family and patient counseling, may lower the expectancy for articulation proficiency, and may support a decision to introduce an augmentative system. With this in mind, as well as the general topic of symptomatology of DAS, the following is a review of the available measurement and assessment tools.

Measurement and Assessment Tools

As the reader has no doubt assumed from the previous section, a differential diagnosis of DAS is complicated and continues to elude many diagnosticians. There are very few tests specific to the assessment of DAS, and none have sufficient norms, standardization, validity, and reliability findings to be considered more than tentative measures which may hold potential. They await empirical data as to their ultimate value.

One such assessment is an unpublished protocol, *Motor Speech Examination* (Logue, Note 10; Note 14), which attempts to identify deficits in a child's motor speech planning. The examination assesses these motor skills and behaviors: (1) nonvolitional oral behaviors, (2) indices of dominance and laterality, (3) cranial nerve function, (4) diadochokinesis or multiple cranial nerve integration, (5) competitive articulatory posturing, (6) motor speech integration, and (7) imitative and spontaneous articulatory production skills.

Another test is the *Screening Test for Developmental Apraxia of Speech* (Blakeley, 1980), developed to aid in differential diagnosis and to suggest when further speech and language assessment and neurologic evaluation is needed. A cluster of symptoms, selected on the basis of the work of authors referred to in this chapter, is thought by Blakeley to have implications for a diagnosis of verbal apraxia. The following 8 subtests make up the test: I. Expressive Language Discrepancy, II. Vowels and Diphthongs, III. Oral-Motor Movement, IV. Verbal Sequencing, V. Articulation, VI. Motorically Complex Words, VII. Transpositions, and VIII. Prosody. A raw score is converted to a total weighted score and applied to a probability graph to determine exclusion from or inclusion into an apraxia group. The test takes approximately 10 minutes to administer.

Guyette and Diedrich (in press) reviewed the *Screening Test for Developmental Apraxia* to point out their concerns over the use of this instrument. Their review explored the literature Blakeley cited as support for the symptomatology which the test is designed to sample, examined the standard parameters of test construction, and presented data summarizing the author's use of this instrument. The review suggested that the references cited by Blakeley offered little empirical support for his claim that the symptoms of developmental apraxia of speech are those sampled in this test, and they concluded that a test to diagnose developmental apraxia of speech is premature and unjustified because there is still no agreement on the symptomatology of the disorder. Guyette and Diedrich further point out that the *Screening Test for Developmental Apraxia of Speech* has yet to be validated and that no test/retest reliability data are reported for the children or the examiners.

Treatment

The literature regarding developmental verbal apraxia addresses symptomatology and differential diagnosis more than it deals with therapy. Therapy is often described as a slow and difficult process, and many clinicians base a diagnosis of developmental apraxia on the lengthy and arduous course of treatment as well as on supposedly characteristically deviant articulatory patterns.

Most early work in the treatment area contained case studies (Dabul, 1971; Daly et al., 1972; Hadden, 1891; Rosenbek et al., 1974; Rosenthal, 1971; Logue & McClumpha, Note 15) or suggestions based on clinical experience (Chappell, 1973; Edwards, 1973; Eisenson, 1972; Morley, Court, Miller, & Garside, 1955; Morley & Fox, 1969; Yoss & Darley, 1974b; McClumpha & Logue, Note 5). They emphasized primarily: capitalizing on the visual modality and reading; association of correct sound production with visual, motor, and auditory cues; introduction of highly contrasted sounds; gradual increase in length and complexity of linguistic units; backward chaining; stimulation for syllable shapes and movement patterns rather than single phonemes; use of intonation and rhythm; decrease in speaking rate by clinician and child; and sensorimotor stimulation or oral motor facilitation. Truly needed are investigations to systematically evaluate the therapeutic effectiveness of a variety of treatment approaches.

Rosenbek (Note 1) suggests that the best current treatment methods for both apraxic children and adults are very similar except for obvious differences such as the selection of therapy material. He lists these methods as Total Communication; Melodic Intonation Therapy; the motokinesthetic approach; contrastive stress drills to exploit the effects of meaning; and pacing methods with intersystemic or gestural reorganization, utilizing movement via pacing boards, syllabic tapping, and the like.

Total Communication

Total Communication, speech combined with all modes of communication, but primarily manual communication, may be a viable treatment approach with some apraxic children. This would probably be because: (1) the child has not experienced a history of failure; (2) the visual channel, which may be a stronger input channel than the auditory one, is utilized, (3) the child can watch his or her own hands for feedback; (4) the fine motor competence required of speech is absent; (5) the hands are easier for the clinician to mold and shape than the mouth; (6) the signs can be extended in time without distortion, while speech is transitory; (7) a degree of iconicity in sign language facilitates language growth, and (8) the sign can help the child's speech by the association of a meaningful gross motor movement with units of speech. An effective Total Communication program emphasizes meaning, spontaneous communication, and consequences of communicative acts rather than imitation, repetition, and drill.

For these reasons, Jaffe (Note 16; Note 17) proposes extensive use of manual sign language and the manual alphabet in a treatment program for young children who are considered to be moderately to severely apraxic. In the early stages of therapy, sign language can be the major communication system, and in the later stages, signs and finger spelling can augment verbal communication. Total Communication is introduced at the onset, not as a last resort. By repeated association, it appears that signs may help the child recall and correctly articulate sound patterns and produce correct syntactic sequences. The use of signs with speech can help the clinician slow the rate of presentation and help the child reduce rate of utterance. The manual alphabet is introduced to establish a meaningful, visual-motor and kinesthetic movement pattern to cue production of the target phonemes and to facilitate blending and sequencing of phonemes.

Over a 9-month period, preliminary data were collected on 4 young apraxic children in individual and group therapy situations and parent-child interactions. All of the children showed a decrease in gestures and unintelligible vocalizations with an increase in signs and intelligible verbalizations, combinations of signs and speech, and total communicative output.

Melodic Intonation Therapy

The recent application of Melodic Intonation Therapy (MIT) with developmentally apraxic children (Doszak, McNeil, & Jancosek, Note 18; Helfrich-Miller, Note 19; in press) may also prove to be an important treatment approach. Melodic Intonation Therapy has been used successfully with adult apraxic patients (Berlin, 1976; Sparks, Helm, & Albert, 1974; Sparks & Holland, 1976). This technique focuses on the formulation of propositional expressive language through use of intoned sequences. Its original intent was to place emphasis on recovery of propositional language (Albert, Sparks, & Helm, 1973) rather than on the motor aspects of speech production. Sparks and Holland (1976), however, noted that while MIT is directed toward language, some clinicians have also reported success adapting it to improve slurred articulation and to reduce the frequency of phonemic errors in some apraxic patients.

The following are suggested as rationales for using this approach with apraxic children: (1) alterations in prosody—rhythm, stress, and intonation—may improve speech production, (2) the emphasis on movement may improve phonemic and linguistic sequencing through intersystemic organization, and (3) the reduced rate of verbal input and verbal output may facilitate correct articulatory placement and inclusion.

Helfrich-Miller (Note 19; in press) adapted procedures, previously described in the literature with adult aphasics, for a treatment program with developmentally apraxic children. In place of tapping out a rhythm, manual sign language was substituted in the MIT hierarchy to facilitate sequencing and language structure. Three levels were hierarchically arranged to move the child in small graded steps toward achieving normal speech prosody. The progression from the first to the third level entailed 4 principles: (1) increased length of unit, (2) increased phonemic, morphologic, and syntactic complexity, (3) decreased dependency on the clinician, and (4) diminished reliance on intoning and signing. It was essentially an imitative program.

Helfrich-Miller has treated children as young as 2 years of age with less formalized adaptations of MIT. The ideal candidate for a formalized program, however, is a 7- to 8-year old, with moderate to marked verbal apraxia, demonstrating poor repetition skills. Such a child would need an MLU of at least 3 to 4 words and an attention span of at least 15 to 20 minutes. Children with accompanying dysarthria are not candidates for this technique.

Data presented on 2 children reported convincing gains in articulation, sequencing abilities, and expressive language. Both children took 11 months to finish the program. Once the formalized program was completed, the use of MIT principles continued throughout therapy. The children were taught to self-cue through intonation and signing to facilitate linguistic sequencing. When the program is used appropriately, Level III is not the end of MIT but the beginning of an internalized cueing system which seeks to normalize sequencing abilities in apraxic children.

Doszak et al. (Note 18) evaluated the effectiveness of MIT in improving prosodic and articulatory features in a single subject, a 10-year-old male diagnosed as having developmental apraxia of speech. A time series withdrawal design (ABAB) was used to determine the effects of MIT versus nontreatment. Data were analyzed by 2 objective and 1 subjective measure: vowel duration (on all CVC productions) and percentage of duration of final contour compared to the entire sentence duration (on sentence productions), and listener judgments (on the same recurrent sentence production during the picture description), respectively. Duration measures were made on a 4-channel oscillograph and a Visipitch. The 2 objective measures revealed significant ANOVA results for the vowel duration measures and no significant change in the duration of the final contour between any test sessions. Listeners judged the later speech samples as "better sounding." The authors concluded that MIT was effective in improving this subject's speech, inferred that MIT or some component of MIT reduced vowel durations, and suggested further research on the efficacy of MIT with developmentally apraxic children and on the relationship between perceptual changes and acoustic or physiologic changes in speech.

Motokinesthetic and motor learning approaches

Emphasizing motokinesthetic techniques is the moto-sequential tactile therapy, or "touch-cue" approach (Bashir, Jones, & Bostwick, Note 20; Jones, Note 21). This is a systematic approach to teaching individual speech sounds and enhancing sound-sequencing abilities. The clinician presents auditory and visual stimuli along with touch-cue points that are designated points on the face which the child touches during production of consonant, consonant-vowel, CVC and VC drills. Therapy is divided into 3 stages, each stage establishing basic skills that will be elaborated in subsequent stages of therapy. Stage I is a collection of articulation drills, arranged in order of difficulty. These drills are to develop self-monitoring and to teach association of auditory, visual, and touch cues. Stage II incorporates the learned sequences from Stage I into the production of real and nonsense words. The phonemic chains increase in complexity to form multisyllabic chains and words. Stage III is concerned with carry-over of these skills into controlled and spontaneous speech. The program depends on the family for cooperation and has a parent-teaching component. Undoubtedly, many therapists are employing such techniques with children who have poor articulation apparently due to a motor planning deficit or hearing impairment, so the approach should be put to empirical test. Motokinesthetic approaches may hold promise for treating developmentally apraxic children.

Another speech-motor training program is the *Monitoring Articulatory Postures* (MAP), developed and refined by Logue (1978; Note 10). The MAP is designed for the child whose breakdown in the programming system seems to occur when integrated movements of phonation, respiration, and articulation are superimposed on nonspeech oral-motor movements.

The premise of MAP is that the apraxic child needs to develop a reliable motor command before concentrating on sound production. The program is in 3 phases. Phase I, Articulatory Posture Training, intends to teach the child to establish and to maintain vowel and consonant associated postures. In Phase II, Speech Shadow Imitation, the clinician first presents a visual model only, then gradually fades the visual emphasis and introduces the auditory model for the first time. Phase III, Competitive Articulatory Posturing, is the most critical phase of the MAP program. It requires considerable anticipatory and reprogramming capability which the author believes is an important prerequisite for articulate speech. The clinician instructs the child to position the articulators to produce a particular vowel, consonant, or word, and then instructs the child to produce a competing vowel, consonant, or word, instead. Thus, the program progresses from simple imitation of vowel postures to the reprogramming necessary to produce a word after assuming the anticipatory posture of a contrasted word. Logue has not yet reported data on the effects of this treatment strategy, including the necessity or helpfulness of each of the stages in the treatment. (One might wonder if the first 2 steps requiring imitation might not be inordinately difficult for an apraxic child, if the inability to voluntarily imitate motor movements is, in fact, a hallmark of the disorder.)

Rate control

One investigation provides an excellent empirical therapy evaluation method which serves as a rare model for the kind of treatment research needed in this confused area of DAS. Rosenthal, Williams, and Ingham (Note 22) conducted an experimental therapy program, the intent of which was to systematically evaluate the effectiveness of certain treatment procedures with 1 female and 3 male apraxic subjects who ranged in age from 10 to 14 years. Subjects were labeled apraxic on the basis of 2 independent diagnoses from qualified speech-language clinicians and on the observation of a history of very slow response to therapy. The treatment program was designed to successively establish correct articulation during slowed oral reading, gradually increase reading rates to a normal level, and then transfer this skill to "monologue" speech.

In Stage I, 6 experimental procedures were sequentially introduced and assessed for each subject. First, the rate of a reading machine was adjusted to approximately 50% of each child's baseline reading rate, established in 6 to 12 5-minute "sessions." The percentage of words correctly articulated was calculated on-line for each subject during alternating 5-minute intervals requiring rate change or returning to baseline conditions. All subjects showed an increase in the percentage of words read correctly under the condition of slowed rate, and this was therefore incorporated into the remaining 5 procedures of Stage I.

Subsequent experimental conditions were introduced in the same fashion and evaluated according to their effect on the percentage of words correctly articulated. Condition 2 introduced response contingent reinforcement wherein subjects earned 1 cent for every 10 correctly articulated words. In Condition 3, following incorrectly articulated words, the experimenter provided the correct production while the subject listened but did not repeat the word. During Condition 4, the clinician again provided a model following incorrectly articulated words and the subject was required to imitate the word immediately. (It is interesting to note that this was ineffective at producing improved articulation for 3 of the 4 subjects.) Because certain subjects had retained particular phonemes in error at this stage of the treatment, in Condition 5 the experimenters implemented phoneme instruction wherein the experimenter demonstrated and described placement and manner of production of the relevant error phonemes and gave the subjects the opportunity to practice words containing those typically misarticulated phonemes. Then Condition 4 was reintroduced so that the effects of specific phoneme instruction could be evaluated. The last experimental treatment procedure introduced during this stage of the treatment—designed to establish correct articulation at slowed reading rates—was to highlight each subject's remaining incorrect phoneme occurrences by contingently providing an explanation of the error; e.g., if the subject read "beat" instead of "beach," the experimenter said, "/tʃ/ at the end: beach"; and the child read the word again.

Following the establishment of 85% correct articulation during slowed oral reading by the end of Condition 6 for all subjects, the next phase gradually moved the reading rate to the subject's normal rate, concurrently providing contingent feedback (a beep) for each incorrectly articulated word. This was followed by a similar progression from slowed to normal speaking rates requiring maintenance of the 85% correct articulation performance in monologue speech. Subsequently, 95% correct production in monologue was required. The final evaluation of the treatment effects occurred when the subjects were required to talk in monologue with no experimenter-controlled feedback of any kind. The data showed maintenance of 95% correct articulation for each subject at that subject's normal speaking rate.

The authors report that 3 procedures appeared to be effective for all 4 subjects: rate control, phoneme production instruction, and the highlighting of error phonemes. They also recommended including reinforcement for correct responding in a therapy program for apraxic children because it produced positive change for all of the subjects (although only marginally for 2), and they believed its presence helped the children persevere in the therapy program. They also pointed out that each condition proved effective for at least 1 of the 4 subjects, so that each might be considered and individually examined with future subjects.

Even though it is, obviously, valuable to know that rate control procedures have been demonstrated to be an effective component of successful treatment for DAS, this study was reported in greater detail than others because it also serves as an example of the careful, systematic, and empirical way in which treatment can be conducted. More research of this nature is required before much of value can be written about the treatment of children diagnosed as DAS.

Final Comments

It was stated earlier that the major works about developmental apraxia of speech have probably yet to be written. These are some of the issues that remain unanswered, with suggestions for further research.

1. Empirical evidence is needed to support all of the clinically defined characteristics of apraxia. Critics have raised the question of whether subjects designated as "apraxic" by one researcher would be "apraxic" by another researcher's criteria. More rigorously designed descriptive studies with larger sample sizes are required to develop an agreed-upon definition of developmental apraxia of speech and to generate hypotheses for careful exploration in experimental studies.

2. Information regarding early developmental nonspeech, prespeech, and speech behaviors that may be indicators of later-appearing DAS would clearly lead to earlier diagnosis and treatment. Kron (1970) found that some infants showed unexplained irregularities of the sucking response and hypothesized that disorganized sucking activities may be related to brain dysfunction. It would be helpful to discover whether verbal apraxia could be predicted in the hospital nursery by studying the earliest infant oral behavior. Eisenson (1972); and Aram and Glasson (Note 2) have suggested other items in supposed apraxic children's histories that may be early signs of DAS and should be systematically investigated.

3. Whether or not neurologic dysfunction can be reliably measured or should be included as a necessary component in the diagnosis of DAS must be resolved.

4. The question of whether verbal apraxia is a motor sequential disturbance which is free from the symbolic aspects of language or whether developmental apraxia in children exists as part of a language disorder remains unanswered.

5. Production of connected speech has been reported and analyzed in a few existing studies (Crary, Note 4; Ekelman, Note 9; Ekelman & Aram, 1983). Analysis of connected speech samples may reveal more and/or different information about the articulatory and linguistic aspects of DAS.

6. There is a need for longitudinal and follow-up studies to help in differential diagnosis, to describe changes over time, and to document the effects of treatment.

7. The aspect of oral perception and sensation and its hypothesized relationship to developmental verbal apraxia needs to be explored further. Some studies (Prichard et al., 1979; Loevner, Note 6) showed

that apraxic children performed significantly more poorly than normal children and articulation-disordered children on tests of oral stereognosis. Are measurements of oral sensory perception of primary importance in etiology and/or differential diagnosis of developmental apraxia of speech?

8. Rosenbek, Wertz, and Darley (1973) noted that certain adult apraxics had a low tolerance for 2-point discrimination tasks. It has been observed clinically that many apraxic children do not tolerate touch well and are especially hypersensitive to touch in and around the mouth. Supporting these clinical reports were the striking differences observed in test-taking behavior between normally speaking and developmentally apraxic children on tests of oral sensory processing (Loevner, Note 6). What is the explanation and significance of these findings?

9. If children with developmental apraxia of speech demonstrate poor tactile/kinesthetic/proprioceptive functioning, could a therapy program based on improving these functions be effective in improving the child's motor programming for speech? Ayres (1973) feels that the tactile system is primarily concerned with the ability to program a skilled motor act, and that dysfunction of the vestibular and other proprioceptive mechanisms may also contribute to the state of generalized apraxia in children. Ayres explains it as a problem in sensory integration. While results of sensory-integrative therapy with children demonstrating overall or verbal apraxia are not well documented, it is an intriguing concept worthy of study that tactile and even vestibular stimulation may improve oral motor and speech programming on a neurologic basis.

10. Sonderman (Note 23) showed that performance on various volitional oral movement tasks was unrelated to articulatory performance but was related to age. We need more studies on normal growth and development of children's ability to perform nonverbal oral motor tasks upon which to base comparisons of children with disordered speech.

11. Finally, there is a need for careful studies comparing a variety of treatment approaches and techniques with this population of children.

Currently, the state of the art relative to verbal apraxia in children is similar to that of acquired apraxia in adults 10 years ago. The writings and investigations of the 1970s, upon which we have based our understanding of developmental apraxia of speech, are being challenged. Speech and language pathologists have an unprecedented opportunity to ask pertinent questions, to share their clinical experiences in evaluation and treatment, and to conduct research in this area. Increased interest in developmental apraxia of speech should generate even more accelerated advances within the next 10 years.

Reference Notes

1. Rosenbek, J.C. Treating apraxia of speech in children and adults. A short course presented at the 4th Annual Three Rivers Conference of Communicative Disorders, Pittsburgh, 1982.

2. Aram, D.M., & Glasson, C. Developmental apraxia of speech. Paper presented at the Annual Convention of the American Speech –Language– Hearing Association, Atlanta, 1979.

3. Saleeby, N.C., Hadjian, S., Martinkosky, S.J., & Swift, M.R. Familial verbal dyspraxia: A clinical study. Paper presented at the Annual Convention of the American Speech and Hearing Association, San Francisco, 1978.

4. Crary, M.A. Developmental verbal dyspraxia: A phonological research perspective. Paper presented at the Annual Convention of the American Speech-Language-Hearing Association, Toronto, 1982.

5. McClumpha, S.L., & Logue, R.D. Approaches to children with motor programming disorders of speech. Paper presented at the Annual Convention of the American Speech and Hearing Association, San Francisco, 1972.

6. Loevner, M.B. An investigation of perceptual abilities in developmental apraxia of speech and comparison with functional articulation disorders. Unpublished doctoral dissertation, University of Pittsburgh, 1979.

7. Glasson, C. Spectrographic analysis of developmental apraxia: Temporal coordination difficulties. Paper presented at the Annual Convention of the American Speech-Language-Hearing Association, Los Angeles, 1981.

8. Crary, M.A. Phonological process analysis of developmental verbal dyspraxia: A descriptive study. Paper presented at the Annual Convention of the American Speech-Language-Hearing Association, Los Angeles, 1981.

9. Ekelman, B.L. Syntactic and semantic findings in developmental verbal apraxia. Paper presented at the Annual Convention of the American Speech-Language-Hearing Association, Los Angeles, 1981.

10. Logue, R.D. Apraxia revisited. Short course presented at the Annual Convention of the Pennsylvania Speech –Language– Hearing Association. King of Prussia, 1983.

11. Aram, D.M. Sequential and nonspeech practic abilities in children with developmental verbal apraxia. Paper presented at the Annual Convention of the American Speech-Language-Hearing Association, Los Angeles, 1981.

12. Comeau, B.S., & Crary, M.A. Developmental verbal dyspraxia: A morphophonemic analysis. Paper presented at the Annual Convention of the American Speech-Language-Hearing Association, Toronto, 1982.

13. Towne, R.L., & Crary, M.A. Syntagmatic distance as a phonological variable in developmental verbal dyspraxia. Paper presented at the Annual Convention of the American Speech-Language-Hearing Association, Toronto, 1982.

14. Logue, R.D. Assessing speech motor behavior: An examination protocol. Presented at the Annual Convention of the American Speech and Hearing Association, Houston, 1976.

15. Logue, R.D., & McClumpha, S.L. Apraxia of speech in children: A case description. Paper presented at the Annual Convention of the American Speech and Hearing Association, New York, 1970.

16. Jaffe, M.B. Treatment approaches with developmentally apraxic children. Paper presented at the Annual Convention of the American Speech-Language-Hearing Association, Detroit, 1980.

17. Jaffe, M.B. Developmental apraxia of speech: Updating clinical skills. Short course presented at the North-East Regional Conference of the American Speech-Language-Hearing Association, Philadelphia, 1981.

18. Doszak, A.L., McNeil, M.R., & Jancosek, E. Efficacy of Melodic Intonation Therapy with developmental apraxia of speech. Paper presented at the Annual Convention of the American Speech-Language-Hearing Association, Los Angeles, 1981.

19. Helfrich-Miller, K.R. The use of Melodic Intonation Therapy with developmentally apraxic children. Paper presented at the Annual Convention of the American Speech-Language-Hearing Association, Detroit, 1980.

20. Bashir, A.S., Jones, F., & Bostwick, R.Y. A touch cue method of therapy with developmentally apraxic children. Paper presented at the Annual Convention of the American Speech-Language-Hearing Association, Detroit, 1980.

21. Jones, F. Moto-sequential tactile therapy. A paper written for Emerson College, 1975.

22. Rosenthal, J., Williams, R., & Ingham, R.J. An experimental therapy programme for developmental articulatory dyspraxia. Paper presented at the Annual Convention of the Australian Association of Speech and Hearing, Launceston, Tasmania, 1978.

23. Sonderman, J.C. The relationship between volitional oral movement production and articulation competence. Unpublished doctoral dissertation, University of Pittsburgh, 1978.

References

Albert, M., Sparks, R., & Helm, N. Melodic Intonation Therapy for aphasia. *Archives of Neurology*, 1973, *29*, 130-131.

Ayres, A.J. *Sensory integration and learning disorders*. Los Angeles: Western Psychological Services, 1973.

Berlin, C.I. On: Melodic Intonation Therapy for Aphasia by R.W. Sparks and A.L. Holland. *Journal of Speech and Hearing Disorders*, 1976, *41*, 298-300.

Blakeley, R.W. *Screening Test for Developmental Apraxia of Speech*. Tigard, Ore.: C.C. Publications, 1980.

Bobath, B. The very early treatment of cerebral palsy. *Developmental Medicine and Child Neurology*, 1967, *9*, 373-391.

Bobath, B. *Abnormal postural reflex activity caused by brain lesions* (2nd ed.). London: William Heinemann Medical Books, 1971. (a)

Bobath, B. Motor development: Its effect on general development and application to the treatment of cerebral palsy. *Physiotherapy*, 1971, *57*, 526-532. (b)

Bobath, K. *The motor deficit in patients with cerebral palsy*. London: Little Club Clinics in Developmental Medicine #23, William Heinemann Medical Books, 1966.

Bobath, K. The normal postural reflex mechanism and its deviation in children with cerebral palsy. *Physiotherapy*, 1971, *57*, 515-525.

Bobath, K., & Bobath, B. Cerebral palsy. Part 1. Diagnosis and assessment of cerebral palsy. Part 2. The neurodevelopmental approach to treatment. In P.H. Pearson & C.E. Williams (Eds.), *Physical therapy services in the developmental disabilities*. Springfield, Ill.: Charles C. Thomas, 1972.

Campbell, P.H. *Problem-oriented approaches to feeding the handicapped child*. Akron, O.: The Children's Hospital Medical Center of Akron, 1982.

Chappell, G.E. Childhood verbal apraxia and its treatment. *Journal of Speech and Hearing Research*, 1973, *16*, 362-368.

Court, D., & Harris, M. Speech disorders in children. Part II. *British Medical Journal*, 1965, *2*, 409-411.

Dabul, B.L. Lingual incoordination-language delay: A case of a lazy tongue? *California Journal of Communication Disorders,* 1971, *2,* 30-33.

Daly, D.A., Cantrell, R.P., Cantrell, M.L., & Aman, L.A. Structuring speech therapy contingencies with an oral apraxic child. *Journal of Speech and Hearing Disorders,* 1972, *37,* 22-32.

Davis, L. Pre-speech. In F.P. Connor, G.G. Williamson, & J.M. Siepp (Eds.). *Program guide for infants and toddlers with neuromotor and other developmental disabilities.* New York: Teachers College Press, Columbia University, 1978.

Edwards, M. Developmental verbal dyspraxia. *British Journal of Disorders of Communication,* 1973, *8,* 64-70.

Eisenson, J. *Aphasia in children.* New York: Harper & Row, 1972.

Eisenson, J. Developmental patterns of non-verbal children and some therapeutic implications. *Journal of Neurological Science,* 1966, *3,* 313-320.

Ekelman, B.L., & Aram, D.M. Syntactic findings in developmental verbal apraxia. *Journal of Communication Disorders,* 1983, *16,* 237-250.

Fawcus, R. Features of a psychological and physiological study of articulatory performance. *British Journal of Disorders of Communication,* 1971, *6,* 99-106.

Ferry, P.C., Hall, S.M., & Hicks, J.L. 'Dilapidated speech': Developmental verbal apraxia. *Developmental Medicine and Child Neurology,* 1975, *17,* 749-756.

Gallender, D. *Eating handicaps.* Springfield, Ill.: Charles C. Thomas, 1979.

Guyette, T.W., & Diedrich, W.M. A critical review of developmental apraxia of speech. In N.J. Lass (Ed.), *Speech and language: Advances in basic research and practice* (Vol.5). New York: Academic Press, 1981.

Guyette, T.W., & Diedrich, W.M. A review of the Screening Test for Developmental Apraxia of Speech. *Language, Speech, and Hearing Services in Schools,* in press.

Hadden, W.B. On certain defects of articulation in children, with cases illustrating the results of education of the oral system. *Journal of Mental Science,* 1891, *37,* 96-105.

Helfrich-Miller, K.R. Melodic Intonation Therapy with developmentally apraxia children. In Aram, D.M. (Ed.) Seminars in Speech and Language: *Developmental Verbal Apraxia.* In press.

Kron, R.E. Prognostic significance of sucking dysrhythmias. In J.F. Bosma (Ed.), *Symposium on oral sensation and perception.* Springfield, Ill.: Charles C. Thomas, 1970.

Logue, R.D. Disorders of motor-speech planning in children: Evaluation and treatment. *Communicative Disorders: An Audio Journal for Continuing Education, Vol. 3.* New York: Grune & Stratton, 1978.

Love, R.J., Hagerman, E.L., & Taimi, E.G. Speech performance, dysphagia and oral reflexes in cerebral palsy. *Journal of Speech and Hearing Disorders,* 1980, *45,* 59-75.

Morley, M.E. *Development and disorders of speech in childhood (3rd ed).* London: E. & S. Livingstone, 1972.

Morley, M., Court, D., Miller, H., & Garside, R. Delayed speech and developmental aphasia. *British Medical Journal,* 1955, *2,* 463-467.

Morley, M.E., & Fox, J. Disorders of articulation: Theory and therapy. *British Journal of Disorders of Communication,* 1969, *4,* 151-165.

Morris, S.E. *Program guidelines for children with feeding problems.* Edison, N.J.: Childcraft Education Corp., 1977.

Morris, S.E. *The normal acquisition of oral feeding skills: Implications for assessment and treatment.* Boston: Therapeutic Media, 1982. (a)

Morris, S.E. *The Pre-Speech Assessment Scale.* Clifton, N.J.: J.A. Preston, 1982. (b)

Mueller, H.A. Facilitating feeding and prespeech. In P.H. Pearson & C.E. Williams (Eds.), *Physical therapy services in the developmental disabilities.* Springfield, Ill.: Charles C. Thomas, 1972.

Mueller, H.A. *Feeding, speech*. In N.R. Finnie (Ed.), *Handling the young cerebral palsied child at home* (2nd ed.), New York: Dutton, 1975.

Mysak, E.D. *Neurospeech therapy for the cerebral palsied* (3rd ed.). New York: Teachers College Press, Columbia University, 1980.

Nicolosi, L., Harryman, E., & Kresheck, J. *Terminology of communication disorders: Speech, language, hearing*. Baltimore: Williams & Wilkins, 1978.

Palmer, M. Studies in clinical techniques. II. Normalization of chewing, sucking and swallowing reflexes in cerebral palsy: A home program. *Journal of Speech Disorders*, 1947, *12*, 415-418.

Perske, R., Clifton, A., McLean, B., & Stein, J. (Eds.). *Mealtimes for severely and profoundly handicapped persons*. Baltimore: University Park Press, 1977.

Prichard, C.L., Tekieli, M.E., & Kozup, J.M. Developmental apraxia: Diagnostic considerations. *Journal of Communication Disorders*, 1979, *12*, 337-348.

Rosenbek, J.C., Hansen, R., Baughman, C.H., & Lemme, M. Treatment of developmental apraxia of speech: A case study. *Language, Speech, and Hearing Services in Schools*, 1974, *5*, 13-22.

Rosenbek, J.C., & Wertz, R.T. A review of fifty cases of developmental apraxia of speech. *Language, Speech, and Hearing Services in Schools*, 1972, *3*, 23-33.

Rosenbek, J.C., Wertz, R.T., & Darley, F.L. Oral sensation and perception in apraxia of speech and aphasia. *Journal of Speech and Hearing Disorders*, 1973, *16*, 22-36.

Rosenthal, J. A token reinforcement programme used in the treatment of articulatory dyspraxia in a nine-year-old boy. *Journal of the Australian College of Speech Therapists*, 1971, *21*, 45-48.

Smartt, J., LaLance, L., Gray, J., & Hibbett, P. Developmental apraxia of speech: A Tennessee Speech and Hearing Association subcommitte report. *Journal of the Tennessee Speech and Hearing Association*, 1976, *20*, 21-31.

Sparks, R.W., Helm, N., & Albert, M. Aphasia rehabilitation resulting from Melodic Intonation Therapy. *Cortex*, 1974, *10*, 303-316.

Sparks, R.W., & Holland, A.L. Method: Melodic Intonation Therapy for aphasia. *Journal of Speech and Hearing Disorders*, 1976, *41*, 287-297.

Westlake, H. *A system for developing speech with cerebral palsied children*. Chicago: The National Society for Crippled Children and Adults, 1951.

Williams, R., Ingham, R.J., & Rosenthal, J. A further analysis of developmental apraxia of speech in children with defective articulation. *Journal of Speech and Hearing Research*, 1981, *24*, 496-505.

Yoss, K.A., & Darley, F.L. Developmental apraxia of speech in children with defective articulation. *Journal of Speech and Hearing Research*, 1974, *17*, 399-416. (a).

Yoss, K.A., & Darley, F.L. Therapy in developmental apraxia of speech. *Language, Speech, and Hearing Services in Schools*, 1974, *1*, 23-31. (b)

Betty Jane McWilliams

Speech Problems Associated with Craniofacial Anomalies

Introduction

Craniofacial malformations, while rare, constitute a major group of handicaps in children. They are usually complex and far-reaching in their life implications. Many are obviously genetically determined, while others occur sporadically. Until recent years, such conditions were considered to be untreatable. Individuals suffering from these problems were often shunted to the margins of society or were institutionalized with the result that speech-language pathologists had only limited experience in the diagnosis and treatment of their communicative deficits. That situation is changing, and speech-language pathologists are now being confronted with new challanges and opportunities in relation to the treatment of the wide variety of craniofacial malformations which have been identified.

Definition

The term "craniofacial malformation" has grown increasingly popular since 1971, when Paul Tessier described the surgical treatment of the severe facial deformities associated with craniofacial synostosis. *Cranio* refers to any skeletal deformity of the head at or above the lower eyelids, and *facial* to any abnormality below that level. *Synostosis* means that there is premature osseous union of bones that are normally distinct. Thus, theoretically, craniofacial malformations are those that affect both the cranium and the face. However, there has been a recent trend to include in the definition malformations affecting any part of the craniofacial complex. The reason for this is that these defects, whether severe or less complicated, are often treated in the same interdisciplinary facilities that once were concerned primarily with cleft lip, cleft palate, or both.

Figure 7-1 shows an infant with Pierre Robin Syndrome, an anomaly that involves only the face. Note the small chin, or *retrognathic mandible*. This is usually associated with a cleft of the soft palate, but the cranium is unaffected. The syndrome is complicated by *glossoptosis*, or retraction of the tongue into the pharyngeal space, rendering normal breathing impossible in many cases. About one-third of these children have learning disabilities ranging from mild to severe (McWilliams, Note 1). The origin of these problems is unclear. They may be logically related to early oxygen deprivation, or there may be prior neurological problems, which also contribute to the infant's inability to manage the tongue in the restricted oral space (Mallory & Paradise, 1979). In addition, the symptoms of Pierre Robin are sometimes just one part of a complex group of disorders comprising at least a dozen other syndromes, some of which do include the cranium (Cohen, 1976). Figure 7-2 shows an open palatal cleft, again a defect involving only the oral structures.

Figures 7-3A and 7-3B present a patient with Crouzon disease, or craniofacial *dysostosis*, which includes an abnormally shaped head, maxillary hypoplasia (midfacial deficiency), prognathism (prominent mandible), hypertelorism (wide-set eyes), exopthalmos (protruding eyes caused by shallow orbits), and low-set ears. These children are not usually mentally retarded. Crouzon is clearly a craniofacial abnormality as is Apert Syndrome (Figures 7-4A and 7-4B). This latter syndrome has many characteristics similar to Crouzon, but they are more severe. In addition, palatal deformities are common. *Syndactly* (webbing or union) of the fingers and toes is always present. While overt palatal clefts are sometimes seen, a more frequent deformity is a very high-arched narrow palate with excessive pile-up of tissue on the maxillary arch. While this often looks like a true cleft, it is not. Mental retardation is more common in Apert Syndrome than in Crouzon and may occur in as many as 50% of those affected.

These examples of representative craniofacial abnormalities should make the reader aware of the wide variety of forms, severity, and life implications of these birth defects. They should also suggest the possibility that similar variations in structure might be acquired as the result of surgical intervention or injury. Figures 7-5A and 7-5B show a young woman with

FIGURE 7-1
An infant with Pierre Robin Syndrome.

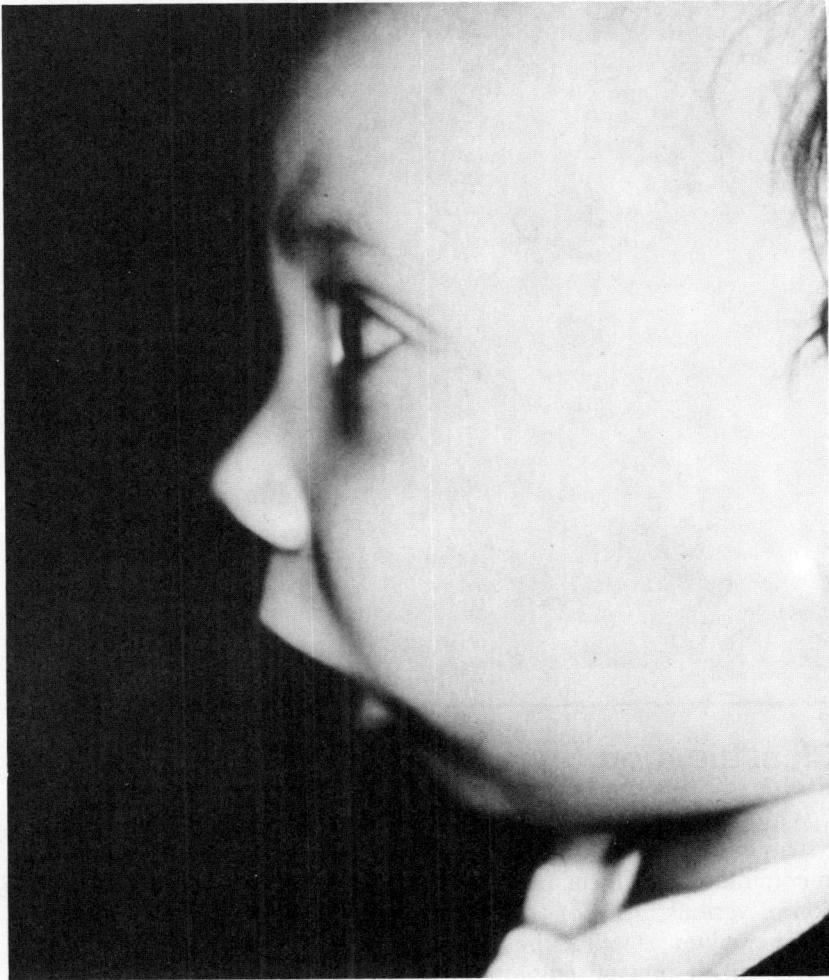

a prognathic mandible and marked open bite, which resulted from a fall from a second-story window at the age of 2½. She is an example of an *acquired* facial defect.

FIGURE 7-2
An open palatal cleft.

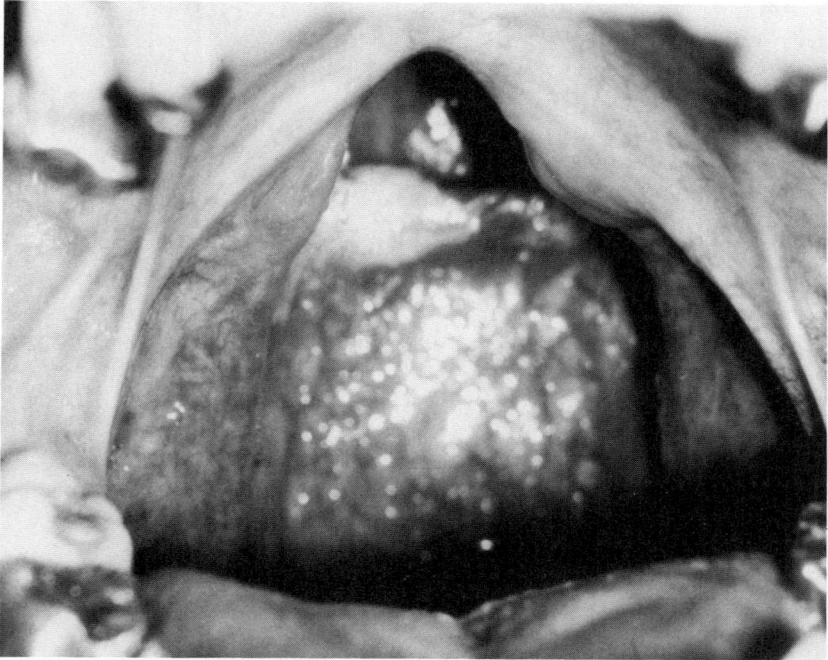

Classification

Whitaker, Pashayan, and Richman (1981) proposed a classification system for these kinds of defects. It takes into account the variations found in craniofacial malformations as described above and permits the inclusion of various forms of clefts and other deficits involving just the face or the cranium, as well as those in which both are malformed in some way. They suggest that all craniofacial anomalies may be classified into 5 categories based on etiology, anatomy, and current treatment principles. The basic system is as follows:

I. Clefts
   Centric (Midline)
   Acentric (Lateral)

II. Synostoses
   Symmetric
   Asymmetric

III.   Atrophy – hypoplasia   V.   Unclassified

IV.   Neoplasia – hyperplasia

The authors point out that any of the malformations may vary from subtle to extreme. The reader is referred to the article for more details on this and other systems of classification (Whitaker et al., 1981).

Occurrence

Extensive malformations of the craniofacial structures are relatively rare. It is estimated that approximately 1,200 babies with profound defects are born each year in the United States. Yet, as better discernment techniques become available, heretofore undiagnosed problems, particularly those with mild degrees of expressivity, are being appropriately described, diagnosed, treated, and studied. The sad designation of "funny looking kid," or "f.l.k.," has now taken its place with other historically used terms that are both cruel and inaccurate. When the speech-language pathologist sees an unusual looking child, however, it is incumbent upon him or her to investigate and learn as much as possible about the condition. Referral to a center for appropriate evaluation may make the difference between a marginal life and a fruitful one.

Syndromes

Many craniofacial deformities can be recognized as discrete syndromes manifested by groups of symptoms regularly occurring together, so that affected children and adults look much alike even though there is no family relationship. This is true of Crouzon (Figures 7-3A and 7-3B) and of Apert (Figures 7-4A and 7-4B), as well as of many other syndromes. There are literally hundreds of such syndromes, not all of which include craniofacial abnormalities, that have already been described, and Gorlin (Note 2) suggested that several new ones were being identified each month. Sparks and Millard (1981) have provided brief descriptions of the speech problems associated with some of these syndromes. Speech pathologists are becoming more and more involved in both the identification and treatment of syndromes, and there are increasing numbers specializing in the communicative disorders of such patients. This represents a new frontier that is expanding slowly but surely.

FIGURE 7-3A
A patient with Crouzon's disease (craniofacial dysostosis).

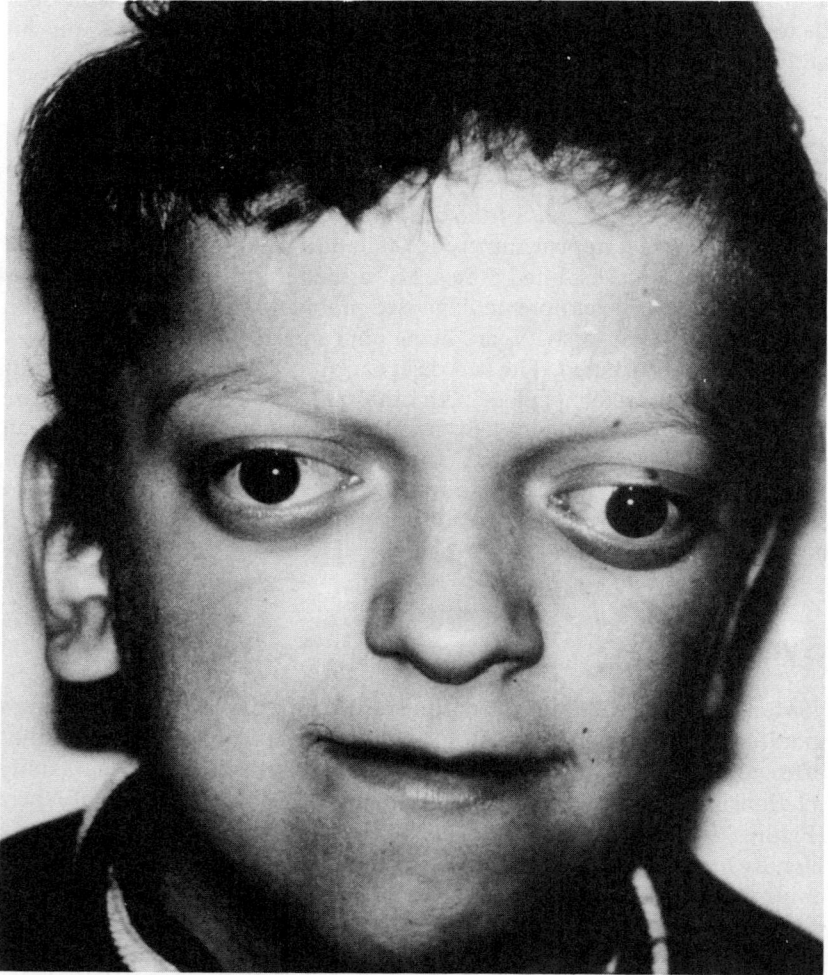

Associated Problems

Syndromes involving craniofacial abnormalities and craniofacial defects not identified as syndromes often include malformations that will affect

FIGURE 7-3B
A patient with Crouzon's disease (craniofacial dysostosis).

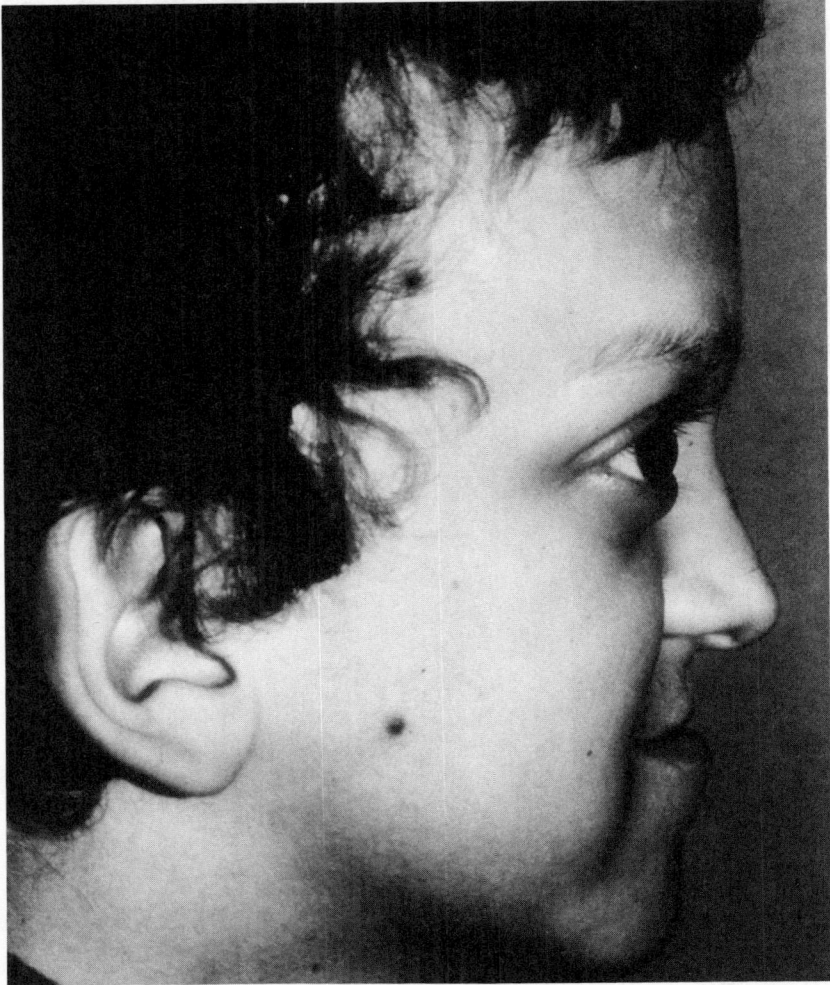

function in some major ways. For example, palatal clefts may occur in approximately 154 syndromes (Cohen, 1978). Smith (1976) includes 55 of these. Thus, children so affected may have all the speech problems that occur if palatal repair does not result in the ability to achieve velopharyngeal

FIGURE 7-4A
A patient with Apert's Syndrome.

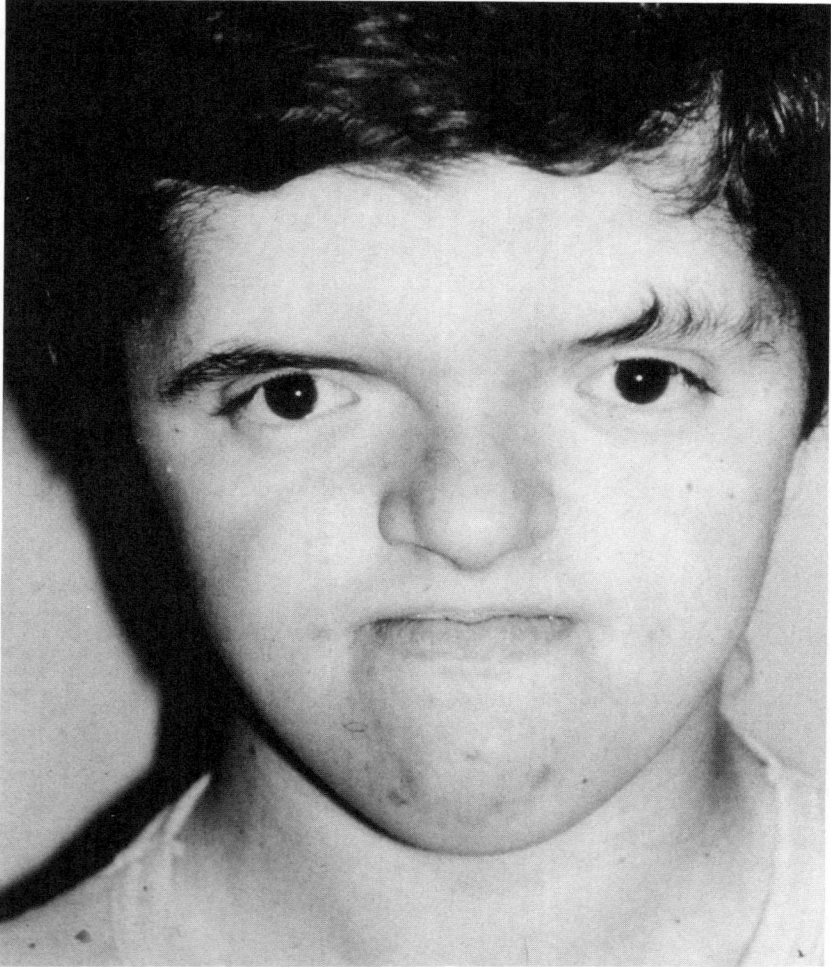

closure. In addition, the other structural deviations may complicate their speech disorders and make them difficult to diagnose and treat. Velopharyngeal incompetency *per se* will not be discussed in this chapter. However, Figures 7-6A and 7-6B show such a patient. This man has

FIGURE 7-4B
Syndactly of Apert's Syndrome.

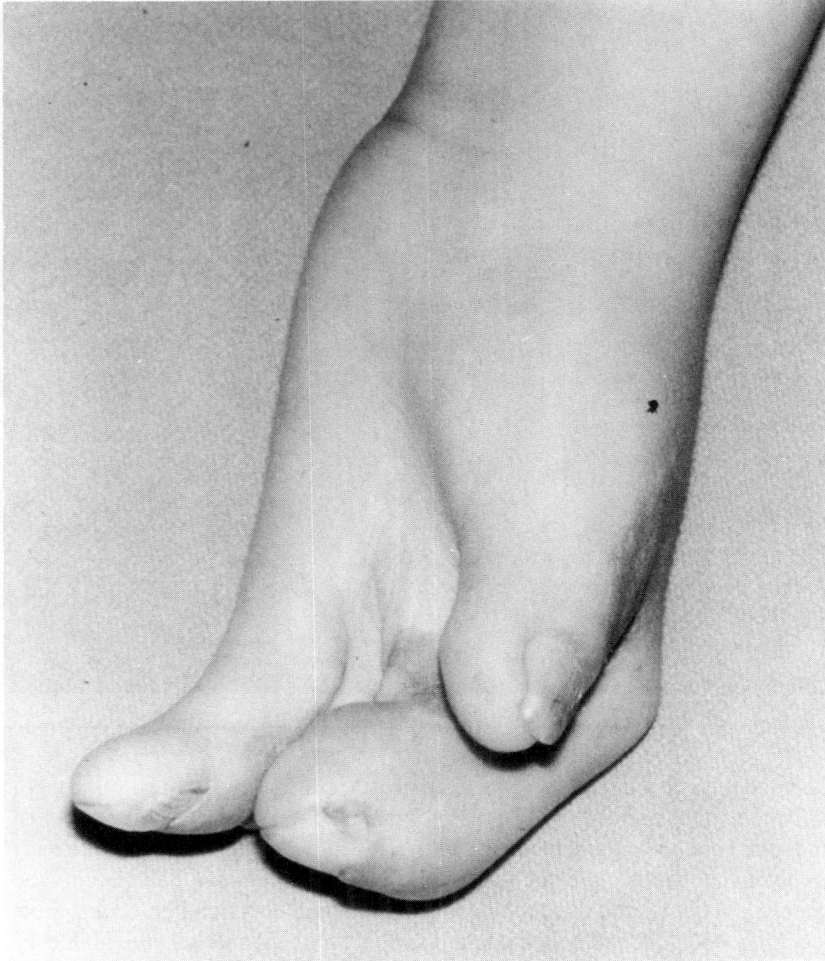

oculoauriculovertebral dysplasia, known also as Goldenhar syndrome. It is thought by some that this may be a variant of hemifacial microsomia (Gorlin, Pindborg, & Cohen, 1976). Birth defects in this patient include *scoliokyphosis* (lateral and posterior curvature of the spine), right upper

FIGURE 7-5A
A patient with a prognathic mandible and marked open bite acquired
as a result of childhood injury.

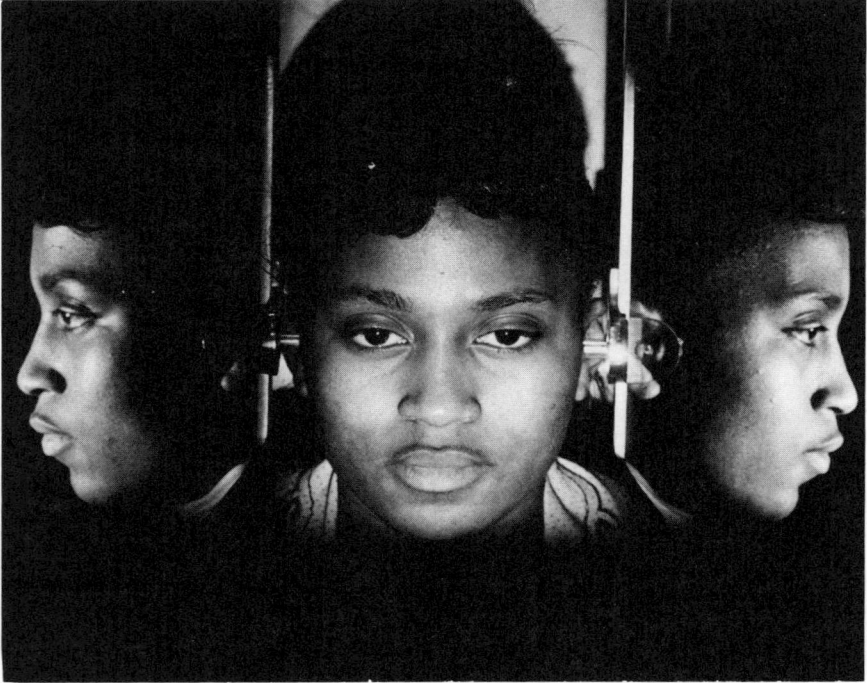

lid ptosis, right auricular tags and microtia, nasal deformities, relative or
real macroglossia, and cleft palate. The problems occurring because of
questionable management of the cleft, and now complicating his already
involved condition, are an oronasal fistula in the soft palate, surgical
removal of the premaxilla, increasing his midfacial deficiency, and a short
upper lip. He also has mild mental retardation but is seen as educable even
though he has spent most of his life in a state institution. Hearing in the
left ear is normal. Speech is unintelligible since he cannot get a lip seal,
cannot produce tongue tip elements, and cannot maneuver his tongue for
consonant production in the limited space available. This man has no consonants that are accurately produced, and he is a poor candidate for therapy
prior to massive facial reconstruction. He is an example of a person who
was probably destined to have disordered speech because of his basic struc-

FIGURE 7-5B
A patient with a prognathic mandible and marked open bite acquired as a result of childhood injury.

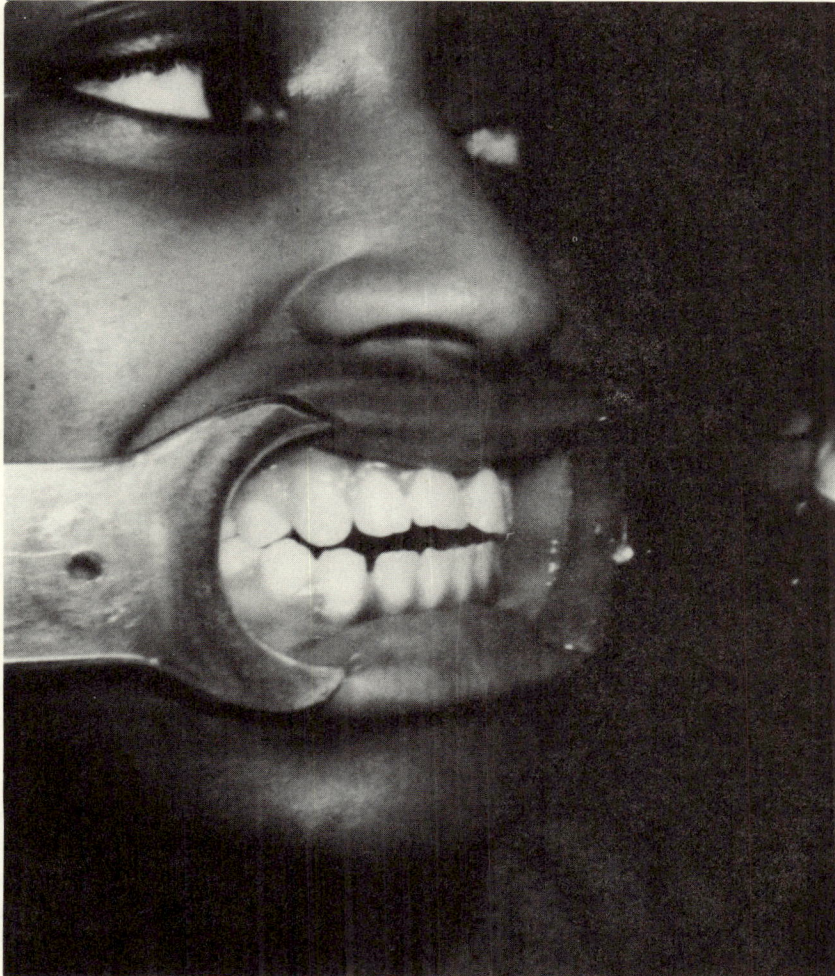

tural deviations but whose problems were exacerbated by the cleft and the way in which it was treated.

Smith (1976) lists various conditions that are associated with specific syndromes. The informed speech-language pathologist should be alerted

FIGURE 7-6A
A patient with Goldenhar Syndrome (oculoauriculovertebral dysplasia).

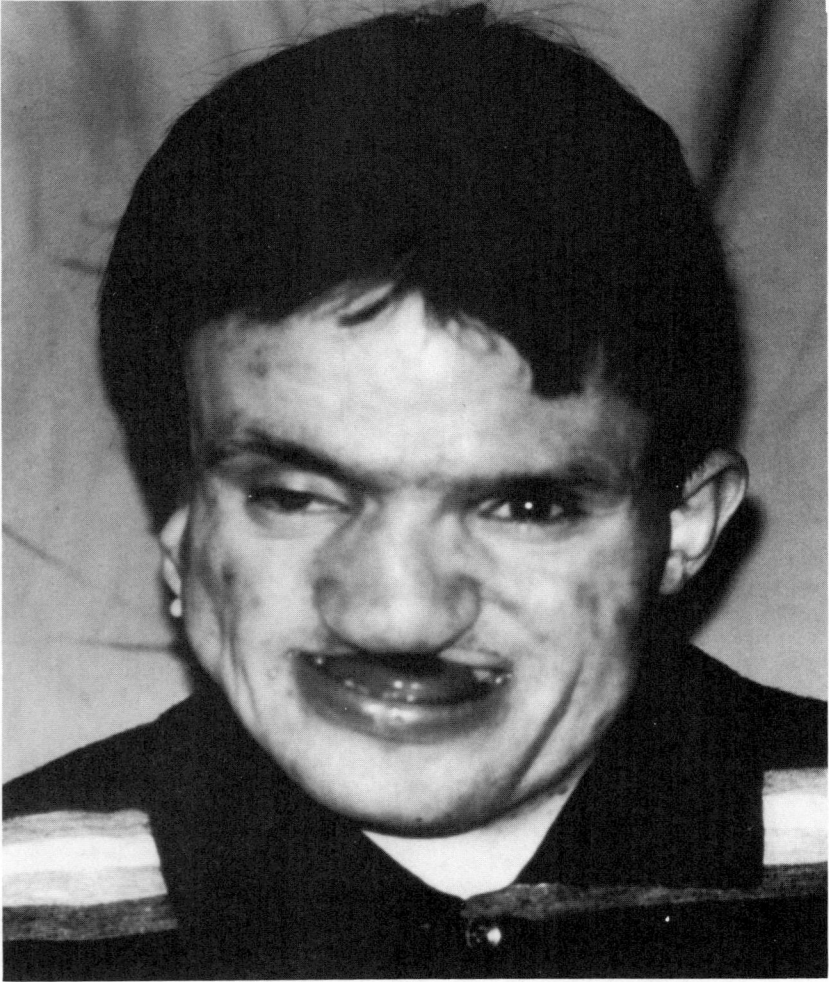

to these symptoms and be ready to investigate them thoroughly. You will note that 36 disorders are associated with "deafness," which includes all degrees of hearing impairment, 73 with some form of ear deformity, and

FIGURE 7-6B
A patient with Goldenhar Syndrome (oculoauriculovertebral dysplasia).

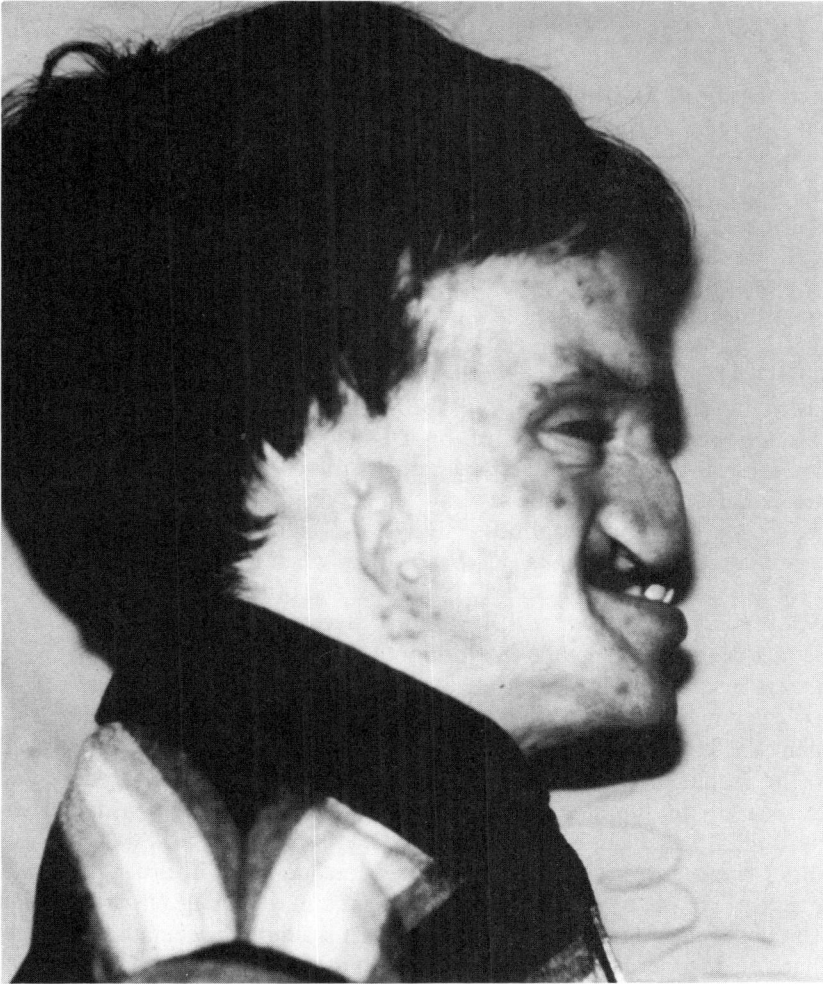

38 with frequent or occasional maxillary hypoplasia, often with a narrow or high-arched palate. Fifty are associated with micrognathia, 6 with prognathism, 4 with *microstomia* (small mouth), 8 with *macrostomia* (greatly

exaggerated mouth width), 7 with cleft or irregular tongue, and 7 with *macroglossia* (excessively large tongue, sometimes filling the oral cavity). Any of these deficits, separately or in combination, may be responsible for communicative defects, especially those involving articulation, even though, within limits, remarkable compensatory ability is demonstrated again and again, clinically. Specifying the exact nature of resulting speech problems is impossible at this time because of the wide range of expressivity seen from one patient to another and, quite simply, because there are a sparsity of published data.

Mental Retardation

The risk of mental retardation in association with craniofacial malformations can be extremely high. Within any given syndrome the degree of retardation may be highly variable, so it is dangerous to make predictions about the intelligence of specific children since they may not be representative of the population trends. However, in Rubinstein-Taybi Syndrome, an IQ range of 17 to 86 suggests that some reduction in intelligence is almost invariable (Smith, 1976) and that the range is from profound retardation through the borderline classification. DeMeyer, Zemon, and Palmer (1964) go so far as to say that "the face predicts the brain." For example, in the median cleft face syndrome, a major characteristic is *hypotelorism* (close-set eyes), and this is almost always associated with brain damage and mental retardation, as is hypertelorism when it is extreme and is the only facial anomaly (DeMeyer, 1967). On the other hand, Russell-Silver syndrome is associated with slow motor development and so may easily be misdiagnosed as mental retardation even though intelligence is almost always normal as, indeed, it is in a number of other syndromes.

When mental retardation is a factor, articulation and language development are likely to reflect the reduced level of functioning, and that aspect of the problem must be weighed against the purely structural components. In view of the hundreds of problems that exist and the high degree of variability present in the expression of these disorders, it is wise to read about the syndrome or anomaly under consideration in order to derive a general picture of the nature of the defect and then to *examine the child* who has it. There is no substitute for that. It is simply inaccurate to assume that *any* disorder is perfectly equated with mental retardation, but it must not be ignored clinically if it exists.

Hearing Impairment

All children who have palatal clefts, whether other abnormalities are present or not, will suffer from otitis media or middle-ear effusions

(Paradise & Bluestone, 1969). Ear deformities are quite common in children with craniofacial variations, and these may result in severe conductive losses or, in some instances, in sensorineural losses. For example, Treacher Collins syndrome, or mandibulofacial dysostosis, is associated with malformation of the auricles, often including atresia, and with defects of the external ear canal. These defects result in conductive hearing losses. Wardenburg syndrome, on the other hand, includes severe bilateral sensorineural hearing loss in about 20% of the cases. When these profound losses are present, the hearing becomes the major problem and tends to diminish the relevance of other abnormalities such as cleft palate or other structural deviations in the oral cavity. Speech and language problems of all kinds will be associated with these syndromes, but they will have multiple causation.

Psychosocial Factors

Communication is an interactional phenomenon and assumes an exchange between and among people. When human relationships are disrupted, communicative skills suffer in some way. A child born with massive defects to which society responds is always at increased risk for psychosocial problems. Society itself may reject him or her in subtle or not-so-subtle ways. If this occurs, the person with the craniofacial malformation may seek partial relief by entering into conversations as infrequently as possible and may refuse to talk at all in some especially threatening situations. The "practice" necessary to perfect speech patterns may not occur if basic human relationships are disrupted. Thus, language delay and articulatory immaturities *may* be accounted for in part by psychosocial immaturity, a sense of worthlessness and loneliness, and inability to handle the social attitudes encountered in day-to-day living. MacGregor (1951) conducted in-depth interviews of 115 patients who required plastic surgery for the correction of varying degrees of facial disfigurement. She concluded that the majority of these patients were dismayed by their own mirror images and that they "saw their handicaps reflected in the reaction of others toward them." They were aware of staring, remarks, curiosity, questioning, pity, rejection, ridicule, whispering, nicknames, and discrimination, all of which made them unhappy and self-conscious. Whether these feelings were based on reality or not is not at issue. They represented the social perceptions of facially disfigured human beings. As such, they cannot be discounted, especially since the majority were viewed also as having adjustment difficulties including feelings of inferiority, self-consciousness, frustration, preoccupation with the deformity, hypersensitivity, anxiety, hostility, paranoia, withdrawal, antisocial states, and psychosis. MacGregor pointed out that the problems of these patients are at least partially traceable to the negative attitudes and prejudices that help both to create and to perpetuate special difficulties for the facially disfigured. Obviously, this is not the most fertile soil in which to nurture communicative skills.

Rusk (1963) also observed that the face is the focus of attention in interpersonal relationships and is the area most closely identified with the intimate, personal entity that one calls "self." He added that people with facial disfigurement encounter countless human and social indignities and deprivations. The literature abounds in similar statements from many other authors (MacGregor, 1951). Nonverbal aspects of communication are also undoubtedly influential since alterations in facial expression may be impaired, and general communicative behavior may be adversely affected.

The speech-language pathologist has a big responsibility to help children with craniofacial deficits find a place in the world and to work with that world to become more caring and accepting. A big job! But perhaps far more relevant than therapy for faulty articulation—important as that is.

Nature of Disordered Speech

Morrees, Burstone, Christiansen, Hixon, and Weinstein (1971) stated that the likelihood of defective speech increases as the number of structural deviations increases. This remains a reasonable statement of the relationship between structure and speech, although that relationship is not a perfect one. Many authors attest to the remarkable ability of speakers to compensate within limits for major structural abnormalities in the vocal tract (Bloomer, 1971; Peterson, 1973). Witzel (Note 3) recognized these compensatory abilities but suggested that there are probably limits beyond which speech will invariably be defective. While these limits are yet to be specified, we recognize the virtual impossibility of normal speech for the young man pictured in Figures 7-6A and 7-6B and previously described.

As noted earlier, one of the barriers to using solid data upon which to make precise determinations is that there is only very limited literature available. Both craniofacial and orthognathic problems (those involving the malpositioning of the bones of the maxilla, mandible, or both) have been incompletely studied, and it has been almost impossible to conduct well-designed prospective studies. Much that has been written is quite general and is plagued by the probability that certain of the patients reported on have been misdiagnosed. This is not surprising when the similarities and subtle differences among many of the syndromes are taken into account (Peterson, 1973). Information about speech has lagged behind that in almost all other areas. In the Smith (1976) work, the word *speech* does not even appear in the index. In Gorlin et al. (1976), the index carries only 2 references under speech and 9 under voice.

Diagnosis

It is clear that the individual suffering from any one of hundreds of craniofacial anomalies associated with speech problems must have a thorough diagnostic evaluation in order to determine as accurately as possible why the speech is in some way defective and if the craniofacial anomaly can be held responsible in whole or in part. Peterson-Falzone (1976) has wisely advised us to keep looking even after we think we have found the answer. In order to decide that the speech is defective because of the structural differences that exist, the speech defect or defects must stand in functional relationship to structure. For example, the protrusion of the tongue during /s/ production in a patient with a marked anterior open bite is reasonable, and the structure and function can logically be related to each other. However, if the same patient had an f/θ substitution, structure would not provide a reasonable explanation for the error, since the tongue is physically capable of articulating with the anterior teeth.

The diagnostic process is essential, too, because given syndromes show wide variations, and the only valid approach to treating resulting speech problems is on an individual basis relating structure and function to the speech pattern that exists. Even if it were possible to describe the speech commonly associated with specific syndromes, a full-length textbook would be necessary to cover the hundreds of variations that would have to be included. In addition, the data are too sparse to make that practical. Instead, the speech-language pathologist is urged to acquire a standard reference on syndromes (Cohen, 1978; Gorlin et al., 1976; Smith, 1981) and to use it diligently as an index of structural variations encountered clinically. Only by very careful case documentation can we ever hope to have more useful data than we have today.

A helpful reference in learning to make significant observations is a 1980 article by Salinas. He points out in the introduction to his systematic examination format that orofacial abnormalities occur in approximately 25% of Mendelian syndromes, in virtually all of the chromosomal disorders, and in several multifactoral disorders. This is an impressive array of disorders that can affect speech, but speech pathologists are only now becoming active in recognizing these important structural variations and in participating on and cooperating with management teams.

Appropriate to this attitude regarding diagnosis is the work of Bloomer and Hawk (1973). They describe the speech mechanism as a tube extending from the laryngopharynx to a bifurcation at the nasopharynx and proceeding via its oral and nasal pathways. Within this simple tubal system, musculoskeletal valves close, constrict, and open to regulate the breathstream and the laryngeally generated sound. These valves influence air pressure, modify and direct energy and airflow, and modify vocal resonance for the production of vowels and consonants. Impairment of the ability to achieve adequate valving anyplace in the system may be responsible for defective speech. Writing about ablative surgery of the face and of the oral and pharyngeal cavities, Bloomer and Hawk (1973) stress the importance of knowing (1) the sites and types of lesions which may impair speech, (2) the nature of the disturbed speech which may follow, and (3) the means for modifying the speech. These same three necessities sum up what is required to understand speech deviations standing in functional relationship to structural deviations. In speech disorders resulting from craniofacial problems, the structures that will be responsible are those to which the important speech pathway is related.

These structures may include the face; the oral, pharyngeal, and nasal cavities; dentition; palate; and tongue. Bloomer (1971), the first to write comprehensively about such problems, refers to them as *orofacial abnormalities*. He includes in his description all the tissues of the orofacial complex—supporting structures of cartilage and bone, teeth, muscles, tendons, motor and sensory nerves, glandular and soft tissue, and skin.

Articulation Errors Associated with Severe Malocclusions

Most of the major craniofacial abnormalities involve some type of serious malocclusion, and it is the malocclusion that appears to be most intimately related to the articulatory problems which occur. These dental and skeletal relationships have been variously classified, often according to Angle (1899). In a Class I occlusion, the mesiobuccal cusp of the maxillary first molar rides comfortably in the buccal groove of the mandibular first molar, and the maxilla is just slightly larger than the mandible. This type of dental relationship is unremarkable and is not usually directly or indirectly responsible for speech problems. The exception to this is when missing or malplaced individual teeth interfere with tongue movement or placement, or when there is an open bite. Angle's Class II occlusion is represented by the mesiobuccal cusp of the maxillary first molar being anterior to the buccal groove of the mandibular first molar. Thus, the maxillary teeth are seen as protrusive to the mandibular. In a Class III relationship, the reverse occurs, and the mandibular teeth are anterior to the maxillary. When there is an opening between the maxillary and mandibular incisors, an *open bite* results. These occlusal patterns may relate only to teeth or to their underlying bony support as well. For example, in mandibular retrognathia the mandible is too small in relation to the maxilla, while in prognathia the mandible is too large to relate well to the maxilla. These problems may also occur as the maxilla interacts with the mandible. Visual examination without cephalometric measurements may be quite misleading. A mandible that appears to be prognathic may actually be of normal size, while a maxilla that is too small is responsible for the "pseudoprognathism." Figures 7-7A (Sassouni, Note 4) and 7-7B (Sassouni, 1969) show variations found in many craniofacial disorders and in orthognathic problems.

It is clear that occlusal variations of minor degree cannot usually be held responsible for speech problems. Many studies have failed to find a relationship (Bernstein, 1956; VanThal, 1935). Others (Bloomer, 1971; Van Riper, 1972) have observed that there is an amazing human ability to compensate even for severe malocclusions.

However, in severe Class II or Class III malocclusions, either with or without open bite, there may be difficulty with lip approximation in connected speech and even with the production of labiodental phonemes. Bilabials may be produced labiodentally if that maneuver can be executed, or /f/ and /v/ may sometimes be produced by action of the lower teeth against the upper lip. In extreme cases, the tongue articulating with the upper teeth may be a substitute gesture. There is a tendency for compensatory efforts to become more bizarre and less successful as the deformities become more and more severe (Bloomer, 1971).

Sibilant phonemes may also be adversely affected in Class II and Class III occlusions and in open bites. The tongue may be carried too low, it may be retruded (Guay, Maxwell, & Beecher, 1978), or the oral port opening may be too large (Klechak, Bradley, & Warren, 1976). Sibilant articulation will obviously be the most sensitive to these occlusal problems as the tongue seeks an appropriate intraoral target that is too far forward, too far back, or altered by an open-bite relationship which destroys the vertical directional behavior of the tongue as well as the horizontal. Bilabial and labiodental consonants appear to have much greater tolerance for these variations than have sibilants.

The majority of orthodontic problems can be treated successfully by the orthodontist without the necessity of extraordinary measures. A small group of such patients, however, and these include those with craniofacial and severe facial anomalies, must be managed surgically, if at all. Witzel (Note 3) reported on 111 such patients prior to and following surgery for

FIGURE 7-7A
Variations found in craniofacial disorders and orthognathic problems.

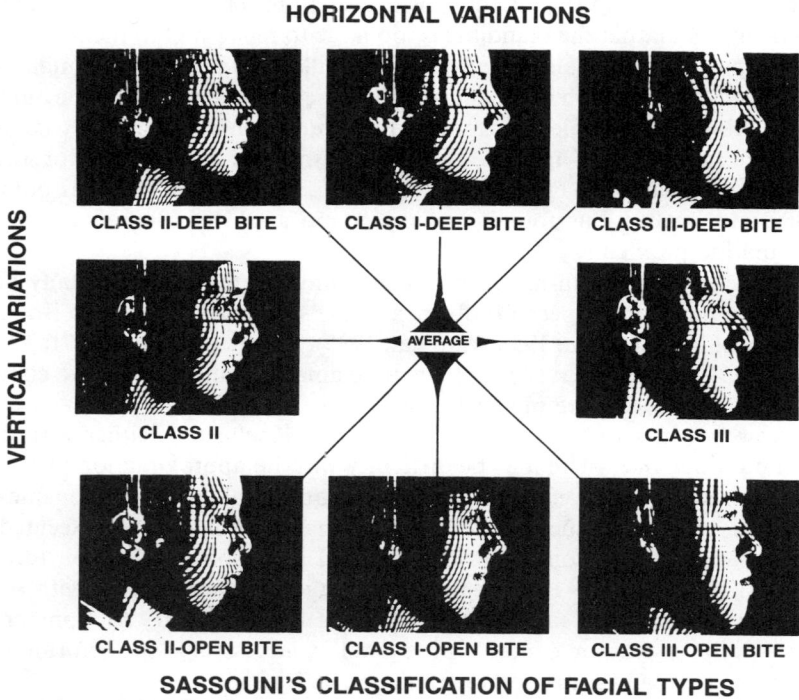

HORIZONTAL VARIATIONS

VERTICAL VARIATIONS

| CLASS II-DEEP BITE | CLASS I-DEEP BITE | CLASS III-DEEP BITE |

AVERAGE

CLASS II   CLASS III

CLASS II-OPEN BITE   CLASS I-OPEN BITE   CLASS III-OPEN BITE

SASSOUNI'S CLASSIFICATION OF FACIAL TYPES

their orthognathic problems of a skeletal nature. None of these was identified as having particular syndromes. She administered the 141-item Templin-Darley Test of Articulation (1969) and, based on the literature indicating most difficulty with sibilants, labiodentals and bilabials, used 3 subtests of 39, 10, and 21 items, respectively. Prior to surgery, 54% of 41 subjects in Group A (patients who did not require Le Fort I osteotomies) had articulation errors of some type. This percentage was reduced to 20% following surgery with no speech therapeutic intervention. Prior to surgery, 46% of the subjects had sibilant errors (most on /s/ and /z/), and this became 17% after surgery, again without speech therapy. Only 15% of the subjects had bilabial errors before their operations and only 3% afterward. Five percent had labiodental errors at the start of treatment and none at its completion.

FIGURE 7-7B
Variations found in craniofacial disorders and orthognathic problems.

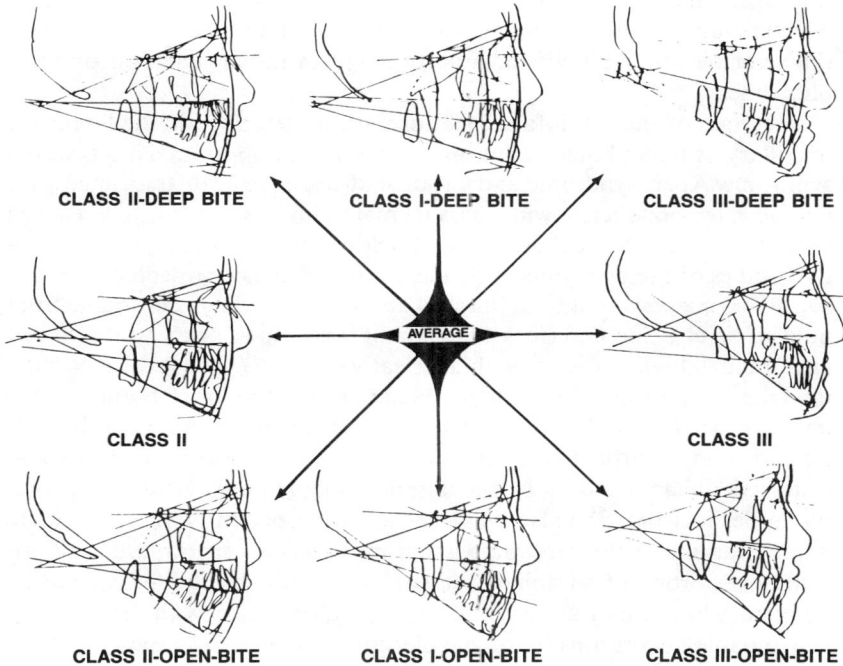

The 70 subjects in Group B required the more complex Le Fort I procedure, which is designed to reposition the maxilla by moving it forward and tilting it appropriately to correct for midfacial deficiency. Seventy-four percent of these subjects had articulation errors prior to surgery, and 36% retained errors following surgery. Sibilants were disordered in 70% before surgery and in 30% afterward. Again labiodental and bilabial errors were infrequent, both occurring in 8.6% of the sample. These latter errors were reduced to 2.7% and 4.3% after surgery.

Forty-two of these 70 subjects also had palatal clefts. It is interesting that 71% of the subjects with clefts had sibilant errors before their Le Fort I procedures and that 43% retained their errors following surgery, as opposed to 21% of the 69% of noncleft subjects with sibilant distortions.

On the other hand, neither labiodental nor bilabial errors occurred either before or following surgery in the cleft subjects.

It is apparent from this study that sibilant articulation, occurring as it does at a valve created normally between the tongue tip and the midportion of the maxillary arch, is highly vulnerable to extreme abnormalities which require surgery and that correcting the structural deficits more often than not results in significant improvement in the articulation of these phonemes.

In certain of the craniofacial malformations described in the literature, maxillary or mandibular deviations, or both, are important aspects of the syndrome. Apert syndrome and Crouzon disease are both associated with midfacial hypoplasia and with Class III malocclusions, often with a reduced oronasal airway. While there are no developmental, or even good descriptive studies of these patients available, clinical evidence presented by Peterson (1973) suggests that both physical and speech findings may range from mild to severe. She describes one patient with Apert who produced /f/ as a lingualabial, /v/ as a bilabial fricative, and /t/ and /d/ by holding the anterior portion of the tongue blade against the lower border of the upper incisors. I would suspect, from the picture incorporated in the article and from the articulation errors described, that he would also have had distorted sibilants caused by the anterior tongue blade articulating with the upper incisors. She also describes a second patient with more severe manifestations of the syndrome and a more serious speech problem, including distortion of all sibilants and affricates, which could be considered obligatory because of the severe Class III malocclusion with the resulting unavoidable aberrations in tongue placement. Figure 7-2 shows a patient with Apert syndrome and the midfacial retrusion leading to these errors.

Crouzon syndrome (Figure 7-3) is a disorder akin to Apert, but is less severe in its manifestations. These patients do not have the syndactyly of hands and feet associated with Apert. They do have similar, but less severe, craniofacial features, however. They may have essentially normal speech, mild disorders with little or no relationship to their abnormal oral features, or defective speech that seems to be directly related to their structural variations. Peterson (1973) describes 2 mildly involved children and 1 severely impaired child who was required to carry his head in an extended position in order to maintain an airway for breathing. He demonstrated oral distortions of sibilants, both fricatives and affricates, and inconsistent distortions of /r/ and /I/—most of which appeared to be related to abnormal tongue placement necessitated by faulty mandible-tongue-maxilla relationships.

We support Peterson's findings from observations of our own cases. A brother and sister and twin brothers all demonstrated anteriorly distorted sibilants. Figures 7-3A and 7-3B show one of the twin boys. Our cases all had denasalized /m/, /n/, and /ŋ/ in association with mouth breathing, necessitated by the reduction in size of the pharyngeal space.

Elfenbein, Waziri, and Morris (1981) reported on the speech characteristics of 6 children, 4 with Apert, 1 with Crouzon, and 1 with Saethre-Chotzen syndrome. One of the subjects with Apert had no speech and appeared to be severely retarded. All of the others had sibilant distortions, and all but 1 had affricate problems. The authors conclude that these articulatory deviations are the logical result of the oral-structural anomalies. It would be difficult to argue otherwise.

The midfacial deficiency seen in both Apert and Crouzon and the forward-riding tongue associated with the poorly related maxilla and mandible, lead almost universally to sibilant errors. While other errors may also be present as previously described, they are far overshadowed by these marked sibilant, which appear to respond minimally to speech therapy as long as the oral structures remain poorly related. Research is needed before we will be able to do more than rely on clinical experience, which can sometimes be misleading.

Two brothers with otopalatodigital syndrome (Figures 7-8A and B and 7-9A and B) serve to highlight the articulation errors associated with this x-linked, recessively inherited disorder. The usual patient is male with a prominent, overhanging forehead, prominent supraorbital ridges, antimongoloid slant, ocular hypertelorism, broad depressed nasal bridge, midfacial flattening, mild retardation, retarded skeletal maturation, malformed fingers and toes with variable curvatures, cleft palate, small oral cavity, and conductive hearing loss. The older of the 2 cases presented here is 18 years old. He demonstrates a severe open bite with malocclusion, midfacial deficiency, incomplete cleft of the secondary palate, small oral opening and oral cavity, and moderate retardation requiring special education. His speech is of low volume and somewhat monotonous, and sibilants are palatalized with the anterior tongue protruding into the space created by the open bite. He is intelligible, but the speech problem is noticeable.

The younger brother is 10 years of age. His physical characteristics are similar to his brother's, but less severe. He retains minor immaturities in his speech pattern, notably f/θ. Aside from those problems, his speech mirrors that of his brother with the addition of "muffling," seemingly a result of the small oral port and cavity. Once again, the relevance of oral structures is emphasized.

It is appropriate to point out here that children born with cleft palates, with or without one of the 154 syndromes which may include some form of clefting, are also prime candidates for these highly complex occlusal

FIGURE 7-8A
Patient, age 18, with otopalatodigital syndrome.

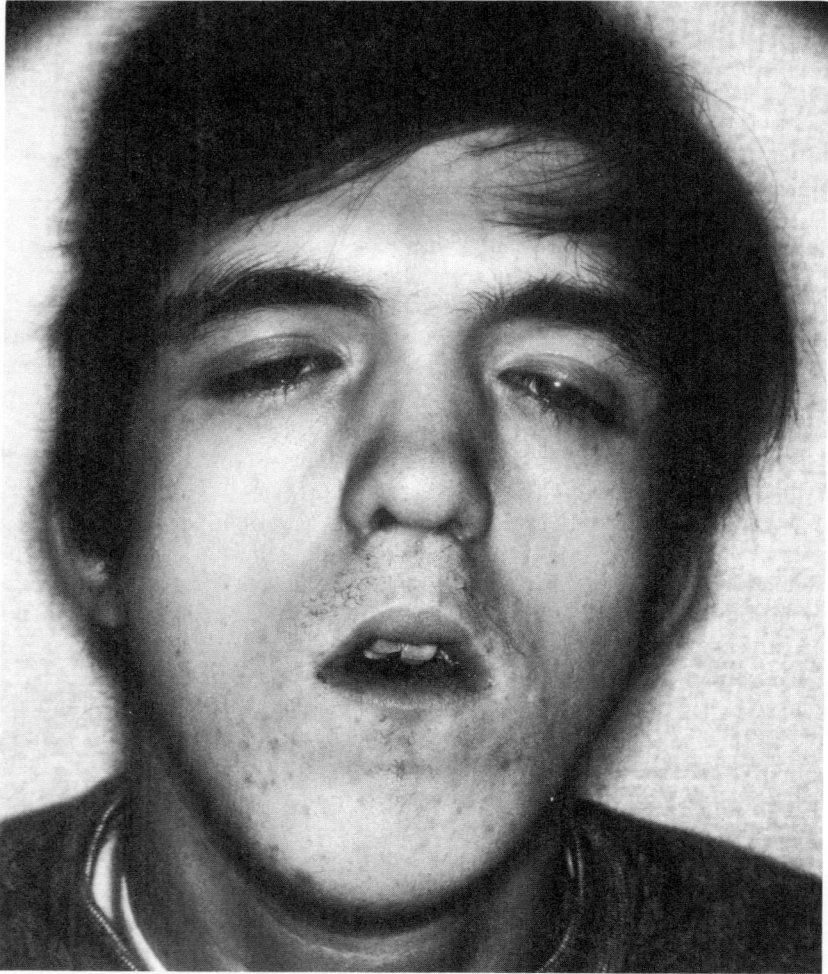

problems, and their speech will have the potential to be similarly affected.
It will be necessary in those cases for the clinician to make the distinction
between distortions caused by velopharyngeal incompetency and those

FIGURE 7-8B
Patient, age 18, with otopalatodigital syndrome.

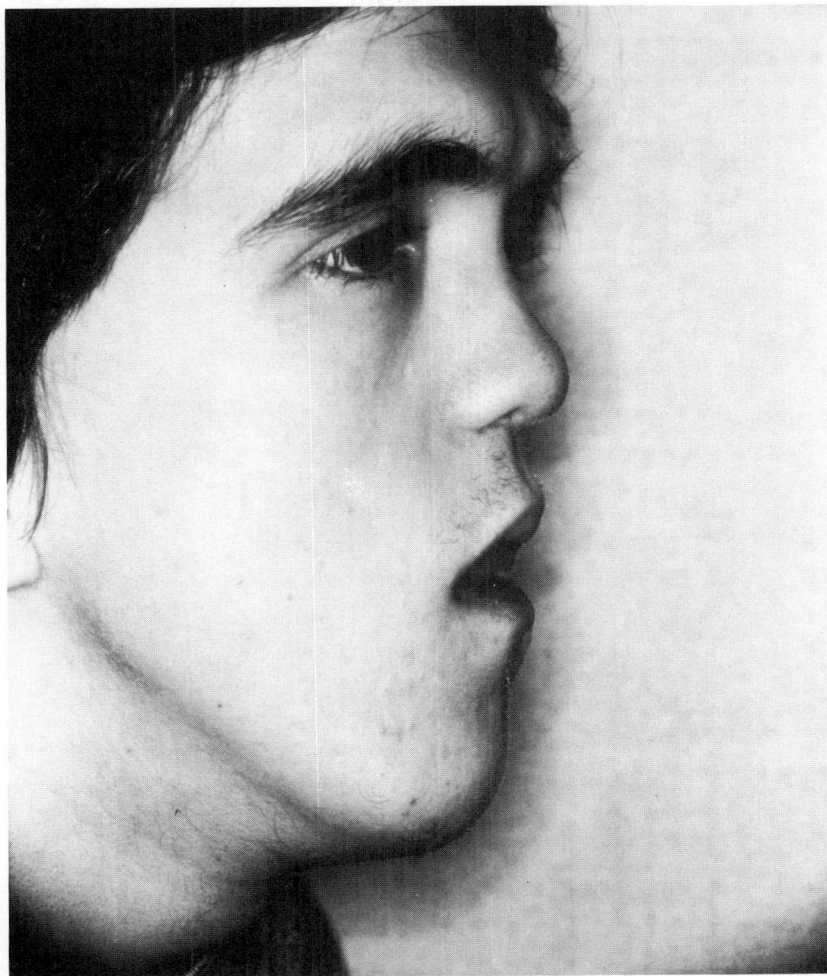

related at least in part to maxillary-mandibular relationships. Complicating the diagnosis and management of such children will also by the high occurrence of cross bite and mising teeth as is seen in Figure 7-10. These dental

FIGURE 7-9A
Patient, age 10, with otopalatodigital syndrome (brother of patient shown in Figures 7-8A and 7-8B).

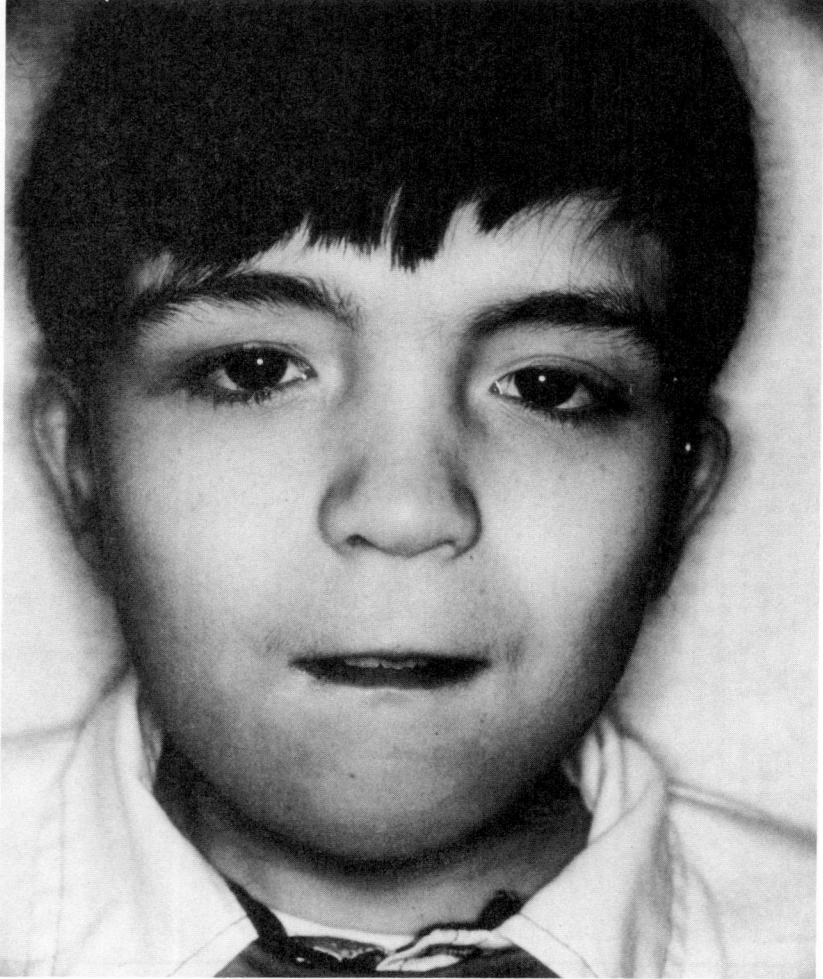

relationships may contribute to frontal distortions of sibilants with the tongue finding its way primarily into the large space on the right and secondarily into the smaller space on the left.

FIGURE 7-9B
Patient, age 10, with otopalatodigital syndrome (brother of patient shown in Figures 8A and 8B).

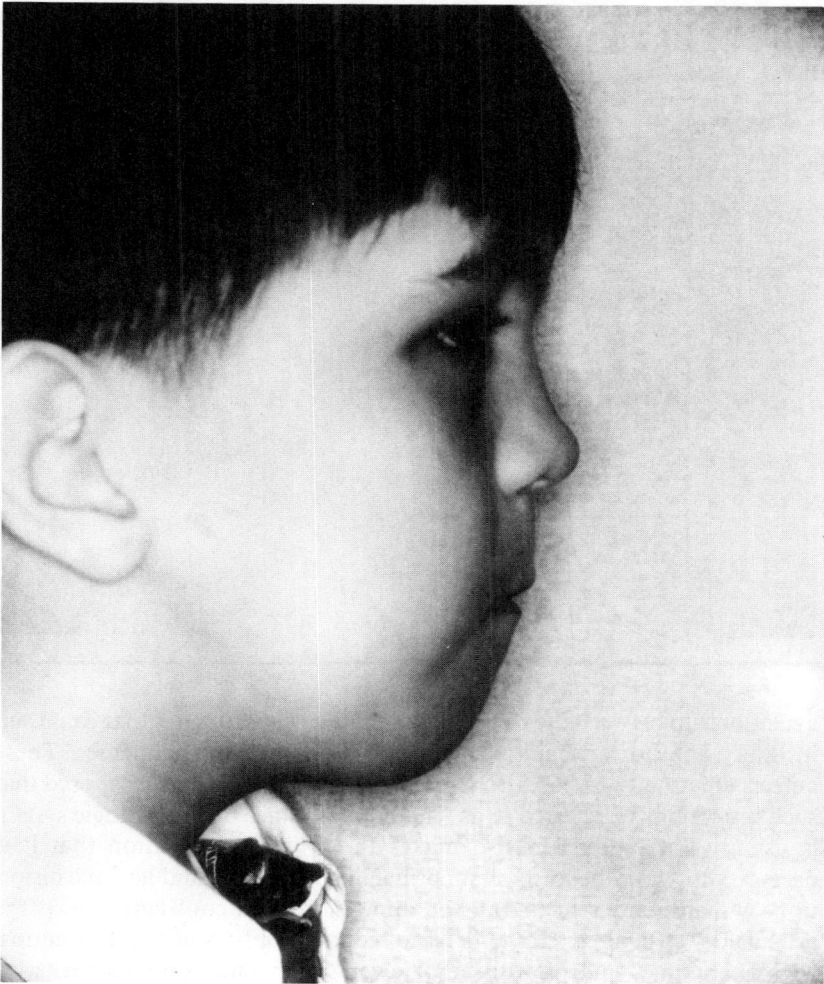

It is important for the student to be aware that any craniofacial or orthognathic abnormality that results in a marked discrepancy between the maxilla and the mandible or in an open bite has the potential for creating

FIGURE 7-10
An example of cross bite and missing teeth.

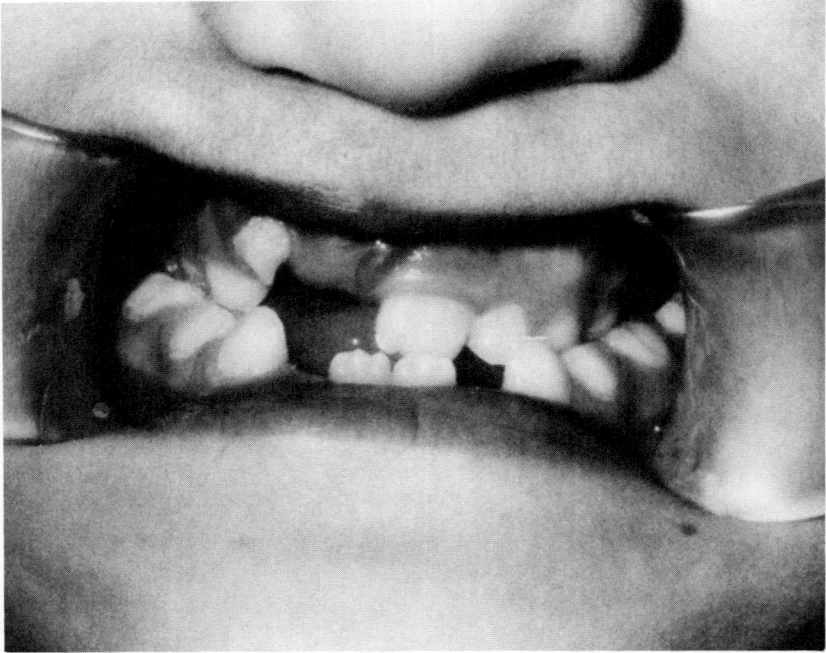

a relationship between the tongue and the aberrant structures that can result in faulty anterior articulation, particularly of sibilant phonemes. These defects are usually of the distortion type. Bloomer (1971) has proposed that such distortions be referred to as "malphones," since the phonologic system is usually not faulty. He also makes the critical observation that it is necessary to know the form of abnormal lingual valving and how the distortion or malphone is related to the dimensions and configuration of the articulatory structures. This requires, of course, careful study and diagnosis; and there is a margin of error even when such instruments as videofluoroscopy are used. However, it is necessary for the speech pathologist to think in far more precise terms than has been true with traditional articulation testing. It is not enough to recognize that there are articulatory distortions in these cases. It is necessary to know as much as possible about the how and why of the deviations under consideration.

Articulation Errors Associated with Lingual Anomalies

Certain of the craniofacial disorders include variations in the structure of the tongue. These are considerably less likely to occur than are the structural deformities discussed in the previous section, and even less is understood about their relationship to speech and how they should be treated.

There is considerable evidence that an absent or rudimentary tongue may have only minimal effects on speech (Bloomer, 1971; Gorlin et al., 1976; Peterson-Falzone, 1976). However, Bloomer notes the distortion of sibilants in a 13-year-old girl with a small tongue. Amazing compensatory behaviors have been described for a tongueless speaker by Eskew and Shepard (1949). Smith (1976) lists no syndromes associated with aglossia or microglossia, while Gorlin et al. (1976) describe two cases of Moebius syndrome, one with a "small tongue" and the other with "atrophy of the tongue" from birth. Since these patients have bilateral facial paralysis, their speech is usually disordered and can be described as dysarthric. It would be difficult to determine the role of the size of the tongue in these cases.

Hemiatrophy of the tongue is usually seen in hemifacial atrophy (Gorlin et al., 1976). This disorder, progressive in nature, also includes atrophy of the face on the affected side with resulting severe malocclusion. These cases are complex and usually are complicated by Jacksonian epilepsy. Speech problems have not been described, but they are likely to relate both to dysarthria and to the often severe occlusal manifestations.

Macroglossia, or an enlarged tongue, appears to pose a greater threat to speech than does a rudimentary or small tongue. Beckwith-Wiedmann syndrome (Gorlin et al., 1976) is characterized by macroglossia as a major symptom which often leads to respiratory and feeding difficulties in infancy. The syndrome is also marked by omphalocele, enlargement of the viscera, cytomegaly of the adrenal cortex, accelerated skeletal maturation, prominent eyes and occiput, mandibular prognathism and open bite (may be secondary to large tongue), hypoglycemia in early infancy, among others. Growth of the oral cavity is sometimes enough to accommodate the tongue, but partial glossectomy may be necessary. In this and other conditions where the tongue fills the oral cavity, speech may be seriously impaired because there is no space for articulation to occur. In addition, the oral cavity may be so constricted that voice will be muffled. Children with macroglossia may be intelligent and have excellent language development. One case known to the writer, however, had unintelligible speech with articulatory variations on all consonants. The tongue filled the entire available space so that the lips could not be approximated for labial consonants, which were produced by action between the upper lip and the massive blade of the tongue. No compensation was possible because of the enormity of the tongue. Surgery is required in these extreme cases.

Certain syndromes with enlarged tongue may be complicated by a high incidence of mental retardation as in several of the mucopolysaccharidoses, mucolipidoses, and related disorders (Gorlin et al., 1976). Hurler syndrome is an example.

Summary

Speech defects emerging out of the complicated craniofacial disabilities now receiving increasing clinical attention may be explained partially on the basis of associated hearing losses, mental retardation, and psychosocial factors including societal responses to the disorders. Speech problems may be related also to the malformation of oral structures, which may be too seriously impaired to permit normal speech.

Articulation disorders associated with congenital malformations of the craniofacial complex tend to be distortions of sibilants related to dental or skeletal malocclusions, particularly when open bit is present. Labials may be affected when the lips cannot be approximated, and nasals may be essentially eliminated when the size of the pharyngeal space is significantly diminished. An excessively large tongue will usually be more of a hazard to speech than will a very small or rudimentary tongue and may seriously reduce intelligibility.

While the human organism is unquestionably capable of amazing feats of compensation, there are physical limitations beyond which speech therapy is not a useful mode of treatment in the absence of surgical alteration of the impaired structures. On the other hand, there is evidence to show speech improvement following such surgery without intervention by the speech pathologist. Thus the speech pathologist must know when to recommend speech therapy, when to refer for consultation and other forms of intervention including surgical and orthodontic, and how to work in concert with specialized clinics providing the necessary care.

Speech Therapy

Introduction

As we have already suggested, speech therapy in the presence of these massive oral deformities is almost never effective. Correction of the defect, insofar as that is possible, is the first stage of treatment. As we have also shown, these alterations are sometimes followed by spontaneous changes of a positive nature in speech. However, such improvement does not occur universally, and speech therapy may be required. Unfortunately, there are almost no data available about speech therapy for communication deficits associated with craniofacial or orofacial anomalies.

Social-Interactional Therapy

Long and Dalson (1982) found that 1-year-old infants with cleft palates, a group not specifically addressed in this chapter, were significantly less likely to pair gestural and vocal behaviors than were noncleft children. The authors speculated that there may be a stage in development when nonspecific vocalizations become attached to gestures of communicative value to the child and that children with clefts are deficient in this regard.

The failure of these children to make transitions of this type could point to early disruption in social interaction. While there is only limited research in relation to children with clefts, and none concerning children with craniofacial problems, the information that is available supports our view that infant stimulation and socialization programs of various sorts are highly desirable for most children with facial disfigurement.

Parent Training

It is our philosophy that therapy should emerge out of a careful diagnostic evaluation and that it should be planned so that the desired goals can be accomplished as simply and quickly as possible. Formal therapy should never be undertaken if informal techniques and encouragement will enable a child to function at his or her maximum capacity. Thus, it is logical to educate parents so that they can help to modify the child's interactive environment, if that is necessary, and can capitalize on opportunities in daily living to enhance communication. Parent training of this type can result in parents who read to their children, understand the advantages of listening and responding when their children "read" or talk to them, parallel talk as their children play, increase life experiences, encourage peer interaction, foster independence, and reinforce and expand on communicative attempts. In short, the child must learn about, and be rewarded for, interacting verbally with others. This *learning* is of both a cognitive and a pragmatic nature and encompasses the child's feeling system.

We know of no formal approaches that have been suggested for the parents of children with craniofacial problems. Hahn (1979) recommended a 4-session series for the parents of children with clefts, and this system has elements in it that can be modified for children with other facial anomalies.

The first session occurs when the child is an infant and is designed to acquaint the parents with the normal speech mechanism and its function and the way in which their child's structure differs. They are helped to understand normal speech and language development and are taught by the speech pathologist to interact and to enter into vocal play with their infant. They are encouraged to allow the child time for response and to reinforce responses when they occur. The parents are taught to use single words strongly, clearly, and repetitiously quite early in the child's life, as the situation determines their appropriateness. The parents are expected to begin verbal stimulation immediately after the first session, and they are informed that the speech pathologist will provide additional help in future sessions.

The second session occurs when the child is 12 months old. The clinician again demonstrates procedures, this time incorporating single key words presented and stressed in the context of simple statements and questions. At this time the parents are encouraged to widen the child's experiences and to describe them in simple terms. Since infants with clefts often have palatal surgery at about 1 year of age, the surgery and its effects on speech development are also discussed.

The third session is 6 to 8 weeks after surgery, and it stresses the child's imitation of initial consonants. The parents stimulate single words until the baby uses a few words spontaneously. Then they are instructed to stimulate 2-word combinations. The parents are taught to use reinforcers such as words of approval, candy, or kisses. We prefer social reinforcers since communication is a social function.

The fourth session is planned when the child is about 3½, at which time the importance of a peer group is emphasized along with planning to help the child understand the nature of his or her physical impairment. (We prefer both of these latter activities to be ongoing from birth.) If formal speech therapy is required, it is implemented at this time.

The important aspects of this program for those with craniofacial anomalies lie in its stress on the normal developmental patterns of children. The program can be modified for children according to their needs and extended for parents who cannot manage without regular support from the speech pathologist. On the other hand, extreme care must be exercised to avoid conditioning parents to respond to their children as if speech problems are inevitable. This attitude can be detrimental rather than helpful. In reality, the goal is to assist parents to do well what all parents should be doing with young children. If the parents are doing well on their own, reinforce their efforts! Avoid intervention that may lead them to think they are not handling the situation satisfactorily.

Other detailed programs of this type have been described by Philips (1979) and Brookshire, Lynch, and Fox (1980). All of these systems of therapy relate to the developmental landmarks seen in normal children. It is essential that undue anxiety not be triggered in parents whose children are developing slowly. Thus, any activities undertaken should begin at the child's own developmental level and should not be too demanding too early. For this reason, it is necessary to provide for a complete developmental assessment before deciding to undertake any therapy. In addition, the goal is always to help the child derive satisfaction out of communicative experiences so that he or she will be comfortable and at ease in any situation. Avoid any activity which the parents and child do not enjoy!

Play Groups
Irwin and McWilliams (1974) and Tisza, Irwin, and Scheide (1973) used various types of play therapy, including a great deal of creative dramatics with cleft children. They learned that the children had initial difficulty with expression of feelings but that they were finally able to reveal unconscious conflicts, which could then be treated or controlled in a make-believe world so that helplessness was minimized. This approach to improving communicative skills and to increasing verbal output can and should be incorporated into the techniques regularly used by speech pathologists.

Preschool Programs
Preschools of various sorts are highly desirable for children with facial disfigurement provided the teachers are informed, understanding people who will encourage and provide opportunities for children to relate to each other and who understand the semantics of disfigurement and the subtle ways in which children who are different can be rejected completely or maneuvered into marginal positions within the group. A skillful teacher assisted by informed parents and insightful speech pathologists can minimize the negative potential that is always present and create, instead, a warm, understanding environment in which communicative skills are nurtured and fostered.

Articulation Therapy
When articulation errors remain 3 months postoperatively, diagnostic evaluation should be carried out to be certain that the structure, often falling short of the ideal, is compatible with improved articulation. If it

is, then articulation therapy, usually stressing placement, is indicated. Postoperatively, articulation therapy for these patients does not differ from articulation therapy for any other group, with the possible exception of the stress on placement. This emphasis is essential since the original speech pattern was acquired in an abnormal oral environment to which the speaker had to adapt as well as he or she was able. With the change in the oral environment, it is not unusual for the individual to maintain, sometimes with difficulty, the preoperative pattern. Thus, the old habits must be eliminated and replaced by new articulatory behaviors—a far-from-easy task, especially in children over the age of 8 and in adults.

A word of caution is necessary relative to the outcome of articulation therapy for individuals with defects of oral structures. Prognosis is always dependent on anatomy and physiology, and it is often necessary to accept less than perfect speech as the best that can be achieved. It is incumbent on the speech pathologist, therefore, to understand the relationship of function to structure and to learn early to make valid judgments. Otherwise, people who are doing as well as they can will be subjected to useless therapy, or those who can improve may be denied the help they require.

Therapy for Resonance Disorders

Hyponasality

Hyponasality is usually caused by resistance in the nasal airway or at its entrance. When this occurs in association with such problems as a shallow pharynx and midfacial deficiency, it is often eliminated when the airway is opened up by maxillary advancement, adenoidectomy, or any other procedure designed to enlarge the space. Speech therapy is not the solution prior to surgery, and it is not usually required after surgery. If, in rare cases, an individual has a patent airway but continues to close off the airway during the production of nasals in an effort to maintain speech as it was preoperatively, articulation therapy may be safely undertaken. The warning here is that the speech pathologist must be secure in the knowledge that the airway *is* open.

Hypernasality

After midfacial advancement, some patients may develop hypernasality as the result of the deepening of the pharyngeal space. When this occurs, it is necessary that there be a complete assessment of the velopharyngeal valve. This can best be done in a multidisciplinary cleft palate clinic equipped to evaluate the valve during function. If incompetence is present, surgical correction will be required. If speech was normal prior to the maxillary advancement, the prognosis is favorable.

Sometimes, following a pharyngeal flap, residual incompetence remains. If it is unequivocal, there is very little that can be accomplished by speech therapy, and a secondary surgical procedure may be required. If closure is inconsistent, that is, if the valve is successful in separating the oral from the nasal cavity on some speech tasks but not on others, or if closure can be obtained during blowing or whistling as observed on multiview videofluoroscopy or through a transnasal endoscope, speech therapy can *sometimes* be helpful. The therapy procedures described by Shprintzen, McCall, and Skolnick (1975) are recommended. This is a detailed therapy program which makes use of operant procedures performed systematically, moving from the task on which closure is achieved to speech activities at increasing levels of difficulty, until the hypernasality has been eliminated and the inconsistent valving has become consistent. This therapy is suitable only for those subjects who meet the criteria and may be unsuccessful even for some of them. However, it is worth trying under the proper circumstances.

Speech pathologists should understand that speech therapy should probably not be undertaken at all for at least 3 months following a pharyngeal flap procedure and that spontaneous speech improvement may continue for about 1 year after surgery.

Concluding Remarks

Individuals with craniofacial and orofacial malformations are often not candidates for speech therapy either before or after corrective surgery. Therapy, when it is indicated, must be based on evidence that the structure is compatible with better speech than is being produced. If that is the case, therapy for these patients does not differ in any remarkable way from speech therapy in general.

Reference Notes

1. McWilliams, B. J. Learning disorders in children with Pierre Robin syndrome. In preparation.

2. Gorlin, R. J. Clefts in syndromes. Paper presented at the Annual Convention of the American Cleft Palate Association, Phoenix, 1972.

3. Witzel, M. A. Orthognathic defects and surgical corrections: The effects on speech and velopharyngeal function. Unpublished doctoral dissertation. The University of Pittsburgh, 1981.

4. Sassouni, V. Sassouni's classification of facial types, University of Pittsburgh, Unpublished.

References

Angle, E. H. Classification of malocclusion. *Dental Cosmos,* 1899, *41,* 248–264.

Bernstein, M. Relation of speech defects and malocclusion. *Alpha Omegan,* 1956, *50,* 90–97.

Bloomer, H. H. Speech defects associated with dental malocclusions and related abnormalities. In L. E. Travis (Ed.), *Handbook of speech pathology and audiology.* New York: Appleton-Century-Crofts, 1971.

Bloomer, H. H., & Hawk, A. M. Speech considerations: Speech disorders associated with ablative surgery of the face, mouth, and pharynx—Ablative approaches to learning. *ASHA Reports No. 8.* Washington, D. C.: American Speech and Hearing Association, 1973.

Brookshire, B. L., Lynch, J. I., & Fox, D. R. *A parent-child cleft palate curriculum: Developing speech and language.* Tigard, Ore.: C. C. Publications, 1980.

Cohen, M. M. The Robin Anomalad—Its nonspecificity and associated syndromes. *Oral Surgery,* 1976, *34,* 587–593.

Cohen, M. M. Syndromes with cleft lip and cleft palate. *Cleft Palate Journal,* 1978, *15,* 306–328.

DeMeyer, W. The median cleft face syndrome: Differential diagnosis of cranium bifidum occultum, hypertelorism and median cleft nose, lip and palate. *Neurology,* 1967, *17,* 961–971.

DeMeyer, W., Zeman, W., & Palmer, C. O. The face predicts the brain: Diagnostic significance of median face anomalies for holoprosencephaly (arrhinencephaly). *Pediatrics,* 1964, *34,* 256–263.

Elfenbein, J. L., Waziri, M., & Morris, H. L. Verbal communication skills of six children with craniofacial anomalies. *Cleft Palate Journal,* 1981, *18,* 59–64.

Eskew, H. A., & Shepard, E. E. Congenital aglossia. *American Journal of Orthodontia,* 1949, *35,* 116–119.

Gorlin, R. J., Pindborg, J. J., & Cohen, M. M. *Syndromes of the head and neck* (2nd ed.). New York: McGraw-Hill, 1976.

Guay, A. H., Maxwell, D. L., & Beecher, R. A radiographic study of tongue posture at rest and during phonation of /s/ in Class III malocclusion. *Angle Orthodontia,* 1978, *48,* 10–22.

Hahn, E. Directed home training program for infants with cleft lip and palate. In E. R. Bzoch (Ed.), *Communicative disorders related to cleft lip and cleft palate.* Boston: Little, Brown, 1979.

Irwin, E., & McWilliams, B. J. Play therapy for children with cleft palates. *Children Today,* 1974, *3,* 18–22.

Klechak, T. L., Bradley, D. P., & Warren, D. W. Anterior open bite and nasal port constriction. *Angle Orthodontia,* 1976, *46,* 232–242.

Long, N. V., & Dalston, R. M. Paired gestural and vocal behavior in one-year-old cleft lip and palate children. *Journal of Speech and Hearing Disorders,* 1982, *47,* 403–406.

MacGregor, F. C. Some psychosocial problems associated with facial deformities. *American Sociological Review,* 1951, *16,* 629–638.

Mallory, S. B., & Paradise, J. L. Glossoptosis revisited: On the development and resolution of airway obstruction in the Pierre Robin syndrome. *Pediatrics,* 1979, *64,* 946–948.

Morrees, C. F., Burstone, C. J., Christiansen, R. L., Hixon, E. H., & Weinstein, S. Research related to malocclusion, A state-of-the-art workshop, the oral-facial growth and development program, N.I.D.R. *American Journal of Orthodontia,* 1971, *59,* 1–18.

Paradise, J. L., & Bluestone, C. D. Diagnosis and management of ear disease in cleft palate infants. *Transactions of the American Academy of Ophthalmology and Otolaryngology,* 1969, *73,* 709–714.

Peterson, S. J. Speech pathology in craniofacial malformations other than cleft lip and palate. *Asha Reports No. 8.* Washington D. C.: American Speech and Hearing Association, 1973.

Peterson-Falzone, S. J. Speech and language problems in selected craniofacial anomalies. *Communicative disorders: An audio journal for continuing education.* New York: Grune and Stratton, 1976.

Philips, B. J. Stimulating syntactic and phonological development in infants with cleft palate. In K. R. Bzoch (Ed.), *Communicative disorders related to cleft lip and palate* (2nd ed.). Boston: Little, Brown, 1979.

Rusk, H. A. *Conference on facial disfigurement: A rehabilitation problem.* U. S. Department of Health, Education, and Welfare, V. R. A., 1963.

Salinas, C. F. An approach to an objective evaluation of the craniofacies, birth defects: *Original Article Series,* Volume XVI, 1980, *5,* 47–74. March of Dimes Birth Defects Foundation.

Sassouni, V. A classification of skeletal facial types. *American Journal of Orthodontia,* 1969, *55,* 109–123.

Shprintzen, R. J., McCall, G. N., & Skolnick, M. L. A new therapeutic technique for the treatment of velopharyngeal incompetence. *Journal of Speech and Hearing Disorders,* 1975, *40,* 69–83.

Smith, D. W. *Recognizable patterns of human malformation* (2nd ed.) *(Vol. VII): Major problems in clinical pediatrics.* Philadelphia: W. B. Saunders, 1976.

Smith, D. W. *Recognizable patterns of human deformation: Identification and management of mechanical effects on morphogenesis (Vol. XXI): Major problems in clinical pediatrics.* Philadelphia: W. B. Saunders, 1981.

Sparks, S. N., & Millard, S. Speech and language characteristics of genetic syndromes. *Journal of Communication Disorders,* 1981, *14,* 411–419.

Templin, M. C., & Darley, F. L. *Templin-Darley Tests of Articulation.* Seattle: University of Washington Press, 1969.

Tessier, P. The definitive plastic surgical treatment of the severe facial deformities of craniofacial synostosis. *Plastic Reconstructive Surgery,* 1971, *48,* 419–442.

Tisza, V. B., Irwin, E., & Scheide, E. Children with oral-facial clefts: A study of the psychological development of handicapped children. *Journal of the American Academy of Child Psychiatry,* 1973, *12,* 292–313.

Van Riper, C. *Speech Correction: Principles and methods* (5th ed.). Englewood Cliffs, N.J.: Prentice-Hall, 1972.

VanThal, J. H. The relationship between faults of dentition and defects of speech. *Proceedings of the Second International Congress of Phonetic Science.* Cambridge: Cambridge Press, 1935.

Whitaker, L. A., Pashayan, H., & Richman, J. A proposed new classification of craniofacial anomalies. *Cleft Palate Journal,* 1981, *18,* 161–176.

Section Two

STUTTERING

Richard F. Curlee

Stuttering Disorders: An Overview

An extraordinary amount of information about stuttering and stutterers has been published in the past several decades. Recent research has significantly advanced our understanding of the nature of stuttering and of its treatment. Nevertheless, much of what we know comes from isolated studies, many of which have lacked satisfactory experimental controls or have employed small, perhaps unrepresentative, samples. Such methodological limitations particularly characterize the studies on children who stutter. Consequently, our information about stuttering is somewhat fragmentary and rarely will support unqualified conclusions. This chapter will summarize current information on stuttering in children and will attempt to evaluate its scientific credibility. Tentative conclusions will be drawn when warranted, and potential areas of fruitful inquiry will be suggested.

The Nature of Stuttering

Objective standards of fluency are not available, and there is still substantial uncertainty regarding the specific nature of the types of disruptions in speech that should be considered as stuttering. For the most part, fluent speech has been defined as the absence of disfluencies, and data on the perceptual or acoustic characteristics of fluency are extremely limited. In contrast, there have been many studies of stutterers' and nonstutterers' speech disruptions and of listeners' reactions to such disfluencies. As a result, information on the nature of stuttering must be synthesized from many different studies that have posed a variety of questions. For example: What types of speech disruptions, if any, distinguish stutterers' speech? Which disfluencies are listeners most likely to judge as stuttering? How consistent are listeners in identifying stuttering? Are behavioral and perceptual definitions of stuttering similarly useful? How comparable are the fluent portions of stutterers' and nonstutterers' speech? Succeeding paragraphs will briefly summarize the findings from a number of such studies as we consider characteristics which differentiate the speech of stutterers from that of nonstutterers.

It is apparent from casual observation and data from a number of controlled studies that stutterers evidence more speech disruptions than nonstutterers. Still, nonstutterers have many of the same types of disfluencies as stutterers, and some nonstuttering talkers are more disfluent than some stutterers. Such overlap may best be illustrated by Johnson's (1961a) comparisons of 100 stutterers with 100 nonstutterers. There was some overlap between the two groups on each of 8 types of disfluency. For example, 30% of the nonstutterers uttered more phrase repetitions than 30% of the stutterers, while 20% of the stutterers had fewer word repetitions than 30%-40% of the nonstuttering group. Nevertheless, overlap in the two groups' part-word repetitions approximated only 10%, and few nonstuttering talkers evidenced any sound prolongations or broken words. Johnson concluded that interjections, revisions, and phrase repetitions are likely to be considered by listeners as normal disfluencies, while part-word repetitions have the highest probability of being classified as stuttering. These conclusions were supported by Young's (1961) findings that ratings of stuttering severity increased with slowed speech rate and the frequency of part-word repetitions, sound prolongations, and broken words. Similarly, Schiavetti (1975) reported that severity ratings of feigned part-word repetitions ranked higher than sound prolongations, followed by interjections and word repetitions. The overlap in disfluency types observed among nonstuttering and stuttering adults has also been found in several empirical studies with children (Johnson & Associates, 1959; Yairi, 1972; F.H. Silverman, 1974). In addition, differences in the relative frequency of children's disfluency types have also been reported. For example, Voelker (1944) found that children who stuttered evidenced significantly more sound prolongations, syllable repetitions, and word repetitions than did their nonstuttering peers. Similarly, Floyd and Perkins (1974) found no overlap in the frequency of syllable disfluencies of preschool stutterers and nonstutterers.

Speech disruptions that occur within words are more likely to be judged by listeners as stuttering than are other types of disfluencies.

Williams and Kent (1958) compared a variety of feigned disfluencies and found that listeners judged syllable repetitions and sound prolongations as instances of stuttering more consistently than they did revisions, interjections, or word and phrase repetitions. Using recorded speech samples of stutterers and nonstutterers, Boehmler (1958) obtained similar findings with both naive and experienced listeners. More recently, Huffman and Perkins (1974) studied the reactions of school teachers to audio recordings of various types of disfluencies that were simulated with and without tension. They found that part-word repetitions, sound prolongations, and hesitations were identified as stuttering more often than were other disfluency types. In addition, those disfluencies produced with audible stress or tension were judged as stuttering more often than were the same types of disfluencies without simulated effort. It also seems noteworthy that judges without special training or instruction appear to classify speech disfluencies similarly to expert professional judges. Because school-age children evidence similar perceptual standards when listening to adult speakers (Giolas & Williams, 1958), it is unlikely that such standards result from either training or personal experiences. Comparable studies with child speakers have not been completed, but it seems likely that similar results would be found. Thus, the types of disfluencies that listeners most often identify as stuttering are the same types that occur more frequently in stutterers' speech than in that of nonstuttering talkers.

Much of what we know about the nature of stuttering relies heavily on listeners' judgments, and listeners are often inconsistent in their judgments. Boehmler (1958) reported that listeners classified part-word repetitions of nonstuttering talkers as instances of stuttering about as often as they did those of stutterers. It may also be noteworthy that listeners readily identify nonstutterers' feigned disfluencies as stutterings or as having been spoken by a stutterer (William & Kent, 1958; Huffman & Perkins, 1974). Such findings are consistent with the view that normal disfluencies and instances of stuttering occupy the same perceptual continuum, with the speech disruptions judged consistently as stutterings or as normal disfluencies at the opposite extremes of the continuum. If so, people may be classified as stutterers as the frequency of their unambiguous instances of stuttering increases or becomes a substantial proportion of all their disfluencies. Although MacDonald and Martin (1973) concluded that stuttering and disfluency were separate, unambiguous response classes that can be differentiated reliably by listeners, a follow-up study (Curlee, 1981) that controlled for independence of listener judgments could not replicate their findings. Indeed, the latter study found overlap in listeners' judgments on more than 70% of all the disfluencies and stutterings identified. Thus, a substantial proportion of the speech disruptions observed in the utterances of chronic adult stutterers are likely to be judged inconsistently by listeners and may reflect, in part, the instructions, the context, and the conditions under which such judgments are made. The extent to which these findings can be generalized to children who stutter is not known, but it seems plausible that a large proportion of children's speech disruptions would be judged ambiguously as stuttering or as normal disfluencies. These speculations, and others, may have important practical and theoretical implications and warrant systematic study.

There is ample evidence from a number of different studies that listener agreement on frequency of stuttering is high. It usually exceeds .80 and often averages above .90 (Young, 1969; Young & Downs, 1968; Curlee, Perkins, & Michael, Note 1). Such agreement has been demonstrated consistently among both naive and experienced listeners (interjudge agreement) and between different judging sessions with the same listeners (intrajudge) agreement). There is substantially less agreement, however, on the specific words or the loci of speech disruptions that are identified as disfluencies or as instances of stuttering, an issue that warrants further discussion. In an early study of listener agreement, Tuthill (1946) remarked that only 37% of all words judged as stuttered had been marked by all listeners. Likewise, Williams and Kent (1958) noted that there was considerable disagreement about which words were stuttered among listeners judging taped utterances of simulated disfluencies. Young (1975a) described a systematic study of interjudge agreement across a variety of listening conditions. He found high agreement among judges ($r \geq .90$) for frequency of stuttering; however, listener agreement on which words were stuttered was substantially lower, approximating .50 regardless of practice, training, or instructions. Similarly low levels of listener agreement were reported recently by Martin and Haroldson (1981) when the words judges had identified as stuttered were compared on a word-by-word basis.

Young suggested that having listeners mark only words and not allowing them to identify stuttering on intervals between words could affect agreement adversely. This possibility was explored as part of a study in which listeners' ability to differentiate between instances of stuttering and disfluencies was studied (Curlee, 1981). As in previous investigations, interjudge agreement on frequency of stuttering during speaking and reading tasks yielded correlation coefficients in the .90s. These same listener judgments, when analyzed in terms of specific words and intervals marked as stuttered, yielded interjudge agreements which averaged less than .30. Intrajudge agreement on specific units marked as stuttered, though somewhat higher, still averaged only in the .50s. Instead of improving agreement, allowing listeners to select both words and intervals between words resulted in less consistent judgments of stuttering. Thus, data from several studies yield relatively high estimates of reliability when analyzed in terms of agreement on frequency of stuttering; however, when agreement is evaluated on a unit-by-unit basis, listeners' uncertainty about specific instances of stuttering becomes apparent.

Studies of listener agreement usually instructed judges to use one of two basic ways of defining stuttering. One type of definition asks listeners to count specific types of behaviors, such as part-word repetitions and audible or silent prolongations, as stuttering. The other type asks listeners to count any type of speech disruption which they personally perceive to be an instance of stuttering. The former instructions can be considered as a behavioral definition of stuttering, the latter as a perceptual definition. Two recent studies have compared listener agreement using each type of definition (Curlee, 1981; Martin & Haroldson, 1981). Both studies asked listeners to use Wingate's (1964) definition and their own personal perceptual standards of stuttering during alternate listening sessions. Both studies found unit-by-unit agreement comparably low for both types of definitions. Apparently, a substantial proportion of judged instances of stuttering are not agreed on by most judges, or by the same judge on different occcasions, when satisfactory controls assure that judgments are made independently.

Frequent, repeated judgments by the same listener of the same speech sample, or by several listeners working collaboratively, likely violate requirements of observational independence, and the reliability of such judgments cannot be estimated satisfactorily. Since behavioral and perceptual definitions are comparable in identifying frequency of stuttering, both can be used satisfactorily as an index of severity or of change. Indeed, it is an enormous practical advantage to clinicians that frequency counts of stuttering are relatively stable and reliable across a variety of listening conditions for both naive and experienced listeners. Unfortunately, the observed disagreement among independent observers regarding specific instances of disfluencies poses a significant methodological problem for researchers interested in behavioral, physiological, or acoustical correlates of stuttering or other speech disruptions. Moreover, such disagreements suggest that the isolation of specific disruptions in the flow of stutterers' speech may also be of questionable validity.

In view of listeners' apparent difficulty in distinguishing between normal disfluencies and stuttering and in identifying specific instances of stuttering reliably, it may be surprising that stutterers' and nonstutterers' fluent utterances can be differentiated. Wendahl and Cole (1961) compared the fluent portions of 8 stutterers' aloud readings with comparably edited recordings of the same passage read aloud by 8 nonstutterers who had been matched for age and reading proficiency. Groups of unsophisticated judges who listened to these matched utterances rated stutterers' speech as less normal in rate and rhythm and as evidencing more force or strain. Moreover, the fluent samples of each stutterer were identified as those of a stutterer significantly more often than those of the nonstutterer with whom the subject was matched. Using the same matched recordings, Young (1964) asked different listeners to identify which samples were those of stutterers; however, their judgments about a talker's utterances were made without benefit of a comparison to those of the talker's matched control. Young found that 3 of the 16 talkers were identified as stutterers by a significant majority of listeners, although 1 of the 3 was a nonstutterer. Similarly, of the 8 talkers who were identified by listeners as nonstutterers, 2 were stutterers. The remaining 5 speakers, all of whom were stutterers, were not consistently classified by listeners as either stutterers or nonstutterers. These findings led Young to conclude that stutterers' fluent speech cannot be readily differentiated from that of nonstutterers. Methodological and analytical differences between these two studies likely account for the differences in their outcomes. Paired-stimulus presentations of stutterers with nonstutterers often provide listeners with sufficient cues to distinguish nonstuttering from stuttering talkers. For example, even when the fluent utterances of treated, adult stutterers and nonstutterers are paired, listeners are usually able to differentiate most stutterers reliably (Ingham & Packman, 1978; Runyan & Adams, 1978, 1979). In contrast, recent studies with children who stutter indicate that most cannot be reliably differentiated from their matched, nonstuttering peers, even when paired presentations of fluent utterances are employed (Colcord & Gregory, Note 2; MacIndoe & Runyan, Note 3). Additional studies are needed to determine if these findings can be replicated.

What, then, should be concluded from the literature we have just reviewed? It is obvious that most of what we know about stutterers' speech comes from studies of chronic adult stutterers. These studies indicate that there are quantitative and qualitative differences in the speech disruptions of stutterers when compared to those of persons who are not stutterers. Listeners count the frequency of stuttering in adults in a reliable manner, even though there may be considerable disagreement regarding which interruptions in speech are instances of stuttering. In addition, listeners are comparably reliable using a perceptual or a behavioral definition of stuttering. While there may be substantial overlap between groups of stutterers and nonstutterers, stutterers typically evidence more frequent speech disruptions, particularly part-word repetitions, prolongations, and, possibly, hesitations. The latter type of disfluency has not been investigated as thoroughly as other speech disruptions, however. Evidence is also accumulating regarding differences in the perceptually fluent utterances of adult stutterers. Such differences have been demonstrated perceptually in several paired-stimulus studies, although the acoustic bases of such differences are uncertain. In any event, it seems clear that most listeners can reliably identify who is a stutterer and how often he stutters; considerable difficulty is encountered, however, in determining exactly when each instance of stuttering occurs.

Comparable objective studies of children's speech are not available. We do not know how reliable listeners are in assessing children's disfluencies because empirical studies are lacking. Based on clinical reports about the difficulty involved in determining whether some young children have begun to stutter or not, it seems doubtful that listeners would evidence better agreement on the speech disruptions of young children. Intuitively, it seems more likely that perceptual distinctions between children's normal disfluencies and stuttering may be more ambiguous than between those of adults. Recent comparisons of the fluent speech of stuttering and nonstuttering children suggest that only a small proportion of young stutterers may evidence perceptually distinctive fluency, and follow-up longitudinal studies are warranted to determine if such differences are related to severity or to subsequent remissions. Much of what has been written about stuttering in children has been based on reports of clinical observations or brief studies of small groups of children who stutter. Consequently, the empirical foundation of our information on the speech of children who stutter is not secure, particularly with regard to younger children who have not been stuttering long.

In view of the apparent perceptual ambiguity between stutterers' normal disfluencies and instances of stuttering and the apparent distinctiveness of the "fluent" segments of their utterances, it is of questionable validity to view adult stutterers' speech as consisting of intermittent instances of stuttering which occur during the flow of ongoing, normal speech. If the perceptual boundaries of instances of stuttering are uncertain, and if stutterers' fluent utterances are distinctive from those of nonstutterers, classifying stutterers' speech into discrete segments of stuttered, disfluent, or fluent speech may distort the inherent continuity of their speech characteristics or of disordered dimensions that should be studied. While instances of stuttering can serve as a reliable index of stuttering severity, and may have many practical clinical applications, its use as a unit of study in research that is directed at understanding the nature of stuttered speech clearly limits the perspective of such research. Indeed, different perspectives may yield more fruitful insights.

Speech Characteristics of Young Stutterers

Data Obtained by Direct Observation

Much of the data on how stuttering begins has been obtained retrospectively through questionnaires or interviews with parents and with older stutterers. Data based on direct observations made by trained observers have usually involved cross-sectional studies of children who have been stuttering for some time; ascertainment of children shortly after they begin to stutter is probably biased by severity of onset, with the more severe being seen sooner. In addition, there have been few empirical studies of the fluency characteristics of nonstuttering children during the course of speech and language development. Indeed, adequate normative data on the fluency or disfluency of normally developing children, of children with suspected fluency problems, or of confirmed young stutterers do not exist. Systematic longitudinal studies are needed to resolve many important questions concerning stuttering onset.

Two longitudinal studies pertinent to the onset of stuttering are available. Epidemiological data from a study of 1,000 families in England have been summarized by Andrews and Harris (1964), and the findings of a larger, more recent study completed in the United States have been reported by LaBenz and LaBenz (1980). Unfortunately, both of these studies provided only limited information on speech characteristics, accessory behaviors, and associated features of beginning stutterers. As a result, it is not clear how the speech of those children who were identified as having fluency problems specifically differed from that of other children in the studies. Moreover, neither study provided the type of data needed to identify patterns of progression or remission of stuttering among the children studied. Consequently, the findings from these studies cannot help us identify the empirical bases on which beginning stutterers may be differentiated from their normally disfluent peers.

What is known about the disfluencies of normally developing young children comes mainly from a few cross-sectional investigations. The number of children observed at different age levels has been relatively small, thereby severely restricting our appreciation of how the characteristics studied vary within the population. Limitations in our data base hinder clinicians trying to identify children who are beginning to stutter, and perpetuate theoretical disagreements about the nature of stuttering. In spite of the paucity of normative data, there is substantial agreement among independent reviewers about a number of findings (Adams, 1980; Bloodstein, 1981; Curlee, 1980a; Johnson, 1980; Van Riper, 1982). Unfortunately, such agreement among authors of disparate theoretical persuasions may generate more confidence in the available information than the data warrant, and probably, does not encourage additional research that is needed.

Repetitions are common characteristics of preschoolers' speech. Winitz (1961) observed infants' vocalizations during 30 consecutive breaths at 12 age levels from birth to age 2. The number of infants observed at each age level varied from 31 to 80. He reported that infants' prelinguistic repetitions seemed to peak at around 1 year of age, then to decrease steadily during their second year of life as words began to occur more frequently in utterances. These findings are consistent with those of several other studies with older preschoolers. Metraux's (1950) cross-sectional investigation, involving 207 children between 18 and 54 months of age, developed qualitative speech profiles for six age groups ranging in size from 16 to 42 children. Her descriptions indicated that "developmental stuttering" was evidenced for the first time among 2½-year-olds, even though part-word, word, or phrase repetitions were common characteristics of the 1½- and 2-year-old age groups. How developmental stuttering was differentiated from other disfluencies is not clear; however, it is implied that the frequency and apparent effort associated with a child's speech disruptions may have been involved. In an earlier study of preschoolers' repetitions and language development, Davis (1939, 1940) observed 1-hour speech samples of 62 children from 24 to 60 months of age. She found that word and phrase repetitions decreased with age, but syllable repetitions did not. Based on personal observations of several active and former stutterers in her sample, Davis concluded that syllable repetitions differentiated stutterers from nonstutterers. Correlations between measures of children's language acquisition and their speech repetitions were generally low, and, according to Davis, lacked either theoretical or practical importance. Finally, Yairi's (1981) study of 33 normally talking 2-year-olds found that single-syllable word and part-word repetitions constituted about 39% of all their disfluencies. There was a substantial range in the frequency of disfluency across children, but all types of disfluencies were observed, even tense pauses and sound prolongations. Whole-word repetitions and revisions were the most frequently occurring disfluency types for these 2-year-olds, each accounting for slightly more than 21% of all disfluencies.

In another recent study, Bjerkan (1980) observed essentially no sound prolongations, blocks, or part-word repetitions in the speech samples of 108 nursery school children between 2 and 6 years of age. In contrasting these findings with observations of two preschool children who stutter, Bjerkan concluded that early stuttering typically involves disruptions within word boundaries. This conclusion supports an earlier finding of Floyd and Perkins (1974), who found no overlap in the frequency of syllable disfluencies (which included repetitions, prolongations, and interjections of syllables) between four preschool stutterers and 20 normally speaking peers. Although Yairi (1981) found a relatively high proportion of syllable repetitions among his group of nonstuttering 2-year-olds, he did not, unfortunately, have a comparison group of young stutterers with whom to contrast the frequency of part-word disfluencies.

It is important to note that only a few stutterers have been involved in these studies, and generalizing these findings to other children who may be starting to stutter may not be warranted. Indeed, Bloodstein's (1974; 1981) observations of young stutterers have convinced him that whole-word repetitions characterize the speech disruptions of beginning stutterers more than any other type of disfluency. He has argued that much of the data from other studies reflect the tension and fragmentation which he believes comes to characterize more and more of stutterers' speech the longer they stutter. Still, Van Riper (1982) has reported data on 61 clients, all of whom were seen within 3 weeks of stuttering onset, and in whom he observed more part-word than whole-word repetitions. Obviously, the severity of these onsets may have biased Van Riper's findings, and additional data are needed from better controlled longitudinal studies to resolve these issues. Supporting Van Riper, however, Yairi's (1983) study of 22 2- and 3-year-old children found that syllable repetitions were all but a universal characteristic of stuttering onset reported by parents and that 3 or more units per repetition typified such speech disruptions of 90% of the children studied.

A number of studies report considerable overlap in the type and frequency of disfluencies that are observed among stuttering and nonstuttering children. The most extensive accumulation of such data involved a series of studies by Johnson and Associates (1959). One study compared the disfluencies of 68 boys and 21 girls who stuttered with those of a matched group of nonstutterers. Both groups averaged 5 years of age, ranging from 2½ to slightly above age 8. According to parents' reports, stuttering had begun, on the average, 18 months prior to observation in the study. Thus, speech findings may not be representative of children who are just beginning to stutter. Although Johnson emphasized the overlap between the two groups' speech characteristics, there were a number of reliable group differences found. Stuttering children were disfluent significantly more often than nonstuttering children, with part-word repetitions and sound prolongations showing the least overlap between the 2 groups. In addition, the children who stuttered evidenced substantially more units per repetition than did nonstutterers. Subsequent studies of elementary school-aged children have reported similar patterns of overlap and distinction between stuttering and nonstuttering children (F.H. Silverman, 1974; Yairi, 1972). Likewise, Westby (1979) compared the speech of 10 stutterers, 10 highly disfluent nonstutterers, and 10 typically disfluent nonstuttering children. She found that the highly disfluent nonstutterers' speech disruptions were more similar to those of stutterers than to those of the typically disfluent nonstutterers. Similarly, E.M. Silverman's study (1972) of 10 4-year-old nonstutterers reported frequent observations of the types of disfluencies often identified as stuttering. Apparently, objective differentiation of young stutterers cannot be as straightforward as we would like.

There is considerable evidence that groups of stuttering and nonstuttering children produce the same types of disfluencies. While there is disagreement about how much overlap is found in the frequency of disfluencies, expecially part-word repetitions and sound prolongations, it is apparent that the frequency and pattern of disfluencies evidenced by *some* stuttering children can be quite similar to that of *some* children usually regarded not to be stutterers. For the most part, however, the data indicate that there is little overlap among *most* nonstutterers and *most* stutterers. Moreover, it can also be noted that few studies have included hard articulatory or glottal attacks or hesitations as disfluencies, therby ignoring disruptions in fluency that are commonly observed in many stutterers. Some of the disagreement found in the literature may reflect differences in authors' theoretical perspectives and interpretations of findings rather than differences in data. Furthermore, Westby's study indicates that stutterers can be differentiated from highly disfluent nonstutterers even though the basis for such differentiation may not be apparent.

Data Obtained from Parent Interviews

Information on the speech characteristics of beginning stutterers obtained from parent interviews agrees substantially with the observational studies just summarized. As might be anticipated, there have been similar disagreements about how such data should be interpreted. There seems to be general agreement that repetitions constitute the most frequent types of disfluency observed in children when they first begin to stutter (Glasner & Rosenthal, 1957; Johnson & Associates, 1959; Van Riper, 1982). The largest and most comprehensive of these studies compared reports from parents of 150 stutterers with those from parents of 150 nonstutterers (Johnson & Associates, 1959). The authors emphasized the similarities found in parents' descriptions of their children's speech and argued that the two parent groups had reacted in strikingly different ways to essentially the same types of childhood disfluencies. In short, parents of children who began to stutter were believed to have misdiagnosed their children's normal nonfluencies, thereby initiating the problem of stuttering. Subsequently, however, these interpretations of the study's findings have been challenged by several authors (Curlee, 1980a; McDearmon, 1968; Van Riper, 1982). For example, it has been pointed out that only half of the parents of nonstutterers were able to describe their child as having any speech disruptions, and most of these descriptions consisted of such disfluencies as pauses between words, interjections, difficulties expressing ideas, or repetitions of words or phrases. Thus, approximately 95% of the parents of normally developing children apparently had not noticed any disruptions in their child's speech or reported only those types of disruptions commonly considered to be normal disfluencies. Approximately 4% of nonstutterers' parents indicated they had observed part-word repetitions or prolongations on occasion, and less than 1% reported ever having observed their child hesitate in the middle of a word, block, or not finish sentences. On the other hand, approximately 75% of the parents of stuttering children indicated that sound prolongations, part-word repetitions, blocks, and signs of tension or struggle had characterized their child's speech at the time of their initial concerns. As with studies involving direct observations of stutterers' and nonstutterers' speech, parent reports suggest that overlap in stuttering and nonstuttering children's disfluencies does not involve a majority of either group once a problem is suspected. Nevertheless, accurate identification of some beginning stutterers may present a diagnostic challenge to clinicians, and extensive observations and evaluations of some children's speech in different speaking circumstances may be necessary.

Loci

The speech disruptions of stutterers do not occur randomly and, with few exceptions, are distributed similarly to those of nonstutterers. It has been shown that the disfluencies of adult stutterers and nonstutterers tend to occur on the same words across repeated utterances, and so do those of stuttering and nonstuttering children (Bloodstein, 1960; Bloodstein, Alper, & Zisk, 1965; Neelley & Timmons, 1967; Williams, Silverman, & Kools, 1969). For both stutterers and nonstutterers of school-age and older, speech disruptions occur more frequently, and thereby more consistently, on longer words, content words, words beginning with consonants, and words of lower predictability, but only stutterers have substantially more speech disruptions at the beginning of sentences (Blankenship, 1964; Chaney, 1969; Mann, 1955; F.H. Silverman, 1972; Silverman & Williams, 1967; Williams, Silverman, & Kools, 1969). Preschool-age children, stutterers and nonstutterers alike, also evidence speech disruptions more often while initiating utterances and, in contrast to older age groups, on such function words as pronouns and conjunctions (Bloodstein & Gantwerk, 1967; Helmreich & Bloodstein, 1973; F.H. Silverman, 1974). Recently,

Bloodstein and Grossman (1981) reported that young stutterers' whole-word repetitions occur almost exclusively at the beginning of syntactic units. Obviously, such characteristics represent different ways of classifying linguistic phenomena in a convenient manner, and different characteristics that are related statistically to speech disruptions can also share other common attributes. For example, longer words are more likely to be content words as well as words of lower predictability than are shorter words. Longer words may also differ from shorter words in terms of suprasegmental stress or may require greater motor or linguistic planning. In any event, stuttering appears to be sensitive to the same factors or constraints that affect the speech disruptions of nonstuttering talkers.

Variability

One of stuttering's more puzzling attributes is its seeming variability. Even casual observation indicates that stuttering varies in form, frequency, and severity from situation to situation, listener to listener, or from one moment to another during the same conversation. Yet, groups of stutterers evidence similar reactions to a number of speaking conditions. Unfortunately, we have little empirical information about how groups of children who stutter respond to different conditions, even though it is possible that much of what we know about adult stutterers may apply to children, especially those who are older. Empirical studies of adults have shown, for example, that stuttering is substantially decreased while speaking or reading in time to rhythmical stimuli (Brady, 1969; Fransella & Beech, 1965; Martin & Haroldson, 1979), reading aloud in unison with another (Adams & Ramig, 1980; Ingham & Packman, 1979; Johnson & Rosen, 1937), singing (Bloodstein, 1950; Colcord & Adams, 1979; Healey, Mallard, & Adams, 1976), speaking slowly in a prolonged manner with or without DAF (Curlee & Perkins, 1969; Johnson & Rosen, 1937; Soderberg, 1969b), talking while alone (Bloodstein, 1950; Hood, 1975) speaking during auditory masking (Adams & Hutchinson, 1974; Cherry & Sayers, 1956; Perkins & Curlee, 1969), or talking during response-contingent stimulation of stuttering (Ingham & Andrews, 1973; Martin & Haroldson, 1979; Siegel, 1970). Experimentation has demonstrated that reduction of stuttering with reduced syllable rate depends on prolongation of phones within the syllable (Perkins, Bell, Johnson, & Stocks, 1979). Another experimentally demonstrated relationship, which appears to be invariant and must, therefore, be accounted for in any adequate understanding of abnormal dysfluency, is the reduction of stuttering with whispering, and its elimination with voiceless lipped speech (Perkins, Rudas, Johnson, & Bell, 1976). Conversely, stuttering usually has been found to increase in frequency or severity as audience size increases (Bloodstein, 1950; Siegel & Haugen, 1964), when stuttering is anticipated (Johnson & Sinn, 1937; Milisen, 1938) or in circumstances in which communicative stress or general tension or anxiety appear to be elevated (Bloodstein, 1950; Gray & Brutten, 1965). There is some evidence that the frequency of nonstutterers' disfluency varies similarly. For example, disfluencies of nonstutters are reduced while speaking in time to rhythmical stimulus (F.H. Silverman, 1971), under auditory masking (Silverman & Goodban, 1972), and during repeated readings of the same passage (Soderberg, 1969a; Williams, Silverman, & Kools, 1968).

Although there are numerous clinical reports suggesting that preschool stutterers' speech disruptions vary noticeably across speaking conditions, adequately controlled empirical studies are lacking. There is evidence that preschoolers' stuttering decreases with response-contingent stimulation (Martin, Kuhl, & Haroldson, 1972; Reed & Godden, 1977) or while speaking in time to rhythmical stimulus (Coppola & Yairi, Note 4). Because few empirical studies have been completed with children, especially preschoolers, substantial gaps in our knowledge remain. The weight of available evidence suggests that speech disruptions of stutterers follow patterns of occurrence similar to those observed among persons who do not stutter. An apparent exception is the substantially greater percentage of stuttering among adult stutterers that occurs at the beginning of utterances and syntactic units. Although substantially fewer data are available for children, the disfluencies of young stutterers and nonstutterers appear to vary in loci and in frequency as a function of the same variables, and there are no demonstrably reliable findings to the contrary. Thus, a theory which accounts for the relationships between stuttering and various speaking conditions or psycholinguistic variables may also account for the speech disruptions of nonstutterers.

Onset

Stuttering can be viewed as a developmental problem that begins most often during the course of a child's speech and language development. Onset is usually insidious; both Morley (1957) and Van Riper (1982) found abrupt onsets of stuttering in only a small percentage of clients, even those examined soon after parents had become concerned about fluency. Their observations are supported by most parent reports (Bloodstein, 1981). Indeed, Bloodstein has hypothesized that mild tension and fragmentations are common features of all preschoolers' speech, which can worsen with communicative stress for some and lead to chronic stuttering. Most stutterers are identified during their preschool years (Andrews & Harris, 1964;

Dickson, 1971; Johnson & Associates, 1959), and there are relatively few onsets after age 9 (Young, 1975b). Although some children may start stuttering around the time they begin to speak in short utterances, most have been using sentences a year or more before they begin (Johnson & Associates, 1959). Andrews and Harris (1964) estimated that the risk of stuttering onset is highest between ages 2 and 5 and gradually decreases thereafter until age 12, when future risk approximates zero. Reports of stuttering beginning during adolescence or adulthood are sparse and essentially anecdotal. Van Riper (1982) noted that such reports often describe abrupt onsets that are associated with an emotional shock or physical injury. It is possible that some late onsets may involve recurrences of early stuttering problems that have been forgotten or that some fluency problems, though similar in many ways to stuttering, may differ from developmental stuttering upon more careful observation. As with other areas of uncertainty, additional research is needed.

Stutterer-Nonstutterer Differences

In recent years, increasing importance has been placed on relatively small but consistent differences found in empirical comparisons of groups of stutterers and nonstutterers. Recent reviews of such findings have been presented by Andrews, Craig, Feyer, Hoddinott, Howie & Neilson (1983) and Bloodstein (1981). As might be expected, there is considerable disagreement concerning which differences, if any, result in stuttering, which result from stuttering, and which covary with stuttering or stutterers but are not causally related. For the most part, differences between stutterers and nonstutterers appear to fall within the range of normal variation, and there is extensive overlap between the two groups. It can also be noted that the variability among groups of stutterers is usually substantially greater than that found among comparison groups. The greater heterogeneity of stutterers' data appears to reflect greater variability in performance across different stutterers as well as less consistent performance of individual stutterers on the same task than is found among nonstutterers. Consequently, it should be remembered throughout subsequent paragraphs that generalizations from studies of groups of stutterers are not valid when applied to many individual stutterers.

Cognition

Cognitive abilities or functions of stutterers differ from those of nonstutterers in a number of ways. Stutterers' average performance on intelligence tests falls about one-half a standard deviation below the mean of normal speakers (Andrews & Harris, 1964; Okasha, Bishry, Kamel & Hossan, 1974; Schindler, 1955). Stutterers are also somewhat slower in speech and language development (Andrews & Harris, 1964; Berry, 1938; Darley, 1955) and evidence other speech and language impairments more often (Blood & Seider, 1981; Schindler, 1955; Williams & Silverman, 1968; Winitz & Darley, 1980). As would be anticipated, there is also consistent evidence that stutterers' educational placement and academic achievement, on the whole, lags behind that of nonstuttering children (Darley, 1955; Schindler, 1955; Williams, Melrose, & Woods, 1969). Several well-controlled EEG studies have found differences between stutterers and nonstutterers across a number of different tasks (Moore & Haynes, 1980; Moore & Lang, 1977; Sayles, 1971; Zimmerman & Knott, 1974). Such differences in EEG activities may reflect different cerebral processing activities as well as cerebral dysfunctions. Tests of stutterers' central auditory abilities (Hall & Jerger, 1978; Molt & Guilford, 1979; Toscher & Rupp, 1978), ear preference for meaningful stimuli on dichotic listening tasks (Curry & Gregory, 1969; Sommers, Brady, & Moore, 1975) and auditory tracking skills (Sussman & MacNeilage, 1975) have found, though somewhat less consistently, differences between groups of stutterers and nonstutterers. As might be expected, it is not clear to what extent many of these findings can be applied to children who stutter, particularly those who ultimately recover.

Motor Abilities

Investigations of stutterers' overall motor abilities have found relatively few differences in motor coordination or dexterity. In general, the data are sufficiently inconclusive that one can neither eliminate the possibility of subtle differences between stutterers' and nonstutterers' nonspeech motor abilities nor clearly implicate any specific differences with confidence. Studies of the speed and accuracy with which stutterers use their speech mechanisms have yielded similarly inconsistent results for the most part. Within the past few years, however, a number of different investigators have found reliable differences in voice reaction times. In 1976, Adams and Hayden reported that adult stutterers were significantly slower initiating and terminating phonation of an isolated vowel. Starkweather, Hirshman, and Tannenbaum (1976) found adult stutterers to be similarly slow initiating phonation across a variety of different syllables. Comparable findings have been reported subsequently for both adults and children in a number of different studies (Cross & Luper, 1979; Cullinan & Springer, 1980; Reich, Till, & Goldsmith, 1981; Starkweather, Franklin, & Smigo, Note 5). Several of these studies have also included observations of stutterers' nonspeech vocal and manual reaction times. While all of these studies have found the average reaction times of stutterers slower on speech tasks than that of nonstutterers, nonspeech vocal and manual latencies have differed in some studies but not in others. In addition, Cullinan and Springer (1980) found that when their 20 stuttering children were divided into a group of 11 who had concomitant language or articulation problems and a group of 9 whose only problem was stuttering, only the children with concomitant speech-language problems differed significantly from the nonstuttering comparison group. Since most studies have used fewer than 15 subjects per group, inconsistent reports of statistical reliability should be expected. Some discrepancies among studies are not easily accounted for, however. For example, while Cross and Luper (1979) found a high positive correlation between voice and finger reaction times, Starkweather, Franklin, and Smigo (1981) found a moderate negative correlation.

Such findings are intriguing and clearly warrant further investigation; nevertheless, their significance to stuttering is not clear. Apparently, stutterers' reaction times may be slower for speech and some nonspeech tasks, with speech task latencies differentially slower. Because differences have been found even in relatively young stutterers, it seems unlikely that slower reaction times are a consequence of stuttering. If slower reaction times reflect some type of motor dysfuntion common to stutterers, such problems likely extend beyond the larynx, perhaps even the speech mechanism. It is obvious that longer response latencies do not necessarily result in stuttering, since most people with motor speech impairments do not stutter and since there is considerable overlap in stutterers' and nonstutterers' reaction times. Indeed, it seems more plausible that stutterers' slower reaction times and speech disruptions result from their inability to execute rapid, precise complex motor responses. Data from these studies and those involving fiberoptic (Conture, McCall, & Brewer, 1977) and EMG (Freeman & Ushijima, 1978) investigations of stutterers' laryngeal behavior during stuttering have been used to support the hypothesis that the larynx plays a primary role in stutterers' speech disruptions. Such arguments must be carefully constrained to be credible. Clearly, the larynx is not essential to stuttering. If it were, stuttering could not persist following laryngectomy, and, yet, occasionally it does. Whether or not subsystems of the speech mechanism are hierarchically arranged is debatable. If they are, then it is not clear how one subsystem of the mechanism could be more involved or more responsible for stuttering than other subsystems of the same mechanism. At best, these findings may represent critical keys to our future understanding of stuttering. Only further research can tell.

Personal Adjustment

Several relatively complete reviews of information about stutterers' personal adjustment are available, and specific investigations will not be covered here (Bloch & Goodstein, 1971; Bloodstein, 1981; Goodstein, 1958; Sheehan, 1958; Van Riper, 1982). However, there is general agreement among these reviews that: stutterers fall within the normal range on tests of personality and are more similar to normal persons than to psychiatric comparison groups; that personalities of severe stutterers do not differ reliably from those whose stuttering is mild; that older stutterers' personalities do not differ in significant ways from those of younger stutterers; that parents of stutterers are not substantially more maladjusted than parents of children who do not stutter. Even though many people apparently have a negative stereotype of stutterers' personalities (Turnbaugh, Guitar, & Hoffman, 1979; Woods & Williams, 1976), standardized tests do not reveal a reliable pattern of traits or characteristics for groups of stutterers. The few consistent reports of differences between stutterers' and nonstuttering persons' self-confidence or anxiety usually have been attributed to normal, secondary reactions to a communication disability. It is interesting to note in this regard, however, that Prins (1972) found more prevalent signs of maladjustment among subjects with other communication disorders than among a matched group of stutterers. It is possible, of course, that studies of heterogeneous groups of stutterers have obscured distinctive personality patterns of several different subgroups or that current measures of personal adjustment are not able to differentiate stutterers' abnormal adaptations from normal variations in personality. Because most of what we know comes from studies of adults, such information may not be pertinent to factors which precipitate stuttering onset or which lead to recovery. Nevertheless, it is clear that there is no credible body of evidence which indicates that stutterers' personal adjustments are of significance to either the etiology or the maintenance of stuttering.

Incidence and Prevalence

It has been estimated that about 4% to 5% of the population stutter for some period during their lives (Andrews & Harris, 1964; Bloodstein, 1981; Curlee, 1980a; Van Riper, 1982). In contrast, the prevalence of stuttering, among school-age children approximates 1% or less (Bloodstein, 1981; Brady & Hall, 1976; Hull, Mielke, Williford, & Timmons, 1976; Winitz & Darley, 1980; Young, 1975b). Stuttering may be somewhat less prevalent during high school years than elementary school and is probably more prevalent during preschool years, but adequate documentation is lacking.

Data from several more recent studies (Brady & Hall, 1976; Winitz & Darley, 1980) suggest that stuttering may be less prevalent than was indicated by previous studies; however, different ascertainment procedures and criteria for identifying stutterers do not permit direct comparisons across studies. Although all studies reporting prevalence or incidence estimates can be challenged on the basis of several methodological limitations (Curlee, 1980a; Ingham, 1976; Young, 1975b), their data are relatively consistent. Indeed, even prevalence and incidence differences among different cultures or socioeconomic groups are relatively small and have often been interpreted to accommodate authors' differing theoretical biases.

One of the few findings for which there is complete agreement across studies is that more males than females stutter. While the proportion of male to female stutterers has varied somewhat from study to study, most findings cluster around a 3:1 male-to-female ratio (Bloodstein, 1981; Van Riper, 1982). Males also manifest such other problems as asthma, epilepsy, chorea, spina bifida, or cleft palate more frequently than females and differ from females in terms of stature, longevity, baldness, and education. Bloodstein (1981) believes that the sex ratio may be positively related to age, with the proportion of males to females increasing in older age groups. Recent data reported by Yairi (1983) on stuttering onset among 2- and 3-year-olds indicate an equal sex distribution for children who begin to stutter this young. The data available on this issue are limited, however, and may only reflect sampling errors across studies. If further studies confirm this finding, it would be important to determine if there is a differential recovery rate between males and females or if males begin to stutter at somewhat older ages than females.

The prevalence of stuttering is substantially higher among persons with cerebral damage (Bloodstein, 1981; Bohme, 1968; Van Riper, 1982). For example, among the mentally retarded, prevalence appears to increase with severity of cognitive deficits, and may be even higher among those whose retardation has resulted from organic etiology (Bloodstein, 1981; Boberg, Ewert, Mason, Lindsay, & Wynn, 1978; Brady & Hall, 1976; Van Riper, 1982). These data suggest that incidence may be higher and recovery lower among people with cerebral dysfunction. There have also been a number of reports in the past decade describing fluency impairments that result from cerebral lesions (Farmer, 1975; Helm, Butler, & Benson, 1978; Quinn & Andrews, 1977; Rosenbek, Messert, Collins, & Wertz, 1978). Apparently these stutter-like speech impairments may or may not be accompanied by apraxia, dysarthria, or aphasia, and are often transient, but may persist if cerebral lesions are bilateral (Helm, Butler, & Benson, 1978). Similar types of speech disruptions have also been reported as an early sign of a patient's progressive neurological deterioration following long-term, chronic dialysis (Rosenbek, McNeil, Lemme, Prescott, & Alfrey, 1975). While such patients' speech disruptions obviously resemble stuttering in many ways, systematic studies of their patterns of occurrence or of patients' response to masking, rhythm, or response-contingent stimulation have not been reported. It is still not clear, therefore, to what extent these acquired fluency impairments are identical to stuttering or reflect a distinctive type of motor speech disorder.

Interest in the familial incidence of stuttering has been renewed in recent years, and several current reviews of these findings are available (Bloodstein, 1981; Sheehan & Costley, 1977). The recent work of Kidd (1977), Kidd, Kidd, and Records (1978), Kidd, Oehlert, Heimbuch, Records, & Webster (1980), Gladstein, Seider, and Kidd (1981), and Howie (1981) have extended the findings of earlier studies and strongly implicate the role of genetic factors in stuttering. The evidence can be summarized as follows: The risk of stuttering is at least three times higher among first-degree relatives of active or recovered stutterers than in the general population. Incidence is higher among the offspring of stutterers than among their siblings, while first-degree male relatives of female stutterers are four times more likely to stutter than first-degree female relatives of male stutterers. Concordance of stuttering among monozygotic twin pairs is substantially higher than among dizygotic pairs controlled for age, sex, and independence of classification. Nevertheless, about 25% of monozygotic twin pairs are discordant for stuttering, and both stuttering severity and recovery from stuttering appear to be independent of familial incidence. Consequently, while the evidence for stuttering's genetic transmission is growing steadily, it is also clear that environmental factors play a role in some, if not all, onsets of stuttering. It is important to remember that the contributions of genetic factors to behavioral differences or dysfunctions are likely to be indirect. The structural or organic characteristics transmitted genetically to individuals probably impose only certain limits on behavior. If so, genetically inherited traits or abilities may best be viewed as predisposing conditions in which a given behavior may be manifested. It is also likely that genetically based predispositions limit behavior differently as a function of different environmental factors. Our present state of knowledge, therefore, does not permit us to identify the critical predispositions that may be transmitted genetically or to describe how such predisposing limitations interact with the environment to bring about stuttering. Recent research may help us to ask more important, more critical questions, but much remains to be answered.

Etiological Considerations

Again, there are compelling, albeit indirect, data supporting the hypothesis that a predisposition to stutter is transmitted genetically. An individual's level of susceptibility could result from a single gene or from a number of genes acting in combination (Kidd, 1977). It is tempting to speculate that a polygenic model of inheritance may account for the high variability usually found among groups of stutterers. Regardless, it is apparent that a number of environmental factors may influence whether an individual's predisposition to stutter will, in fact, be manifested in the development of a stuttering problem. This perspective hypothesizes that predispositions to stutter are continuously distributed across all speakers with a developmental threshold dividing the distribution into two discontinuous groups, stutterers and nonstutterers. Current data suggest that one's liability for exceeding this threshold is highest after connected speech begins during the preschool years and decreases with age thereafter. As noted previously, however, many critical questions remain to be answered. For example, what cognitive, motor, or affective functions or abilities are involved in one's predisposition to stutter, what environmental factors increase or decrease one's susceptibility to stutter, and how do predispositional and environmental factors interact to precipitate the onset of stuttering? It should also be acknowledged that factors that precipitate stuttering onset may differ from those that affect stuttering severity or recovery. It has been argued that those characteristics associated with the persistence of chronic stuttering, as well as many of the differences found between adult stutterers and nonstutterers, probably reflect attributes that have functioned as barriers to recovery (Curlee, 1980a). Thus, much of the information available about stutterers may not be representative of most children who stutter. At the present time, all etiological explanations are unsatisfactory, a circumstance which will likely continue until a better understanding of the genetic-neurophysiological bases of fluency and disfluency are available and described in specific operational terms.

Clinical Management of Stuttering Children

It should be apparent from the information reviewed pertaining to the overlap in speech and language characteristics across stutterers and nonstutterers that reliable identification of those children who are just beginning to stutter can be difficult, particularly if the frequency or severity of their speech disruptions is relatively low. For the most part, evaluation strategies and procedures employed with children who are suspected of being incipient stutterers have evolved through the experiences of clinicians rather than through controlled empirical studies. The types of observations made and the characteristics assessed may often reflect practitioners' beliefs regarding the etiology of stuttering. Several recent publications have recommended guidelines for distinguishing beginning stutterers from normally nonfluent children (Adams, 1977; Curlee, 1980a; Gregory & Hill, 1980; Johnson, 1980). For the most part, the guidelines presented by these authors were strikingly similar with part-word repetitions, prolongations, difficulties initiating utterances, and signs of struggle proposed as distinguishing signs of incipient stuttering. While the rationales of these authors have some empirical support, the reliability and validity of the clinical evaluation procedures now used to differentiate normally speaking children from beginning stutterers are essentially unknown.

Prognosis

Information on prognosis comes from two types of studies: investigations of treatment outcomes and of the spontaneous remission of stuttering. Neither type of study will support many conclusions that cannot be challenged. A number of different treatment procedures seem beneficial, at least for adult stutterers (Andrews, Guitar, & Howie, 1980). Few chronic adult stutterers appear to experience complete recoveries, however. Because most remission studies have involved interviews or questionnaire surveys, there is always some uncertainty that those who claim recovery ever really stuttered or that all recoveries from early episodes of stuttering were identified. Second, it is doubtful that the samples studied are representative of the general population of all stutterers. Futhermore, the bases for claiming recovery are not clear, since a substantial proportion of those who claim to have recovered also report occasional recurrences of stuttering. The role of treatment in most studies is also unclear. Ingham (1983) has argued convincingly, for example, that common-sense speech modification practices (e.g., slowing down) used by parents or older stutterers probably account for many of the "spontaneous remissions" reported in the literature. Finally, there is no accepted standard of how long one must be free of stuttering to claim recovery. Despite such limitations, a number of inferences are viable until further research indicates otherwise.

People report recoveries from stuttering at all ages, whether associated with formal treatment or not, but more remissions occur before or during puberty (Andrews & Harris, 1964; Dickson, 1971; Glasner & Rosenthal, 1957; Shearer & Williams, 1965; Sheehan & Martyn, 1970). It is not clear to what extent the duration of subjects' stuttering problems may contribute to these findings, but the chance of either beginning to stutter or of recovering from stuttering are substantially reduced among older adolescents and adults. It has been suggested that these findings may reflect neurophysiological changes that accompany maturation of stutterers' nervous systems during the course of years of severe chronic stuttering which, after a certain age, becomes more resistant to change and to remission of stuttering (Curlee, 1980a). There may also be fewer complete recoveries that occur at older ages. Shearer and Williams (1965) noted less frequent reports of residual stuttering episodes among those subjects whose remissions had occurred by 13 years of age. This finding needs to be replicated with larger, more representative samples, and large scale studies of both active and recovered stutterers are needed to explore stuttering's persistence and its remission past young adulthood. Such studies are essential if we are to determine the conditions under which stutterers recover or if we are to gain a better understanding of the circumstances in which systematic formal treatment procedures are necessary to effect recovery, in contrast to those remissions associated with common-sense practices adopted by parents and older stutterers.

A substantial proportion of people who begin to stutter recover, perhaps as high as 80% (Andrews & Harris, 1964; Cooper, 1972; Dickson, 1971; Glasner & Rosenthal, 1957; Sheehan & Martyn, 1970). Recovery rates of 80% or higher would account for the differences in current estimates of stuttering prevalence and incidence. Wingate's (1976) compilation of remission studies clearly shows that older, recovered stutterers report substantially fewer remissions during their childhood years than might be anticipated from studies of younger recovered stutterers. Such discrepancies could reflect poor ascertainment of recovered stutterers among older age groups or frequent recurrences of stuttering after early reports of remission. The questionable reliability and validity of subjects' reports cannot be discounted, either. For example, approximately two-thirds of the parents of the high school students who had identified themselves as recovered stutterers in Lankford and Cooper's (1974) study denied that their children had ever stuttered. The only longitudinal study in which both stuttering onsets and remissions were determined by direct observation rather than report found a recovery rate of 79% by age 16 (Andrews & Harris, 1964). It seems safe to conclude, therefore, that chances for complete recovery, whether associated with treatment or not, are relatively high, especially among children.

It is believed that most stuttering remissions, whether associated with formal treatment or not, occur gradually (Johnson & Associates, 1959; Shearer & Williams, 1965; Wingate, 1964). These beliefs are based largely on the recollections of self-identified, recovered stutterers. Consequently, the information now available to us is of uncertain reliability and validity.

If stuttering becomes more intermittent and less severe over an extended period of time during recovery, which seems to be the case, it may not be possible to identify subjects' specific ages at remission, and it may be more appropriate to conceive of recovery as representing a continuum of behaviors. If so, there are at least three groups who warrant careful study— completely recovered stutterers, partially recovered stutterers, and active stutterers. Systematic longitudinal investigations of such groups may provide valuable insights for our understanding of both the recovery process and of relapse, two crucial areas of information that are of great practical importance.

Findings from several studies indicate that recovery may be inversely related to severity of stuttering. Sheehan and Martyn (1970) estimated the recovery rates of college students who had rated their stuttering as mild, moderate, or severe at 87%, 75%, and 50%, respectively. In addition, they found that stutterers who reported blockings as their initial symptoms had recovered less frequently than those whose initial problems involved only repetitions. This finding was replicated among elementary and junior high school students by Dickson (1971). Similarly, Glasner and Rosenthal (1975) found that remission was related to the number of disfluency types reported by parents of entering first graders. More than half of the children whose stuttering was limited to one type of disfluency (repetition, prolongation, or hesitation) had stopped stuttering at the time of the study; but only a third of those with two or three disfluency types had stopped. More recently, Panelli, McFarlane, and Shipley (1978) examined 15 preschoolers at onset of stuttering and again several years later. During this time, 12 stopped stuttering. The children who recovered had evidenced substantially fewer speech disruptions and accessory features during their initial evaluation than the 3 whose stuttering had persisted. The notion that less severe stutterers are more likely to recover is intuitively appealing; such is the case for other types of problems and disorders. Still, we could place more confidence in these findings if they were not based largely on self-ratings, parent reports, or recollections of long-passed events. Such measures are of questionable reliability.

Remission of stuttering has not been found to be related to age of onset (Andrews & Harris, 1964; Sheehan & Martyn, 1970), familial incidence (Sheehan & Martyn, 1970), or therapy (Andrews & Harris, 1964; Glasner & Rosenthal, 1957; Shearer & Williams, 1965; Sheehan & Martyn, 1970; Wingate, 1964). It should be noted that the lack of statistical relationship between treatment and recovery may be biased by differences in which severe and mild stutterers are seen for therapy. It is also plausible that these findings could reflect the use of less effective treatment methods than those currently employed. The finding that neither stuttering severity nor recovery are related to familial incidence of stuttering suggests that both severity and remission of stuttering may be determined substantially by environmental factors. Thus, most stutterers recover regardless of severity, family background, or treatment history. These findings, if reliable, have important implications for genetic counseling, counseling of parents of beginning stutterers, and clinical management strategies.

While the odds for recovery clearly favor most young stutterers, it is not possible to determine the prognosis of an individual child with confidence. One of the few prospective empirical studies of prognostic factors was reported by Stromsta in 1965. As part of an initial evaluation, sound spectograms were made of the disfluencies of 63 children who were suspected of stuttering. A follow-up questionnaire 10 years later found that most of the children who continued to stutter had evidenced abnormal formant transitions and abrupt terminations of phonation on the spectographic recordings of their disfluencies made during their initial evaluations. Conversely, most of those who recovered had not. Operational criteria for analyzing these spectograms were not described, and it is not known how many of the children received therapy. Consequently, additional study is needed to determine if these findings are replicable and clinically useful for prognostic purposes.

Treatment of Children Who Stutter

There have been few well-controlled studies of therapy for children who stutter. As a consequence, adequate empirical support for treatment approaches used with young stutterers is lacking. The present discussion will provide only a general overview of current habilitative practices, since following chapters will cover these issues in detail. As might be expected, a variety of techniques have been advocated for stuttering children and their parents. Many seem to reflect authors' etiological biases; most have evolved during trial-and-error experiences of clinical practice; and a few have been developed through preliminary clinical research.

Indirect treatment approaches have been used most often with young stutterers, particularly those who are just beginning to stutter and who are not evidencing accessory or associated features of stuttering (Curlee, 1980b). Intervention under these circumstances can be viewed as an attempt to prevent the development of a chronic stuttering problem. These approaches presume that modifying a child's environment can affect speech and usually involve parent counseling that is intended to reduce environmental pressures or communicative stress experienced by a young stutterer. Some authors (Bar, 1973; Curlee, 1980a; Johnson, 1980) have also advocated that parents deliberately reinforce fluent speech or model slower speech rates (Johnson, 1980). Others have modified more general parent-child interaction patterns (Shames and Egolf, 1976). Thus, some indirect approaches directly manipulate circumstances seemingly associated with more fluent speech. Although indirect approaches seem to be widely accepted and used with young stutterers, their effectiveness is essentially unknown. There have been few single-subject studies completed, and matched treatment groups of untreated young stutterers have not been used to control for spontaneous recoveries which may occur in group studies.

Once a child has begun to evidence accessory and associated features of stuttering with some consistency and is viewed as a confirmed stutterer, direct treatment approaches are used more frequently (Curlee, 1980b). This strategy appears to reflect the belief that a substantial proportion of these children will become chronic stutterers if left untreated and that direct intervention will not be harmful. A number of techniques have been utilized, and most studies report decreases in stuttering. Certainly, most provide sufficient evidence to justify further, more systematic investigation, and there is no evidence that such approaches may be detrimental to young stutterers. Direct approaches have involved contingency management procedures for both instances of stuttering (Costello, 1980; Martin, Kuhl, & Haroldson, 1972; Reed & Godden, 1977) and fluent utterances (Costello, 1983; Leach, 1969; Manning, Trutna, & Shaw, 1976; Peters, 1977; Rickard & Mundy, 1965; Shaw & Shrum, 1972), training of fluency-maintaining speaking behaviors (Ryan, 1971; Shine, 1980; Coppolo & Yairi, Note 3), and teaching of how to stutter with less effort (Gregory & Hill, 1980; Van Riper, 1973; Williams, 1979). In addition, some clinicians also advocate use of an indirect approach with parents and teachers in order to optimize the child's environment for achieving more fluent speech, thereby supplementing direct procedures intended to improve speech (Johnson, 1961b; Van Riper, 1973; Zwitman, 1978). The effectiveness of direct approaches used alone or in combination with counseling is also largely unknown.

The available data indicate that a wide variety of techniques may produce marked decreases in stuttering; however, untreated comparison groups have not been used. Moreover, stuttering may also covary with other behavior, at least in some children. For example, Wahler, Sperling, Thomas, Teeter, and Luper (1970) reported that two children with mild behavior problems, who also stuttered, received contingency management procedures designed to reduce their respective behavior problems. In single-subject ABAB experimental designs, the frequency of each child's problem behavior *and* stuttering decreased concurrently, although there was no evidence that inadvertent contingencies had occurred on stuttering. In this study, stuttering appeared to change in association with the modification of other behaviors, even though the mechanism for such changes is not understood.

In most instances, the permanence of reported decreases or the extent to which stuttering is improved in everyday speaking situations is not known. There are several reports, however, that changes observed in therapy often appear to generalize spontaneously for many young stutterers (Ryan, 1971; Martin, Kuhl, & Haroldson, 1972; Reed & Godden, 1977; Shaw & Shrum, 1972; Shine, 1980). These observations have involved a relatively small number of children, without matched controls for spontaneous recovery. Such findings need replication and more systematic study, since generalization of treatment effects is a major problem for many adult stutterers. While the data are not conclusive, there is reason to suspect that treatment of children who stutter may result in better, longer-lasting results than we can achieve with adults. Consequently, many important advances in our ability to facilitate children's recovery from stuttering seem within reach, awaiting further study and exploration.

Reference Notes

1. Curlee, R., Perkins, W., & Michael, W. Reliability of judgments of instances of stuttering. Paper presented at the Annual Convention of the American Speech and Hearing Association, New York, 1970.
2. Colcord, R., & Gregory, H. A perceptual analysis of fluency in stuttering and nonstuttering children. Paper presented at the Annual Convention of the American Speech-Language-Hearing Association, Los Angeles, 1981.
3. MacIndoe, C.A., & Runyon, C.M. A perceptual comparison of stuttering and nonstuttering children's nonstuttered speech. Paper presented at the Annual Convention of the American Speech-Language-Hearing Association, Los Angeles, 1981.
4. Coppola, V., & Yairi, E. Rhythmic speech training with preschool stuttering children. Paper presented at the Annual Convention of the American Speech and Hearing Association, Atlanta, 1979.
5. Starkweather, C.W., Franklin, S., & Smigo, T. Voice-finger reaction-time difference: Correlation with severity. A paper presented at the Annual Convention of the American Speech-Language-Hearing Association, Los Angeles, 1981.

References

Adams, M. A clinical strategy for differentiating the normally nonfluent child and the incipient stutterer. *Journal of Fluency Disorders,* 1977, *2,* 141-148.

Adams, M. The young stutterer: Diagnosis, treatment and assessment of progress. *Seminars in Speech, Language, and Hearing,* 1980, *1,* 289-299.

Adams, M.R., & Hayden, P. The ability of stutterers and nonstutterers to initiate and terminate phonation during production of an isolated vowel. *Journal of Speech and Hearing Research,* 1976, *19,* 290-296.

Adams, M.R., & Hutchinson, J. The effects of three levels of auditory masking on selected vocal characteristics and the frequency of disfluency of adult stutterers. *Journal of Speech and Hearing Research,* 1974, *17,* 682-688.

Adams, M.R., & Ramig, P. Vocal characteristics of normal speakers and stutterers during choral reading. *Journal of Speech and Hearing Research*, 1980, *23*, 457-469.

Andrews, G., Craig, A., Feyer, A. M., Hoddinott, S., Howie, P., & Neilson, M. Stuttering: A review of research findings and theories circa 1982. *Journal of Speech and Hearing Disorders*, 1983, *48*, 226-246.

Andrews, G., Guitar, B., & Howie, P. Meta-analysis of the effects of stuttering treatment. *Journal of Speech and Hearing Disorders*, 1980, *45*, 287-307.

Andrews, G., & Harris, M. *The syndrome of stuttering*. Clinics in Developmental Medicine, No. 17. London: Spastics Society of Medical Education and Information Unit in association with Wm. Heinemann Medical Books, 1964.

Bar, A. Increasing fluency in young stutterers vs. decreasing stuttering: A clinical approach. *Journal of Communication Disorders*, 1973, *6*, 247-258.

Berry, M.F. The developmental history of stuttering children. *Journal of Pediatrics*, 1938, *12*, 209-217.

Bjerkan, B. Word fragmentations and repetitions in the spontaneous speech of 2-6-year-old children. *Journal of Fluency Disorders*, 1980, *5*, 137-148.

Blankenship. J. "Stuttering" in normal speech. *Journal of Speech and Hearing Research*, 1964, *7*, 95-96.

Bloch, E.L., & Goodstein, L.D. Functional speech disorders and personality: A decade of research. *Journal of Speech and Hearing Disorders*, 1971, *36*, 295-314.

Blood, G.W. & Seider, R. The concomitant problems of young stutterers. *Journal of Speech and Hearing Disorders*, 1981, *46*, 31-33.

Bloodstein, O. A rating scale study of conditions under which stuttering is reduced or absent. *Journal of Speech and Hearing Disorders*, 1950, *15*, 29-36.

Bloodstein, O. The development of stuttering: I. Changes in nine basic features. *Journal of Speech and Hearing Disorders*, 1960, *25*, 219-237.

Bloodstein, O. The rules of early stuttering. *Journal of Speech and Hearing Disorders*, 1974, *39*, 379-394.

Bloodstein, O. *A handbook on stuttering* (3rd ed.) Chicago, Ill.: National Easter Seal Society, 1981.

Bloodstein, O., Alper, J., & Zisk, P.K. Stuttering as an outgrowth of normal disfluency. In D.A. Barbara (Ed.), *New directions in stuttering*. Springfield, Ill.: Charles C. Thomas, 1965.

Bloodstein, O., & Gantwerk, B.F. Grammatical function in relation to stuttering in young children. *Journal of Speech and Hearing Research*, 1967, *10*, 786-789.

Bloodstein, O., & Grossman, M. Early stutterings: Some aspects of their form and distribution. *Journal of Speech and Hearing Research*, 1981, *24*, 298-302.

Boberg, E., Ewart, B., Mason, G., Lindsay, K., & Wynn, S. Stuttering in the retarded: II. Prevalence of stuttering in EMR and TMR children. *Mental Retardation Bulletin*, 1978, *6*, 67-76.

Boehmler, R.M. Listener responses to non-fluencies. *Journal of Speech and Hearing Research*, 1958, *1*, 132-141.

Bohme, G. Stammering and cerebral lesions in early childhood. Examinations of 802 children and adults with cerebral lesions. *Folia Phoniatrica*, 1968, *20*, 239-249.

Brady, J.P. Studies on the metronome effect on stuttering. *Behavior Research and Therapy*, 1969, *7*, 197-204.

Brady, W.A., & Hall, D.E. The prevalence of stuttering among school-age children. *Language, Speech, and Hearing Services in Schools*, 1976, *7*, 75-81.

Chaney, C.F. Loci of disfluencies in the speech of nonstutterers. *Journal of Speech and Hearing Research*, 1969, *12*, 667-668.

Cherry, C. & Sayers, B. Experiments upon the total inhibition of stammering by external control, and some clinical results. *Journal of Psychosomatic Research*, 1956, *1*, 233-246.

Colcord, R.D., & Adams, M.R. Voicing duration and vocal SPL changes associated with stuttering reduction during singing. *Journal of Speech and Hearing Research,* 1979, *22,* 468-479.

Conture, E.G., McCall, G.N., & Brewer, D.W. Laryngeal behavior during stuttering. *Journal of Speech and Hearing Research,* 1977, *20,* 661-668.

Cooper, E.B. Recovery from stuttering in a junior and senior high school population. *Journal of Speech and Hearing Research,* 1972, *15,* 632-638.

Costello. J. Operant conditioning and the treatment of stuttering. *Seminars in Speech, Language, and Hearing,* 1980, *1,* 311-325.

Costello, J.M. Current behavioral treatments for children. In D. Prins & R.J. Ingham (Eds.), *Treatment of stuttering in early childhood: Methods and issues.* San Diego: College-Hill, 1983.

Cross, D.E., & Luper, H.L. Voice reaction time of stuttering and nonstuttering children and adults. *Journal of Fluency Disorders,* 1979, *4,* 59-77.

Cullinan, W.L., & Springer, M.T. Voice initiation and termination times in stuttering and nonstuttering children. *Journal of Speech and Hearing Research,* 1980, *23,* 344-360.

Curlee, R. A case selection strategy for young disfluent children. *Seminars in Speech, Language, and Hearing,* 1980, *1,* 277-287.(a)

Curlee, R. Assessment and treatment strategies for young stutterers. *Communicative Disorders,* 1980, *5,* 11. (b)

Curlee, R. Observer agreement on disfluency and stuttering. *Journal of Speech and Hearing Research,* 1981, *24,* 595-600.

Curlee, R., & Perkins, W.H. Conversational rate control therapy for stuttering. *Journal of Speech and Hearing Disorders,* 1969, *34,* 245-250.

Curry, F.K.W., & Gregory, H.H. The performance of stutterers on dichotic listening tasks thought to reflect cerebral dominance. *Journal of Speech and Hearing Research,* 1969, *12,* 73-82.

Darley, F.L. The relationship of parental attitudes and adjustments to the development of stuttering. In W. Johnson & R.R. Leutenegger (Eds.), *Stuttering in children and adults.* Minneapolis: University of Minnesota Press, 1955.

Davis, D.M. The relation of repetitions in the speech of young children to certain measures of language maturity and situational factors: Part I. *Journal of Speech Disorders,* 1939, *4,* 303-318.

Davis, D.M. The relation of repetitions in the speech of young children to certain measures of language maturity and situational factors: Part II and III. *Journal of Speech Disorders,* 1940, *5,* 235-246.

Dickson, S. Incipient stuttering and spontaneous remission of stuttered speech. *Journal of Communication Disorders,* 1971, *4,* 99-110.

Farmer, A. Stuttering repetitions in aphasic and nonaphasic brain damaged adults. *Cortex,* 1975, *11,* 391-396.

Floyd, S., & Perkins, W.H. Early syllable dysfluency in stutterers and nonstutterers: A preliminary report. *Journal of Communication Disorders,* 1974, *7,* 279-282.

Fransella, F., & Beech, H.R. An experimental analysis of the effect of rhythm on the speech of stutterers. *Behavior Research and Therapy,* 1965, *3,* 195-201.

Freeman, F.J., & Ushijima, T. Laryngeal muscle activity during stuttering. *Journal of Speech and Hearing Research,* 1978, *21,* 538-562.

Giolas, T.G., & Williams, D.E. Children's reactions to nonfluencies in adult speech. *Journal of Speech and Hearing Research,* 1958, *1,* 86-93.

Gladstein, K., Seider, R., & Kidd, K. Analysis of the sibship patterns of stutterers. *Journal of Speech and Hearing Research,* 1981, *24,* 460-462.

Glasner, P.J., & Rosenthal, D. Parental diagnosis of stuttering in young children. *Journal of Speech and Hearing Disorders,* 1957, *22,* 288-295.

Goodstein, L.D. Functional speech disorders and personality: A survey of the research. *Journal of Speech and Hearing Research*, 1958, *1*, 359-376.

Gray, B.B., & Brutten, E.J. The relationship between anxiety, fatigue and spontaneous recovery in stuttering. *Behavior Research and Therapy*, 1965, *2*, 251-259.

Gregory, H., & Hill, D. Stuttering therapy for children. *Seminars in Speech, Language and Hearing*, 1980, *1*, 351-363.

Hall, J.W., & Jerger, J. Central auditory function in stutterers. *Journal of Speech and Hearing Research*, 1978, *21*, 324-337.

Healey, E.C., Mallard, A.R., & Adams, M. Factors contributing to the reduction of stuttering during singing. *Journal of Speech and Hearing Research*, 1976, *19*, 475-480.

Helm, N.A., Butler, R.B., & Benson, D.F. Acquired stuttering. *Neurology*, 1978, *28*, 1159-1165.

Helmreich, H.G., & Bloodstein, O. The grammatical factor in childhood disfluency in relation to the continuity hypothesis. *Journal of Speech and Hearing Research*, 1973, *16*, 731-738.

Hood, S.B. Effect of communicative stress on the frequency and form-types of disfluent behavior in adult stutterers. *Journal of Fluency Disorders*, 1975, *1*, 36-47.

Howie, P.M. Concordance for stuttering in monozygotic and dizygotic twin pairs. *Journal of Speech and Hearing Research*, 1981, *24*, 317-321.

Huffman, E.S., & Perkins, W.H. Dysfluency characteristics identified by listeners as "stuttering" and "stutterer." *Journal of Communication Disorders*, 1974, *7*, 89-96.

Hull, F.M., Mielke, P.N. Williford, J.A., & Timmons, R.J. National Speech and Hearing Survey, Final report. Project No. 50978, Office of Education, Bureau of Education for the Handicapped, U.S. Department of Health, Education and Welfare, 1976.

Ingham, R.J. "Onset, prevalence, and recovery from stuttering": A reassessment of findings from the Andrews and Harris study. *Journal of Speech and Hearing Disorders*, 1976, *41*, 280-281.

Ingham, R. Spontaneous remission of stuttering: When will the emperor realize he has no clothes on? In D. Prins & R. Ingham (Eds.), *Treatment of stuttering in early childhood: Methods and issues*. San Diego: College-Hill, 1983.

Ingham, R.J., & Andrews, G. Behavior therapy and stuttering: A review. *Journal of Speech and Hearing Disorders*, 1973, *38*, 405-441.

Ingham, R.J., & Packman, A.C. Perceptual assessment of normalcy of speech following stuttering therapy. *Journal of Speech and Hearing Research*, 1978, *21*, 63-73.

Ingham R.J., & Packman, A. A further evaluation of the speech of stutterers during chorus- and nonchorus-reading conditions. *Journal of Speech and Hearing Research*, 1979, *22*, 784-793.

Johnson, L. Facilitating parental involvement in therapy of the disfluent child. *Seminars in Speech, Language, and Hearing*, 1980, *1*, 301-309.

Johnson, W. Measurements of oral reading and speaking rate and disfluency of adult male and female stutterers and nonstutterers. *Journal of Speech and Hearing Disorders, Monograph Supplement No. 7*, 1961, 1-20. (a)

Johnson, W. *Stuttering and what you can do about it*. Minneapolis: University of Minnesota Press, 1961. (b)

Johnson, W., & Associates. *The onset of stuttering*. Minneapolis: Univeristy of Minnesota Press, 1959.

Johnson, W., & Rosen, L. Studies in the psychology of stuttering: VII. Effect of certain changes in speech pattern upon frequency of stuttering. *Journal of Speech Disorders*, 1937, *2*, 105-109.

Johnson, W., and Sinn, A. Studies in the psychology of stuttering: V. Frequency of stuttering with expectation of stuttering controlled. *Journal of Speech Disorders*, 1937, *2*, 98-100.

Kidd, K.K. A genetic perspective on stuttering. *Journal of Fluency Disorders*, 1977, *2*, 259-269.

Kidd, K.K., Kidd, J.R., & Records, M.A. The possible causes of the sex ratio in stuttering and its implications. *Journal of Fluency Disorders*, 1978, *3*, 13-23.

Kidd, K.K., Oehlert, G., Heimbuch, R.C., Records, M.A., & Webster, R.L. Familial stuttering patterns are not related to one measure of severity. *Journal of Speech and Hearing Research,* 1980, *23,* 539-545.

LaBenz, P., & LaBenz, E.S. *Early correlates of speech, language, and hearing.* Littleton, Mass.: PSG Publishing, 1980.

Lankford, S.D., & Cooper, E.B. Recovery from stuttering as viewed by parents of self-diagnosed recovered stutterers. *Journal of Communication Disorders,* 1974, *7,* 171-180.

Leach, E. Stuttering: Clinical application of response-contingent procedures. In B.B. Gray & G. England (Eds.), *Stuttering and the conditioning therapies.* Monterey, California: Monterey Institute of Speech and Hearing, 1969.

MacDonald, J.D., & Martin, R.R. Stuttering and disfluency as two reliable and unambiguous response classes. *Journal of Speech and Hearing Research,* 1973, *16,* 691-699.

Mann, M.B. Nonfluencies in the oral reading of stutterers and nonstutterers of elementary school age. In W. Johnson & R.R. Leutenegger (Eds.), *Stuttering in children and adults.* Minneapolis: University of Minnesota Press, 1955.

Manning, W.H., Trutna, P.A. & Shaw, C.K. Verbal versus tangible reward for children who stutter. *Journal of Speech and Hearing Disorders,* 1976, *41,* 52-62.

Martin, R., & Haroldson, S.K. Effects of five experimental treatments on stuttering. *Journal of Speech and Hearing Research,* 1979, *22,* 132-146.

Martin, R., & Haroldson, S.K. Stuttering identification: Standard definitions and moment of stuttering. *Journal of Speech and Hearing Research,* 1981, *24,* 59-63.

Martin, R.R., Kuhl, P., & Haroldson, S. An experimental treatment with two preschool stuttering children. *Journal of Speech and Hearing Research,* 1972, *15,* 743-752.

McDearmon, J.R. Primary stuttering at the onset of stuttering: A re-examination of data. *Journal of Speech and Hearing Research,* 1968, *11,* 631-637.

Metraux, R.W. Speech profiles of the pre-school child 18 to 54 months. *Journal of Speech and Hearing Disorders,* 1950, *15,* 37-53.

Milisen, R. Frequency of stuttering with anticipation of stuttering controlled. *Journal of Speech Disorders,* 1938, *3,* 207-214.

Molt, L.F., & Guilford, A.M. Auditory processing and anxiety in stutterers. *Journal of Fluency Disorders,* 1979, *4,* 255-267.

Moore, W.H., Jr., & Haynes, W.O. Alpha hemispheric asymmetry and stuttering: Some support for a segmentation dysfunction hypothesis. *Journal of Speech and Hearing Research,* 1980, *23,* 229-247.

Moore, W.H., Jr., & Lang, M.K. Alpha asymmetry over the right and left hemispheres of stutterers and control subjects preceding massed oral readings: A preliminary investigation. *Perceptual Motor Skills,* 1977, *44,* 223-230.

Morley, M.E. *The development and disorders of speech in childhood,* Edinburgh: Livingstone, 1957.

Neelley, J.N., & Timmons, R.J. Adaptation and consistency in the disfluent speech behavior of young stutterers and nonstutterers. *Journal of Speech and Hearing Research,* 1967, *10,* 250-256.

Okasha, A., Bishry, Z., Kamel, M., & Hassan, A.H. Psychosocial study of stammering in Egyptian children. *British Journal of Psychiatry,* 1974, *124,* 531-533.

Panelli, C.A., McFarlane, S.C., and Shipley, K.G. Implications of evaluating and intervening with incipient stutterers. *Journal of Fluency Disorders,* 1978, *3,* 41-50.

Perkins, W.H., Bell, J., Johnson, L., & Stocks, J. Phone rate and the effective planning time hypothesis of stuttering.. *Journal of Speech and Hearing Research,* 1979, *22,* 747-755.

Perkins, W.H., & Curlee, R.F. Clinical impressions of portable masking unit effects in stuttering. *Journal of Speech and Hearing Disorders,* 1969, *34,* 360-362.

Perkins, W.H., Rudas, J., Johnson, L., & Bell, J. Stuttering: discoordination of phonation with articulation and respiration. *Journal of Speech and Hearing Research,* 1976, *19,* 509-522.

Peters, A.D. The effect of positive reinforcement on fluency: two case studies. *Language, Speech, and Hearing Services in Schools,* 1977, *8,* 15-22.

Prins, D. Personality, stuttering severity and age. *Journal of Speech and Hearing Research,* 1972, *15,* 148-154.

Quinn, P.T., & Andrews, G. Neurological stuttering—a clinical entity? *Journal of Neurology, Neurosurgery and Psychiatry,* 1977, *40,* 699-701.

Reed, C.G., & Godden, A.L. An experimental treatment using verbal punishment with two preschool stutterers. *Journal of Fluency Disorders,* 1977, *2,* 225-233.

Reich, A., Till, J., & Goldsmith, H. Laryngeal and manual reaction times of stuttering and nonstuttering adults. *Journal of Speech and Hearing Research,* 1981, *24,* 192-196.

Rickard, H.C., & Mundy, M.B. Direct manipulation of stuttering behavior: An experimental-clinical approach. In L.P. Ullmann & L. Krasner (Eds.), *Case studies in behavior modification.* New York: Holt, Rinehart, & Winston, 1965.

Rosenbek, J.C., McNeil, M.R., Lemme, M.L., Prescott, T.E., & Alfrey, A.C. Speech and language findings in a chronic hemodialysis patient: A case report. *Journal of Speech and Hearing Disorders,* 1975, *40,* 245-252.

Rosenbek, J., Messert, B., Collins, M., & Wertz, R.T. Stuttering following brain damage. *Brain and Language,* 1978, *6,* 82-96.

Runyan, C.M., & Adams, M.R. Perceptual study of the speech of "successfully therapeutized" stutterers. *Journal of Fluency Disorders,* 1978, *3,* 25-39.

Runyan, C.M., & Adams, M.R. Unsophisticated judges' perceptual evaluations of the speech of "successfully treated" stutterers. *Journal of Fluency Disorders,* 1979, *4,* 29-38.

Ryan, B.P. Operant procedures applied to stuttering therapy for children. *Journal of Speech and Hearing Disorders,* 1971, *36,* 264-280.

Sayles, D.G. Cortical excitability, perseveration, and stuttering. *Journal of Speech and Hearing Research,* 1971, *14,* 462-475.

Schiavetti, N. Judgments of stuttering severity as a function of type and locus of disfluency. *Folia Phoniatrica,* 1975, *27,* 26-37.

Schindler, M.D. A study of educational adjustments of stuttering and nonstuttering children. In W. Johnson, & R.R. Leutenegger (Eds.), *Stuttering in children and adults.* Minneapolis: University of Minnesota Press, 1955.

Shames, G., & Egolf, D. *Operant conditioning and the management of stuttering.* Englewood Cliffs, N.J.: Prentice-Hall, 1976.

Shaw, C.K., & Shrum, W.F. The effects of response-contingent reward on the connected speech of children who stutter. *Journal of Speech and Hearing Disorders,* 1972, *37,* 75-88.

Shearer, W.M., & Williams, J.D. Self-recovery from stuttering. *Journal of Speech and Hearing Disorders,* 1965, *30,* 288-290.

Sheehan, J.G. Projective studies of stuttering. *Journal of Speech and Hearing Disorders,* 1958, *23,* 18-25.

Sheehan, J.G., & Costley, M.S. A reexamination of the role of heredity in stuttering. *Journal of Speech and Hearing Disorders,* 1977, *42,* 47-59.

Sheehan, J.G., & Martyn, M.M. Stuttering and its disappearance. *Journal of Speech and Hearing Research,* 1970, *13,* 279-289.

Shine, R.E. Direct management of the beginning stutterer. *Seminars in Speech, Language, and Hearing,* 1980, *1,* 339-350.

Siegel, G.M. Punishment, stuttering, and disfluency. *Journal of Speech and Hearing Research,* 1970, *13,* 677-714.

Siegel, G.M., & Haugen, D. Audience size and variations in stuttering behavior. *Journal of Speech and Hearing Research,* 1964, *7,* 381-388.

Silverman, E. -M. Preschoolers' speech disfluency: Single syllable word repetition. *Perceptual Motor Skills,* 1972, *35,* 1002.

Silverman, E. -M. Word position and grammatical function in relation to preschoolers' speech disfluency. *Perceptual Motor Skills,* 1974, *39,* 267-272.

Silverman, F.H. The effect of rhythmic auditory stimulation on the disfluency of nonstutterers. *Journal of Speech and Hearing Research,* 1971, *14,* 350-355.

Silverman, F.H. Disfluency and word length. *Journal of Speech and Hearing Research,* 1972, *15,* 788-791.

Silverman, F.H. Disfluency behavior of elementary-school stutterers and nonstutterers. *Language, Speech, and Hearing Services in Schools,* 1974, *5,* 32-37.

Silverman, F.H. & Goodban, M.T. The effect of auditory masking on the fluency of normal speakers. *Journal of Speech and Hearing Research,* 1972, *15,* 543-546.

Silverman F., & Williams, D. Loci of disfluencies in the speech of stutterers. *Perceptual Motor Skills,* 1967, *24,* 1085-1086.

Soderberg, G.A. A comparison of adaptation trends in the oral reading of stutterers, inferior speakers and superior speakers. *Journal of Communication Disorders,* 1969, *2,* 99-108. (a)

Soderberg, G.A. Delayed auditory feedback and the speech of stutterers: A review of studies *Journal of Speech and Hearing Disorders,* 1969, *34,* 20-29. (b)

Sommers, R.K., Brady, W.A., & Moore, W.H., Jr. Dichotic ear preferences of stuttering children and adults. *Perceptual Motor Skills,* 1975, *41,* 931-938.

Starkweather, C.W., Hirschman, P., & Tannenbaum, R.S. Latency of vocalization onset: Stutterers versus nonstutterers. *Journal of Speech and Hearing Research,* 1976, *19,* 481-492.

Stromsta, C. A spectrographic study of dysfluencies labeled as stuttering by parents. *De Therapia Vocis et Loquelae, Vol. I,* XIII Congress, International Society of Logopedics and Phoniatrics, 1965.

Sussman, H.M. & MacNeilage, P.F. Hemispheric specialization for speech production and perception in stutterers. *Neuropsychologia,* 1975, *13,* 19-26.

Toscher, M.M., & Rupp, R.R A study of the central auditory processes in stutterers using the Synthetic Sentence Identification (SSI) test battery. *Journal of Speech and Hearing Research,* 1978, *21,* 779-792

Turnbaugh, K.R., Guitar, B.E., & Hoffman, P.R. Speech clinicians' attribution of personality traits as a function of stuttering severity. *Journal of Speech and Hearing Research,* 1979, *22,* 37-45.

Tuthill, C. A quantitative study of extensional meaning with special reference to stuttering. *Speech Monographs,* 1946, *13,* 81-98.

Van Riper, C. *The treatment of stuttering.* Englewood Cliffs N.J.: Prentice-Hall, 1973.

Van Riper, C. *The nature of stuttering* (2nd ed.). Englewood Cliffs, N.J.: Prentice-Hall, 1982.

Voelker, C.H. A preliminary investigation for a normative study of fluency: A clinical index to the severity of stuttering. *American Journal of Orthopsychiatry,* 1944, *14,* 285-294.

Wahler, R., Sperling, K., Thomas, M., Teeter, N. & Luper, H. The modification of childhood stuttering: Some response-response relationships. *Journal of Experimental Child Psychology,* 1970, *9,* 411-428.

Wendahl, R.W., & Cole, J. Identification of stuttering during relatively fluent speech.. *Journal of Speech and Hearing Research,* 1961, *4,* 281-286.

Westby, C.E. Language performance of stuttering and nonstuttering children. *Journal of Communication Disorders,* 1979, *12,* 133-145.

Williams, D. A perspective on approaches to stuttering therapy. In H. Gregory (Ed.), *Controversies about stuttering therapy.* Baltimore: University Park Press, 1979.

Williams, D.E., & Kent, L.R. Listener evaluations of speech interruptions. *Journal of Speech and Hearing Research,* 1958, *1,* 124-131.

Williams, D.E., Melrose, B.M., & Woods, C.L. The relationship between stuttering and academic achievement in children. *Journal of Communication Disorders,* 1969, *2,* 87-98.

Williams, D.E., & Silverman, F.H. Note concerning articulation of school-age stutterers. *Perceptual Motor Skills,* 1968, *27,* 713-714.

Williams, D.E., Silverman, F.H., & Kools, J.A. Disfluency behavior of elementary-school stutterers and nonstutterers: The adaptation effect. *Journal of Speech and Hearing Research,* 1968, *11,* 622-630.

Williams, D.E., Silverman, F.H., & Kools, J.A. Disfluency behavior of elementary-school stutterers and nonstutterers: Loci of instances of disfluency. *Journal of Speech and Hearing Research,* 1969, *12,* 308-318.

Wingate, M.E. A standard definition of stuttering. *Journal of Speech and Hearing Disorders,* 1964, *29,* 484-489.

Wingate M.E. *Stuttering: Theory and treatment.* New York: Irvington, 1976.

Winitz, H. Repetitions in the vocalizations of children in the first two years of life. *Journal of Speech and Hearing Disorders, Monograph Supplement No. 7,* 1961, 55-62.

Winitz, H. & Darley, F.L. Speech production. In P.J. La Benz & E.S. La Benz (Eds.), *Early correlates of speech, language, and hearing.* Littleton, Mass.: PSG Publishing Company, 1980.

Woods, C.L., & Williams, D.E. Traits attributed to stuttering and normally fluent males. *Journal of Speech and Hearing Research,* 1976, *19,* 267-278.

Yairi, E. Disfluency rates and patterns of stutterers and nonstutterers. *Journal of Communication Disorders,* 1972, *5,* 225-231.

Yairi, E. Disfluencies of normally speaking two-year-old children. *Journal of Speech and Hearing Research,* 1981, *24,* 490-495.

Yairi, E. The onset of stuttering in two- and three-year-old children: A preliminary report. *Journal of Speech and Hearing Disorders,* 1983, *48,* 171-177.

Young, M.A. Predicting ratings of severity of stuttering. *Journal of Speech and Hearing Disorders, Monograph Supplement, No. 7,* 1961, 31-54.

Young, M.A. Identification of stutterers from recorded samples of their "fluent" speech. *Journal of Speech and Hearing Research,* 1964, *7,* 302-303.

Young, M.A. Observer agreement: Cumulative effects of repeated ratings of the same samples and of knowledge of group results. *Journal of Speech and Hearing Research,* 1969, *12,* 144-155.

Young, M.A. Observer agreement for marking moments of stuttering. *Journal of Speech and Hearing Research,* 1975, *18,* 530-540 (a)

Young, M.A. Onset, prevalence, and recovery from stuttering. *Journal of Speech and Hearing Disorders,* 1975, *40,* 49-58. (b)

Young, M.A., & Downs, T.D. Testing the significance of the agreement among observers. *Journal of Speech and Hearing Research,* 1968, *11,* 5-17.

Zimmerman, G.N., & Knott, J.R. Slow potentials of the brain related to speech processing in normal speakers and stutterers. *Electroencephalographic Clinical Neurophysiology,* 1974, *37,* 599-607.

Zwitman, D.H. *The disfluent child: A management program.* Baltimore: University Park Press, 1978.

Martin R. Adams

The Differential Assessment and Direct Treatment of Stuttering

During the past 10 to 12 years, there have been several significant developments in the assessment and treatment of children who stutter. We have seen emergence of behavioral criteria that can be used for the purpose of discriminating between the incipient or beginning stutterer and the normally disfluent child. Furthermore, findings have shown that speech and other behavioral problems associated with the stuttering of one youngster may differ appreciably from the behavioral deviations evident in another. Mindful of the existence of these disparities, some clinicians have developed differential assessment procedures to probe for them. The responses of a young stutterer tested in this way are then used as a basis for planning therapy. Since children will present diverse assessment profiles, it follows that a treatment regimen constructed for one patient might be quite unlike the remediation program established for another. Whatever form the therapy takes, the chances are good that a direct approach to clinical intervention will be employed. This direct involvement of youngsters in treatment surely represents the most profound change in our orientation to the management of stuttering in children. It hardly need be said that for years there was a strong preference for indirect methods such as parent counseling and play therapy. While these techniques are still viable treatment options, they are less popular today.

Here then, summarized, are the 3 key developments cited thus far: (1) the formulation of behavioral criteria for discriminating between the incipient stutterer and the normally disfluent child; (2) the generation of differential assessment techniques to probe for dimensions of stuttering in children; and (3) the construction and application of direct approaches to the treatment of young stutterers. In the next sections of this chapter, we shall take a rather detailed look at each.

Behavioral Criteria for Discriminating Between the Incipient Stutterer and the Normally Disfluent Child

One of the most intimidating problems that confronts the speech-language pathologist involves making clinical discriminations between the incipient stutterer and the normally disfluent child. This differentiation is made formidable by what is at stake: If a child is inappropriately identified as a beginning stutterer, then he or she would presumably be inserted into a treatment program. At the least, his time and that of the clinician would be wasted because therapy is simply not needed; and some believe that such unnecessary treatment might serve to create a problem where one does not in fact exist. Of course, clinicians would not want to mistakenly identify an incipient stutterer as being normally disfluent since such an error would lead to the withholding of remediation where it was actually needed. In the absence of this treatment, there would be a greater opportunity for various aspects of the stuttering pattern to become habituated. That would make the problem more difficult to modify in the future when a correct evaluation was finally rendered. Obviously, there are serious potential consequences associated with mistakenly viewing a normally disfluent child as an incipient stutterer, or with the faulty evaluation of an incipient stutterer as a normally disfluent youngster.

Less than 20 years ago, little had been done to delineate guidelines that might be used to make this crucial differentiation. Thus, clinicians were forced to rely mainly on their intuitions and past experiences when confronted with a child suspected of being an incipient stutterer. If, on those occasions, these workers paled before the task of differentially evaluating the youngster, we can understand why. Fortunately, this situation has now taken a decided turn for the better. Reference is made here to the fact that during the last 5 years, several attempts have been made to identify and describe behavioral criteria that might be used to accurately discriminate between the incipient stutterer and the normally disfluent child. Pertinent are the efforts of such individuals as Adams (1977; 1980), Curlee (1980), Gregory and Hill (1980), Johnson (1980) and Conture (1982). The differential evaluation profiles formed by these workers were developed from their clinical experience and research efforts, and those of still other professionals.

What is remarkable about these profiles is how similar they all are. Granted that the speech-language pathologists who developed the profiles have been influenced by one another. Yet, to a significant extent, these clinicians established their profiles independently. This is a matter of some import because it means that without biasing each other, these professionals have come to similar conclusions about what characteristics to associate with early stuttering and normal disfluency. This high degree of agreement gives some credence to the profiles themselves.

Since the profiles are so much alike, it would be wasteful to examine each of them separately. Instead, descriptions of the fluency behavior characteristics that are common to the profiles that have been developed are presented.

Common Profile Characteristics

In judging a child to be an incipient stutterer, it is now believed that the presence of the following signs or symptoms is crucial: (1) Part-word repetitions and prolongations make up in excess of 7% of all words spoken; (2) the part-word repetitions are marked by at least 3 unit repetitions (e.g., "bee-bee-bee-beet" vs. "bee-bee-beet"); (3) the part-word repetitions are also perceived as containing the schwa in place of the vowel normally found in the syllable that is being repeated (e.g., "buh-buh-buh-beet" vs. "bee-bee-beet"); (4) the prolongations last longer than 1 second; and (5) difficulty in starting and/or sustaining voicing or air flow is heard in association with the part-word repetitions and prolongations. As more and more of these 5 signs are noted in a child's speech, a clinician can be increasingly confident that he or she is dealing with an incipient stutterer. Contrariwise, the fewer of these symptoms that are noted, the more likely that the youngster is normally disfluent. Whichever choice is made, it ought to be based on the foregoing and other behavioral data, be compatible with case history information that bears on the incidence of stuttering in the child's family, take into account any current trends in the frequency of occurrence of the youngster's disfluency (i.e., has it been steadily increasing or decreasing?), and address such other considerations as the presence or absence of emotional and behavioral reactions to the fluency failures by the child, as well as parental attitudes toward their offspring and his fluency irregularities. A final differential evaluation would then be based on the sum of the behavioral evidence and case history information just cited.

Acting on the Outcomes of Differential Evaluations

Based on the foregoing review, there would appear to be 3 possible outcomes of the differential evaluation process. First, a child may present an unequivocal picture of *normal disfluency.* That is, he exhibits none or just one of the signs of incipient stuttering mentioned in the previous section. Or, a youngster might evince what Adams (1980) has referred to as an *ambiguous clinical picture,* or what Gregory and Hill (1980) have described as *borderline atypical disfluency.* That is, the youngster exhibits just 2 or perhaps 3 of the 5 signs of incipient stuttering cited earlier. Finally, the child could reveal a clear pattern of *incipient stuttering.* That is, a clinical picture that includes 4 or all 5 of the symptoms of beginning stuttering could be presented. In this section we shall examine the approaches that have been recommended for dealing with members of each of these 3 groups.

The Normally Disfluent Child

Youngsters identified as being normally disfluent are certainly not candidates for therapy, even in some indirect form. Instead, it is widely agreed that parental counseling is the essential next step to take once a clinician is confident that the child in question is normally disfluent. Within counseling, parents are provided with the assessment of normal disfluency and are given general information about the development of dimensions of speech and language in children. The danger signs of incipient stuttering are identified so that the parents can monitor any hints of these behaviors that might later appear in their child's utterances. In addition, the parents are offered guidance designed to neutralize any lingering concerns they might have over their offspring's development of fully normal speech and are assured of the clinician's ongoing willingness to be of help should the child's fluency development take a negative turn. Lastly, a recheck of the child is usually scheduled for some future date.

Typically, all of the foregoing steps can be accomplished in a brief period of time after the youngster's evaluation. On occasion, however, parents may exhibit such an excess of anxiety about their child's speech development that one or more return visits to the clinic for further counseling will be required. The completion of counseling, however long it might take, marks the end of the clinician's involvement with the child and parents. Nothing else need be done unless a future reevaluation has been set up or is requested.

The Child with an Ambiguous Clinical Picture or Borderline Atypical Disfluency

If there is consensus over how to deal with the normally disfluent child, there is some disagreement over the approach to take with the youngster who presents an ambiguous clinical picture (Adams, 1980) or borderline atypical disfluency (Gregory & Hill, 1980).

As was noted earlier, Adams (1980) has suggested that when a youngster evinces an ambiguous clinical picture, it is best to be cautious and conservative. Direct therapy is bypassed in favor of indirect methods. These take the form of parental counseling if it is needed, and a program for monitoring the child's speech. Specifically, the parents observe their offspring's fluency on a day-by-day basis and then report to the clinician at a prearranged time each week. This tack is taken for up to 6 months. During that period it is expected that the child's speech pattern will change, either for better or worse. Whatever the case, the alterations that do occur should make the youngster easier to evaluate *unequivocally*. If a clear picture of incipient stuttering does materialize, then a direct treatment program is immediately set into motion. In contrast, if the child has gravitated into a clear pattern of normal disfluency, then that assessment is made and the parental monitoring regimen is gradually phased out. On rare occasions, a youngster's ambiguous clinical picture will not change within the 6 months allotted for the counseling and monitoring program. When that happens it should be assumed that the negative features of the child's ambiguous pattern are starting to become habituated and thus require direct and immediate treatment.

Gregory and Hill (1980) are far more prompt and direct in their dealings with the child who they refer to as exhibiting borderline atypical disfluency. To begin with, they will conduct a comprehensive evaluation of this youngster to see if he exhibits other behavioral irregularities and/or disorders of speech and language. Even if the results of this far-reaching assessment show the child to be free of other defects, the borderline atypical disfluency is subject to a combined direct and indirect treatment program. The specifics of this dual approach will be presented in a subsequent section. For the present it suffices to say that this regimen involves interactions between the clinician and the youngster, between the clinician and the parents, and between the parents and their offspring. Upon completion of therapy, procedures for monitoring the child's fluency are set up and reevaluations are scheduled for the future. Even more elaborate rehabilitative measures are taken with the youngster who evinces borderline atypical disfluency *and* other disturbances in speech and language behavior. Again, we shall defer comment on Gregory and Hill's specific rehabilitative tactics until later.

The Incipient Stutterer

There is now wide agreement that once a firm evaluation has been made, therapy should be routinely recommended for the incipient stutterer. Yet, before treatment can begin, the clinician must decide whether intervention should be direct or indirect, and what should be included in a child's rehabilitative program. However, before we can develop answers to these inquiries it is necessary to come to some understanding of what the terms "indirect" and "direct" therapy mean. In this chapter, and elsewhere in this book (see Guitar, Chapter 10), a relatively narrow meaning has been applied to the label "indirect therapy." That is, we shall consider as "indirect" any therapy in which a professional strives to enhance a client's fluency by means *other* than stimulating speech responses and applying consequences to them. Within the boundaries of this definition, indirect treatment does not require that the child be placed in a formal treatment setting or even be dealt with at all for that matter. For example, parent counseling is a form of indirect therapy wherein the child is excluded from the rehabilitative process. Anxiety deconditioning through systematic desensitization, play therapy, and drug tranquilization are also types of indirect treatment. In these latter 3 cases, the client is involved, being seen by a speech-language pathologist, psychologist, or physician. However, the youngster's speech responses are not actively evoked for the purpose of manipulating them through orderly application of consequences.

In sharp contrast to this definitional posture, we shall attach a very broad meaning to the term "direct therapy." That is, we will refer to as "direct" any regimen that, at the least, places a child in a treatment setting with a qualified speech-language clinician who actively evokes speech responses and then applies consequences to one or more aspects of the client's ensuing utterances, all for the purpose of augmenting fluency. Within this framework, a clinician could work directly on stuttering in an effort to reduce or eliminate it. Of course, neither stuttering nor fluency need be the focus of therapeutic stimulation. Rather, fluency might be increased (and stuttering decreased) as a by-product of the clinician's direct modification of other dimensions of communication such as speaking rate, or the length and complexity of the child's utterances.

Starting several years ago, and continuing until about 1970, it was commonplace for clinicians to employ indirect therapy in the form of parent counseling as the *sole* means of treating young stutterers. By the 1970s some speech-language pathologists (Ryan, 1971) began to deviate from this approach and make *exclusive* use of a rather circumscribed set of direct operant methods in their work with child stutterers. Questions have been raised, however, about this pattern of making exclusive use of a single indirect or direct rehabilitative approach with most, if not all, clients. It has been pointed out that to employ just one treatment tactic, and no other, requires the assumptions that the form of therapy being used is superior to other methods, and that this one treatment program is well suited to essentially all young stutterers. As an alternative to the "single method" view, several clinicians have suggested that differences between young stutterers must be identified and taken into account when planning and conducting therapy. The process by which disparities among stutterers may be uncovered is herein referred to as a "differential assessment."

Differential Assessment of the Incipient Stutterer

The idea that differential assessment was even necessary grew out of a view that is 25 years old; namely, that stuttering may be a multidimensional disorder (Van Riper, 1958). Conceiving of stuttering in this way raises the possibility that dimensions of the problem may differ from stutterer to stutterer. In turn, this would mean that persons who stutter could be segregated into subgroups on the bases of different background characteristics and/or behaviors. With the notable exception of studies by Berlin (Note 1) and Andrews and Harris (1964), this line of thinking received scant attention until the 1970s. At that point a steady increase in efforts to identify and describe dimensions of stuttering began (cf., Canter, 1971; Prins & Lohr, 1972; Van Riper, 1971). The most recent contributors to this work have been Glyndon and Jeanna Riley, and Aaron Smith and David Daly.

The Rileys hypothesized that problems in attending, perceiving, comprehending, encoding, and executing a speech response could function separately, together, or in combination with various environmental factors to promote stuttering. To look into this possibility, they started to collect data from young stutterers through formal tests, informal probes, and longitudinal observations. They also have taken extensive case histories, interviewed parents, and observed parent-child interactions. Occasionally, as this work progressed, these researchers reported on their findings (Riley & Riley, Notes 2 and 3). Then in 1979, the Rileys published a compilation of results they culled from a much larger pool of data drawn from 176 children who stuttered. Portions of the data presented in this article came from 76 young stutterers between the ages of 3 and 12 years. Using factor analysis [1], they were able to identify 4 factors that they believed represented "neurologic components" (Riley & Riley, 1979, p. 283) of stuttering. They also described 2 "intrapersonal components" and 3 "interpersonal components" (Riley & Riley, 1979, p. 282). Subsequently, each member of this total of 9 components was studied among 54 stuttering children who ranged in age from 3 to 11 years. This subset of the larger groups of 176 and 76 youngsters was singled out for study because of the availability of more complete and analyzable test results and other forms of pertinent information. Table 9-1 contains a distillation of some of the major findings provided by the Rileys in their 1979 publication. The table includes the identification and the more prominent behavioral characteristics of each of the 9 components. Also found in Table 9-1 are figures showing the percentages of the 54 children that exhibited clinically significant levels of each component.

Several additional comments need to be made regarding the distribution of components across the 54 children studied. First, all of these youngsters exhibited as least 1 of the 9 components. However, 9.2% of these stutterers were free of neurologic components. Slightly more than 90% of the children evinced at least 1 neurologic component, with over 18% of them showing 3 or all 4 of these components. Seventy-four percent of the children were considered to have neurologic components, the behavioral indices of which were judged to be significant enough to warrant therapeutic attention.

What is missing from the Rileys' 1979 report is some indication of the various ways in which the components might cluster together. This matter was dealt with in a more recent investigation. In this follow-up study (1980), they applied factor analysis to the data gathered from the larger subgroup of 76 stutterers. The results of this study provide insights into the interrelationships that appear to exist among the neurologic components. The more important of these findings indicated that: (1) Stutterers who exhibited reduced linguistic ability were also likely to possess relatively poor auditory perceptual skills and motor problems, as well; (2) children with poor scores on the motor component were good candidates to exhibit some of the characteristics of the attending component (i.e., hyperactivity, perseveration, and/or distractibility), though the motor difficulties of these same children could exist independent of linguistic and auditory perceptual deficits; and (3) youngsters exhibiting auditory processing problems could nonetheless present better-than-average overall language, oral, and fine motor abilities.

As was noted in Table 9-1, the Rileys identified what they believe are four components of a more general neurologic dimension of stuttering. Striking support for this view has evolved out of the experimental work of Smith and Daly (Note 4). During the summers of each year from 1973 to 1980, they have had the opportunity to conduct extensive tests and behavioral observations on youngsters who were attending a residential stuttering therapy program.

During their summers of data collection, Smith and Daly screened 128 stutterers. Twenty-eight of these children exhibited cluttering, cleft palate, cerebral palsy, epilepsy, mental retardation, hearing loss, aphasia, or

TABLE 9-1
Nine components of stuttering identified by Riley and Riley (1979).

Component/Key Behavioral Correlates	Percentages of 54 Children Exhibiting Each Component
Neurologic Components	
Attending problems as evidenced by distractibility, perseveration, hyperactivity, inability to concentrate on tasks, and low frustration tolerance.	36%
Auditory processing problems as evidenced by delayed responses to tasks, need to have directions repeated, clarified, or presented in some other way; self-corrections by the child after he has started to respond.	27%
Sentence formulation problems as evidenced by inability to formulate a sentence from a stimulus word; utterances made up of short, fragmented phrases; utterances marked by word reversals and transpositions; use of verbs and other grammatic elements that lack appropriate complexity; poor sentence repetition ability.	31%
Oral-motor problems as evidenced by poor performance on diadochokinetic tasks; errors during syllable repetition; anywhere from mild to severe articulatory inaccuracy.	69%
Intrapersonal Components	
High self-expectations on the part of the child as evidenced by the youngster's apparent difficulty in accepting anything other than "top" performance from himself; child spontaneously makes unfavorable comments about himself or to peers.	38%
Manipulative stuttering as evidenced by the child's ability to direct parental behavior and/or gain parental attention with stuttering.	25%
Interpersonal Components	
Disruptive communicative environment as evidenced by adult-child conversations that are too rapidly paced; pressure on the child for prompt responding, thus denying him the chance to organize his thoughts; interruptions of the child as he speaks; and adults acting rushed as they wait for the child to speak.	53%
High expectations of the child by his elders as evidenced by adults' expressions of perfectionistic attitudes; adults' fostering of competitiveness; adults' unrealistically high assessment of child's true ability.	51%
Abnormal parental need for the child to stutter as evidenced by their demonstrable rejection of the child because of the stuttering; parental rejection of several other aspects of child's behavior.	5%

emotional difficulties in addition to their stuttering. These individuals were excluded from further testing on the grounds that they were not typical members of the stuttering population. The remaining 100 youngsters, ranging in age from 8 to 19 years, and with a mean age of 13 years, were exposed to a wide-ranging battery of tests that included the entire Wechsler Intelligence Scale, the Benton Visual Retention and Design Copy Test, Raven's Progressive Matrices, the Purdue Pegboard, the Smith Symbol Digits Written and Oral Substitutions, the Memory for Unrelated Sentences, and tests for articulation, language, and stuttering severity.

Based on test results, 12 youngsters were identified as possessing both stuttering and an articulation defect. Another 14 children were identified as being stutterers and learning disabled. The third and largest group contained 74 youngsters, whose stuttering was not attended by either errors of articulation or learning disabilities.

Having identified these 3 subgroups of stutterers, Smith and Daly probed within each subject's test data for indications of "neuropsychological deficits" (Smith & Daly, Note 4). Among the largest group of 74 youngsters, 32 of them (43%) presented evidence of anywhere from 3 to 9 signs indicating organic cerebral dysfunction. Twenty of the 74 stutterers evinced 2 signs. Another 12 of the 74 exhibited 1 sign. That left just 10 youngsters who were free of any signs of organic cerebral dysfunction. In the stuttering + defective articulation subgroup, 9 of the 12 children (75%) provided 3 or more signs of organic cerebral dysfunction. One individual showed 2 signs, another child revealed 1 sign, and the twelfth youngster exhibited no signs. Even more skewed was the incidence of signs in the stuttering + learning disability subgroup. Therein, 13 of the 14 youngsters (93%) evinced 3 or more signs. The remaining stutterer presented 2 signs. Thus, when the findings for the 3 subgroups are taken together, 54 of the 100 children exhibited what Smith and Daly refer to as a "strong indication" of organic cerebral dysfunction; that is, 3 or more signs. Twenty-two of the 100 youngsters evinced 2 signs; that is, what Smith and Daly label as "equivocal" signs of cerebral involvement. Twenty-four of the 100 young stutterers revealed "no compelling evidence of organicity" (Smith & Daly, Note 4); that is, 1 or no signs.

The findings of the Rileys (1979; 1980) and Smith and Daly (Note 4) could well be the strongest evidence that stutterers may have multiple disorders, and that the total clinical picture of one individual may differ from that of another. Still, we must recognize that the work of these two teams of researchers was descriptive of correlations among the variables they chose to study. These sorts of results do not allow us to draw inferences or implications regarding causality. Nonetheless, within their frame of reference the Rileys, Smith and Daly, and other workers

Table 9-2
Recommended Minimum Contents of a Differential Assessment Battery for Children Diagnosed as Incipient Stutterers.

1. Observation of the child's ability to direct, focus, and sustain attention on diagnostic materials and tasks.
2. Observation of the child's verbal and nonverbal activity levels.
3. Observation of any perseverative tendencies.
4. Formal testing of auditory retention span.
5. Formal testing of auditory discrimination ability.
6. Formal testing of auditory verbal comprehension.
7. Formal or informal testing of object naming.
8. Elicitation of story telling from the child in order to estimate (a) mean length of utterance; (b) level of grammar and syntax; (c) word retrieval ability; (d) vocabulary development and usage.
9. Formal language testing.
10. Testing of the motor speech mechanism with tasks that include (a) simple syllable repetition; (b) syllable sequence repetition; (c) alternating lateralization of the tongue; (d) articulatory accuracy during connected speech; (e) sustained phonation; and (f) measurement of voice onset time.
11. Case history taking including inquiries into parents' attitudes towards the child and his stuttering.
12. Observation of any behaviors reflecting the child's awareness of his stuttering.
13. Observation of any behaviors reflecting negative reactions by the child to the stuttering.
14. Testing of the child's ability to effectively increase his fluency.
15. Observation of verbal and nonverbal interactions between parent(s) and child.

(Adams, 1980; Gregory & Hill, 1980) have stressed that, clinically, children who exhibit incipient stuttering should be exposed to a differential assessment. Gregory and Hill have even extended this position to include youngsters who evince borderline atypical disfluency. Recommendations as to the minimum contents of a differential assessment "package" are presented in itemized form in Table 9-2. The tasks and techniques suggested for use are modeled after many of those used by the Rileys (1979, 1980) and, to a lesser extent, by Gregory and Hill (1980).

The contents of Table 9-2 do not represent an all-encompassing statement on what functions to test or what behaviors should be specially noted in the differential assessment of young stutterers. Nonetheless, what has been offered should provide clinicians with a good general idea of the depth and breadth of this sort of evaluation. If sufficient in scope, the differential assessment can produce data that will guide the clinician in forming answers to the questions, "Should therapy be indirect or direct?" and "What should be included in a child's rehabilitative program?" In the next 2 sections we shall address these inquiries and show in each how key results from the differential assessment can be used to make clinical decisions that pertain to the planning and implementation of treatment.

Indirect or Direct Therapy?

In the view of some, this author included, the choice between indirect and direct therapy can be made on the basis of 4 bits of differential assessment data. They are: (1) The clinician's judgment of the child's degree of awareness of stuttering; (2) the apparent extent of the youngster's negative reaction(s) to the problem; (3) the presence of other complicating behavioral problems; and (4) the existence of disturbances in the parent-child relationship. Two guidelines, loosely applied, fit here. First, one might give serious consideration to indirect therapy when the child exhibits little awareness of his stuttering, no negative reactions to it, and no other behavioral problems. Here, indirect rehabilitation might well be preferred because it ought to minimize the chances of focusing the patient's attention on the speech production process and drawing attention to stuttering. The second guideline provides for indirect therapy in circumstances where an hypothesized immediate cause[2] of the stuttering seems to involve an agent *external* to the youngster's speech system; for example, a breakdown in the parent-child relationship, anxiety, or psychological difficulties in some other form. In cases fitting these descriptions, indirect treatment in the forms of parent counseling, anxiety deconditioning, drug tranquilization, and/or psychotherapy would seem wise choices.

In opposition, some sort of direct therapy strategy could be recommended when a child demonstrates negative reactions to the stuttering or, at least, acknowledges its existence. Many children who respond in these ways feel relief and support when a helping adult deals with the stuttering in a calm and open manner. Moreover, some sort of straightforward approach is almost obligatory because the child's demonstrable awareness of the problem makes it pointless to try to avoid focusing on the speech production process as indirect methods do.

Others might suggest that a direct approach should also be selected in cases where the immediate cause of the stuttering seems attributable to an agent operating within the child's speech system. Remember, tests of auditory retention, auditory discrimination, language, and the like were included in the differential assessment because of the possibility that disorders of these functions could promote stuttering. If such does seem to be a possibility, then the deficient function might be treated directly with the view that fluency may improve as a by-product of this intervention.

Up to this point, we have talked as though clinicians must employ either some indirect tactic or a direct methodology on an exclusive basis. In actuality, the vast majority of contemporary therapies for children who stutter include both indirect and direct manipulations, with a decided emphasis on the latter. As was noted early in this chapter, the trend toward use of more direct treatments can be viewed as perhaps the most significant change in our orientation to the management of stuttering in children. We turn now to a description of these primarily direct protocols.

Direct Therapy Programs for Young Stutterers Group Studies

The Gregory and Hill Program

Gregory and Hill view children's disfluencies as falling at various points along a continuum that ranges from typical or usual disfluencies through borderline atypical disfluencies to the most atypical disfluencies. Here, we shall concentrate on the primarily direct treatment regimen that Gregory and Hill (1980) recommend for the child who exhibits the most atypical disfluencies. Once a youngster is observed exhibiting the most unusual disfluencies, Gregory and Hill proceed with a differential assessment. Their purpose here is to uncover any variables that are impeding, or could hamper, a child's development of normal fluency. Results of the differential assessment are then used to construct an individualized therapy program that deals with the salient factors identified in the assessment. This specially tailored regimen involves 2 hours of one-to-one contact and a half hour in a therapy group each week. The program is designed to meet 5 key objectives.

The first objective is to "avoid creating or increasing the child's awareness of a speech problem or stuttering" (1980, p. 357). This is accomplished by describing the treatment as having children attend "school" instead of therapy. In school they will have their own "teacher" who will engage them in enjoyable talking and listening games and other sorts of activities. By proceeding in this way, the focus of therapy is allowed to fall on fluency and behaviors that facilitate fluent speech. With youngsters who exhibit high levels of awareness of their speech disturbance, a more pointed approach can be taken. Specifically, Gregory and Hill follow Williams's lead and recommend talking with the child about "bumpy and smooth speech," and "talking hard and talking easy" (Williams, 1971, pp. 1073-1093; 1979, pp. 241-268).

The second objective is "to increase the amount of fluency that the child experiences" (1980, p. 358). Principally, this is accomplished by having the clinician model for the child an effortless, comfortable, flowing speech pattern that also involves smooth and gradual articulatory transitions into a word, through it, and then onto the following word.[3] Several steps can be taken to facilitate the child's acquisition of the target speech pattern that the clinician has modeled. Smooth, flowing speech can be exemplified by rolling a ball or small car across a table. Articulatory gestures can be slowed to an even greater extent. An edible or tangible reward for proper speech patterning can be introduced to heighten motivation. If bodily tension seems to be interfering with the child's success, then the role playing of such effortless activities as walking in space or floating on water can be interjected into treatment. The target speech pattern is to be used by the youngster as he responds to a series of verbal tasks that have been arranged from the nonpropositional to the propositional. It is considered to be stabilized if the youngster produces the pattern on 90% of the responses across 20 trials in each of 4 consecutive treatment sessions. When this high level of proper response has been achieved, opportunities can be contrived for the child to use the target pattern on propositional single-word responses outside the therapy room and with the parents. For instance, the clinician might offhandedly prompt the child to "tell Mommy one thing you would like for dinner tonight."

Generalization of fluent single-word, target speech responses to settings outside the clinic marks the point where work can begin on utterances of somewhat longer length. This advancement in the Gregory and Hill program could be to 2-, 3-, or even 4-word utterances. The length of responses, their degree of propositionality, and the types of cues introduced to prompt a child are not rigidly fixed. Rather, clinicians are encouraged to use data from the differential assessment and from the phases of treatment already completed to determine the next level in the child's program. For example, imagine a young child who, in spite of his stuttering, presents an otherwise normal differential assessment profile and has responded promptly and positively in the first stage of rehabilitation. With such a child it might well be appropriate to skip the 2-word level and imitative responding and go immediately to 3-word responses that would be evoked with questions posed by the clinician. In contrast, consider a stutterer with an identified deficit in auditory verbal comprehension who first responded slowly and erratically at the 1-word level. To accelerate this child's program by omitting 2-word imitative responding might be risky. Gregory and Hill's obvious thrust here is toward flexibly tailoring steps in treatment to each patient's abilities. This approach to increasing the length of the child's utterances and then transferring them to extraclinical speech situations can be pursued until the mean length of the youngster's responses are within normal limits.

Work on transfer and generalization at each stage of a child's regimen is accompanied by the introduction of techniques for "building tolerance toward fluency disrupting influences" (Gregory & Hill, 1980, p. 359). The establishment of this "tolerance" is Gregory and Hill's third objective. To achieve it the clinician reviews the stutterer's case history and observes the child in the therapy setting and in interactions with the parents. This is done for the purpose of forming a list of factors that appear to be associated with the disruption of fluency. The factors identified on the list are then arranged in a rank order from seemingly least to apparently most disruptive of fluency. To increase a youngster's tolerance for these disruptive stimuli, the clinician systematically introduces them into treatment, starting with the least fluency-disrupting cue and gradually working up to the most disorganizing influence. For example, suppose that a loss of listener attention and being interrupted in midsentence have been identified as the cues that are least and most disruptive of fluency, respectively. Once fluent use of the target speech pattern is well established, the clinician could start to occasionally shift attention away while the child is speaking. If the youngster starts to stutter, then the clinician returns the attention and encourages resumption of the target speech pattern. As fluency stabilizes at a high level once more, the clinician's inattention is introduced again. This process of interjecting, removing, and then reinserting the fluency disrupter is sustained until the child's vulnerability to that stimulus has been lowered. At that point, the clinician would move on to the next disruptive stimulus on the rank-ordered list and proceed in the same way until the most disruptive influence (being interrupted, in our example) had been dealt with effectively.

The fourth objective is to help the child "gain competence in all areas judged to be potential hazards to fluency" (Gregory and Hill, 1980, p. 359). From the contents of Table 9-2 we can see that this might involve weaving into the fabric of treatment procedures for dealing with problems such as a short attention span, reduced auditory verbal comprehension, and slow and inaccurate word retrieval.

We come now to the fifth and final objective, that being "to increase a child's self-confidence or self-acceptance in areas judged to have a potential impact on fluency" (Gregory and Hill, 1980, p. 360). Here, Gregory and Hill endeavor to deal with personality variables and attitudes that could affect fluency. Thus, inappropriate behaviors such as perfectionism, withdrawal, aggressiveness and irrational fears, identified in the case history and/or during the child's presence in the clinic, would become targets for modification.

At this juncture, one other aspect of the Gregory and Hill program needs to be mentioned. That involves 1 hour per week of parent counseling that is run in parallel with the child's therapy. Often, this counseling is conducted as the parents observe their child in treatment. The goals of the counseling regimen are to help parents: (1) identify and discriminate between the various types of disfluency; (2) observe and make accurate written records of their offspring's episodes of atypical disfluency; (3) develop the ability to identify and appropriately modify environmental forces that are disrupting their child's fluency; (4) acquire good models of those behaviors that promote the development of normal fluency; (5) form reasonable expectations for their child and the child's behavior; and (6) comprehend features of their youngster's behavior that may intrude on the generalization of fluency to extraclinical settings, or interfere with the maintenance of higher levels of generalized fluency.

Gregory and Hill (Note 5) provided individual data for a group of 20 children who completed their therapy program. These youngsters ranged in age from 3;6 to 6;3 years. All of them had been given a differential assessment. Deficits identified in some of these youngsters included trouble in attending, learning disabilities, language disorders, combined language-learning disabilities, errors of articulation, voice pathology, and psychological difficulties. Thus, whenever possible, treatment was planned so as to deal not only with fluency, but with these other problems as well. Duration of treatment ranged from 24 to 64 weeks with an average duration of approximately 40 weeks. All of the subjects were tested in 2 conditions both prior to treatment and then immediately after the therapy period ended. The 2 conditions were speaking in a dialogue with a clinician, and speaking during a play activity as the clinician applied various sorts of "pressure" to the child.

From the foregoing description it is clear that the Gregory and Hill regimen contains many parts. Therefore, the assignment of improvement of fluency or any other aspect of performance to any particular aspect of the therapy is virtually impossible. Treatment effects are so intermixed that we cannot decide with any certainty what caused what. With that constraint in mind, Table 9-3 shows that as a group, the 20 children treated

TABLE 9-3
Pre- and posttherapy mean percentage and range of disfluency values across 2 conditions for children treated in Gregory and Hill's program.

	Dialogue		Speech During Play With Clinician Applying Pressure on Patient	
	Pretherapy	Posttherapy	Pretherapy	Posttherapy
Less typical disfluencies*				
Mean % disfluencies:	12.34	1.51	10.45	1.62
Range:	.60–40.7	0.00–7.1	1.60–32.0	0.00–7.0
More typical disfluencies +				
Mean % disfluencies:	9.30	4.85	8.51	4.41
Range:	1.90–19.2	0.00–12.5	.53–21.3	0.00–13.6
Total disfluency				
Mean % disfluencies:	10.82	3.18	9.48	3.02
Range:	5.80–48.0	0.00–19.0	2.13–37.3	0.00–14.7

*Sound-syllable repetitions and prolongations included here.
+Word and phrase repetitions, sound-syllable interjections, and revisions included here.

in the Gregory and Hill program experienced sizable pre- to posttherapy reductions in less typical disfluencies, more typical disfluencies, and, quite naturally, total disfluencies across the 2 test conditions. For a group of patients averaging 4.29 years to exhibit means of 3.18% and 3.02% of words disfluent is encouraging. Readers must remember that *normal* children of this age are still exhibiting somewhere between 1% and 5% of words disfluent in their speech (Davis, 1939). Unquestionably, the posttherapy mean percentage disfluency scores of Gregory and Hill's group fall within this acceptable range. Moreover, Gregory and Hill (1980) report that their subjects' progress was maintained when measured anywhere from 9 to 18 months following the end of treatment. In 6 cases, maintenance was rated as "poor" or "uncertain" (Gregory & Hill, Note 5). These less-than-desirable outcomes were attributed to psychological disturbances in the child and/or poor parental involvement and follow-up in the counseling program.

Riley and Riley's Component Program

In view of their work on differential assessment, it is not surprising that Riley and Riley have assembled a multidimensional treatment regimen for young stutterers. Recall that, based on the differential assessment data they gathered, Riley and Riley (1979) identified 9 components of stuttering (Table 9-1). Youngsters exhibiting various combinations of these components along with their stuttering are placed in individualized rehabilitation programs that contain techniques specifically designed to deal with whatever components are present.

Whenever necessary, attending disorders are treated first, primarily by means of behavior modification (e.g., positive reinforcement for sustaining eye contact for progressively longer periods of time). Second, intra- and interpersonal components are targeted for management. Parent counseling is used to reduce disruptive influences in the child's communicative environment, to help the parents develop more realistic expectations of their offspring, and to alter the consequences attached to any stuttering that is thought to be manipulative in nature. Parents who evince a need for their child to stutter are referred for longer term and more systematic psychotherapy. Coincidentally, the stuttering children are guided into adopting more reasonable expectations of themselves and their behavior and are provided with opportunities to build self-esteem.

The neurologic components of auditory processing, sentence formulation, and oral-motor problems are dealt with third. To manage auditory processing deficits, patients are trained to follow directions of increasing length and complexity. Then, children are instructed to postpone responding for progressively longer intervals so as to develop some tolerance for these delays. Also, youngsters are rewarded for suppressing their urges to respond impulsively. Sentence formulation deficiencies are handled by showing a child a word and then guiding him through the generation of increasingly longer and grammatically more complex sentences that include the stimulus word. Further, patients are encouraged to develop a general sense of sentence length and syntax prior to the execution of an utterance. Oral-motor problems are managed in a variety of ways. There are drills on the accuracy of vowel and consonant posturing and on the production of single and then bi- and trisyllabic sequences. Accuracy in all these productions is achieved initially at a reduced rate of speaking. Then, rate is increased progressively through the systematic application of reinforcement. Fourth, starter, postponement, and avoidance behaviors attendant to a child's stuttering are removed by having the child actively engage in their inhibition. This is done prior to the management of stuttering behaviors per se.

The manipulation of stuttering itself is the last step taken in therapy. Techniques used here include teaching a patient the easy onset of voicing or air flow for vowel or consonant production and instruction on how to sustain the breathstream for speech-making purposes. Additionally, the child is taught to "bounce" and "slide" (Riley & Riley, 1979, p. 289), so as to first attain less effortful stuttering and, eventually, normal disfluency.

Readers will remember from the section on differential assessment that the Rileys studied the distribution of their components in a sample of 54 stutterers. Subsequently, these youngsters were inserted into individualized treatment regimens tailored to fit their differential assessment profiles. Forty-four of these children completed therapy and were accessible for re-evaluation as much as 48 months later. Riley and Riley (Note 6) have provided treatment outcome and maintenance data for this group of children.

As a general rule, treatment took less time if the patient entered therapy before age 6. Youngsters aged 3 to 4 years required fewer hours of remediation than did stutterers 6 years old and older. In part, this difference can be accounted for by the fact that 75% of the children who were enrolled in clinic prior to their sixth birthday *"did not need any direct stuttering behavior treatment"*[4] (Riley & Riley, 1979, p. 289). In other words, the successful modification of a child's components was associated with significant spontaneous improvement in stuttering such that it never became the direct target of therapy. The problem here is that we cannot determine how much of this improvement to attribute to spontaneous recovery that would have occurred without treatment, and how much to the treatment itself. Without a no-treatment control group, this issue cannot be settled. Whatever the case, it is interesting that, in contrast to the younger group of stutterers, 91% of the patients 6 years old and older did need direct modification of their stuttering. These older children were also more likely to need management of starter, postponement, and avoidance behaviors. Since these latter responses and stuttering required clinical attention, the older patients were in treatment longer than their younger counterparts.

These across-age-group differences aside, 36 (82%) of the 44 youngsters were reported as exhibiting either no stuttering or mild residual stuttering in clinic, home, and school at the end of rehabilitation. Twelve months later, all but one of the 36 individuals had either maintained their clinical gains or had improved even further. During the 12-to-24-month interval after therapy ended, 2 children who had made major gains in treatment returned to the clinic for additional maintenance work. One had regressed slightly but was able to regain the improvement previously made. The other patient suffered a rather serious relapse and was not able to recoup this lost ground.

In mild contrast to these results, just 8 (18%) of the 44 stutterers reached the end of therapy with significant residual stuttering or only slight improvement. One of these individuals did progress during the 12 months leading to the first follow-up. The remaining 7 stutterers still exhibited their disappointing end-of-treatment status.

In the 24-to-48-month interval since treatment was terminated, the foregoing patterns have remained essentially unchanged. While complete data are not yet available on all 44 patients, about 80% of these children remain significantly improved, while approximately 20% of them show little change from the picture they presented when therapy started. It is also worth mentioning that the parents of the youngsters who made major progress in therapy expressed great satisfaction over their offsprings' improvement. These parents reported that their children's speech "sounded normal with regard to rate, loudness, stress and pitch" (Riley & Riley, Note 6) except during infrequent moments of stuttering.

Bruce Ryan's GILCU Approach

GILCU is an acronym for "Gradual Increase in Length and Complexity of Utterance." This label very accurately describes the basic strategy in Ryan's program (1974). That is, fluency is instated at the single-word level and then at levels of increasing length and linguistic complexity. As conceived by Ryan, the GILCU program is administered across 3 modes of responding: oral reading, monologue, and conversation. To begin, a clinician instructs the child to "speak more slowly and easily" (Ryan, 1974, p. 88), and then to read a list of simple words (e.g., "ball...car...man"). When the child achieves the criterion level of fluency on this task, a list of 2-word responses is introduced. Attainment of the criterion level of fluency at the 2-word level allows for advancement of the stutterer to the oral reading of 3-word phrases. This basic tactic is followed through the reading of 4- , 5- , and 6-word responses, then to a single sentence, and on to 2, 3, and 4 consecutive sentences. After that, response length is determined by unit of time, starting with utterances that are 30 seconds in length, then 1 minute, 1½ minutes, 2, 2½, 3, 4, and, finally, 5 minutes. There are 18 steps altogether in the oral-reading response mode. As soon as the youngster completes the eighteenth step, the treatment is recycled back to Step 1, but now in the monologue mode of responding. When the next 17 steps are finished in monologue, treatment is recycled back to Step 1 in the conversational mode. Through the thoughtful selection and preparation of speech-evoking stimuli (e.g., word lists, two-word phrases, pictures, etc.), a clinician can exercise anywhere from a strict to a modicum of control over the length and complexity of the client's responses.

For Ryan, transfer involves the child's production of fluent speech "in a wide variety of settings and with many different people" (1974, p. 94). This part of treatment is organized and conducted just as carefully and systematically as the establishment phase. Specifically, transfer can start with the clinician and child conversing in the therapy room, but with the door open. To transfer the youngster's fluency beyond the realm of one-to-one conversations, additional people are introduced, one at a time, into the therapy room. Then, to generalize the child's fluency to strangers and new situations in the natural environment, the patient is taken away from the clinic to locales such as neighborhood stores, shops, and the library. The last step in transfer involves the carry-over of fluency to settings in which the child participates routinely (i.e., home and school).

When the client has achieved a specified criterion level of fluency throughout this multi-step transfer program, the time has come for the transition into maintenance. The goal of maintenance is "fluent speech in a wide variety of settings, with many different people over a long period of time" (Ryan, 1974, p. 105). In Ryan's approach, maintenance involves 3 major steps. They are: (1) self-regulation of one's own fluency through careful monitoring; (2) intermittent home practice; and (3) periodic return visits to the clinic for rechecks and any such reinstruction as might be needed.

It can be seen from Table 9-4 that the patients in the GILCU program experienced major reductions in their stuttering. The mean scores shown testify to the efficacy of the GILCU approach with the youngsters treated. It is also worth mentioning that very recently, Ryan, Rustin, and Ryan (Note 7) have reported similar results for the GILCU methodology following its application in England. Finally, there is one other bit of information that

TABLE 9-4
Pretherapy, posttherapy, and follow-up stuttered words-per-minute range and mean values for 6 elementary-age patients treated in Ryan's GILCU program.

	Stuttered Words Per Minute	
	Range	*Mean*
Pretherapy:	2.85–13.35	7.81
End of establishment phase of therapy:	0.00–0.5	.06
Follow-up*:	0.00–0.5	0.2

Note: After B. Ryan, *Programmed Therapy for Stuttering in Children and Adults.* Springfield, Ill.: Charles Thomas, 1974, pp. 89 and 109.

The values shown here were excerpted from a larger data pool published by Ryan. Ryan's data were not offered in their entirety because some of the scores pertained to adult stutterers and obviously do not belong in the chapter.

*Follow-up measures were made an average of 10.4 months after the child had reached the end of the GILCU program. Follow-up data not available on 1 of the original 6 children.

also gives a measure of indirect support to the use of GILCU with children who stutter. That is, the basic GILCU strategy has been integrated into virtually every demonstrably successful stuttering therapy program for children. We found it in the approaches advocated by Gregory and Hill and by the Rileys. It will appear again in the next regimen to be presented, that being the one developed by Richard Shine.

Richard Shine's Treatment

Richard Shine is yet another therapist for stutterers who advocates the administration of a differential assessment prior to the start of treatment (1980). The assessment includes formal testing, observations of parent-child interactions, the taking of a case history, the measurement of stuttering severity, an analysis of the stuttering itself, and an examination of the physiologic and aerodynamic processes that are integral to speech production.

Apropos of the last 2 parts of the assessment, Shine measures stuttering frequency and describes the topography of all observable symptoms.

Note is taken of any struggle behavior the child might be exhibiting. As regards the evaluation of physiologic and aerodynamic processes, it focuses on any abnormal respiratory, phonatory, or articulatory behaviors that are present. Then, Shine attempts to ascertain the locus of speech breathing (e.g., clavicular, thoracic, abdominal), the regularity and timing of respiratory cycles, and the arrangement of breath groups. Phonation is evaluated for the presence or absence of hard glottal attacks and the child's ability to maintain continuous flow throughout an utterance. Vocal sound pressure level, fundamental frequency, the tension and force in articulatory posturing, and the rate of articulatory movement are all assessed. A judgment is rendered on the appropriateness of the youngster's resonance patterns and estimates are made of stress and intonation use. Finally, attention is devoted to studying the effectiveness with which the youngster coordinates respiration, phonation, and articulation while speaking. The findings of the extensive analysis of stuttering and the physiology and aerodynamics of the child's speech behavior play a central role in shaping Shine's fluency-building program. This regimen is rounded out by the insertion of additional techniques suitable for dealing with any problems other than stuttering that were identified during the differential assessment.

Once the differential assessment has been completed, Shine initiates a 5-phase treatment program. He refers to the first phase as the "picture identification prestep" (1980, p. 344). Shine's goal is to identify, in a collection of pictures, about 50 that the youngster can name quickly and with reliable fluency. These pictures and the words that go with them are used as the first set of stimuli in the next 2 phases of treatment. In the second phase, the clinician attempts to establish speaking variables that are compatible with fluency. Initially, this entails developing in the young stutterer a basic understanding of the concept of an "easy speaking voice" (p. 345). The third part provides the child with fluency training during highly structured activities. One crucial aspect of this structure requires that the clinician select stimulus materials and response modes for the child that will strictly control the length and complexity of the youngster's utterances.[5] The fourth phase involves fluency training during conversation in a host of real-life speech situations.[6] The final phase uses procedures that are designed to ease the patient out of therapy, make provision for assessing the stability of progress after treatment has ended, and help the child maintain improved fluency.

As we look back over Shine's methods, we can see that they begin with a differential assessment and are followed by a direct approach to therapy. Although this treatment is presumably based on the differential assessment, what is not evident is the way in which that evaluation's results are used to determine the phases of therapy through which a child must pass.

This would seem to be an instance in which a differential assessment, to be clinically useful, should lead to differential treatment. There is nothing in Shine's writing to indicate that it does, or that a differential assessment is even needed.

One of Shine's students undertook a comprehensive examination of the effectiveness of her mentor's therapy program (Mason, Note 8). At the start of treatment, the 14 children studied ranged in age from 2;9 to 8;0. Therapy for these youngsters lasted from 1 to 28 months. The mean duration of treatment was approximately 10½ months and involved an average of 56.7 sessions, each of which was 40-50 minutes in length. The 14 children were assessed at the start of treatment, at treatment's end, and then at some point following that termination date, but no sooner than 14 months after therapy had been completed. One child was tested 5 years after his treatment program was concluded. The average time lapse between the end of treatment and the follow-up examination was 3 years, 2 months.

Portions of the testing of the 14 children included the gathering of a 200-word sample of their conversational speech, a rating of their stuttering severity, and qualitative ratings by parents of changes in their offspring's speech. The data collected in these ways were first scrutinized on a subject-by-subject basis. From this initial examination, Mason reported that one stutterer's follow-up test results indicated that a significant relapse had occurred. Individual scores for this youngster were presented and discussed, but then removed from the data pool for the larger sample. Results for the remaining 13 children are presented in Table 9-5. As can be seen, they experienced a substantial reduction in their disfluency by the end of treatment. Moreover, this improvement was sustained at least through the date of the follow-up assessment. Consistent with these findings, it is not surprising that estimates of stuttering severity at follow-up ranged from zero (no stuttering) to mild, with 11 youngsters being rated as very mild. Comparable judgments by parents also were reported. Specifically, before treatment, the speech of all 13 children was rated by their parents as either fair or poor. By the end of therapy, four children had speech that was rated as very good. Nine youngsters were rated as good. When follow-up testing was undertaken, nine children were rated as having very good speech, and four were believed to have good speech. Obviously, several of the youngsters had continued to progress in their parents' eyes months after therapy had ended.

Single Case Studies

Dating back to 1965 and continuing to the present, clinically oriented operant researchers have sought to manipulate the stuttering and/or

TABLE 9-5
Pretherapy, posttherapy, and follow-up range and mean values for 14 child stutterers on measures of stuttered words per minute, words spoken per minute, and struggle behaviors.

		Pretherapy	Posttherapy	Follow-Up
Stuttered words per minute				
	Mean:	13.90	1.70	1.30
	Range:	4.00–22.0	0.00–8.40	0.6–2.60
Words spoken per minute				
	Mean:	*	*	129.80
	Range:	*	*	118.0–143.0
Frequency of struggle behaviors				
	Mean:	*	*	0.00
	Range:	*	*	0.00

Note: After D. Mason. Unpublished Master's thesis, East Carolina University, 1981.

*Pre- and posttherapy measures of words spoken per minute and the frequency of occurrence of struggle behaviors were unavailable to Mason.

fluency of young stutterers through the simple expedient of applying various consequences to these behaviors. Experiments of this type number about 20 now (c.f., Rickard & Mundy, 1965, Shaw & Shrum, 1972; Martin, Kuhl, & Haroldson, 1972), rendering a review of each of them far beyond the scope of this chapter; however, the philosophy underlying the view of stuttering and fluency as operant behaviors and some of the treatment procedures that can emerge from that view are described by Costello (1980). These reports are important to us because they fit our definition of "direct" therapy (see p. 8). Therefore, a summary or overview of them is in order.

The studies in question have all attempted to test the hypotheses that stuttering and/or fluency are operant behaviors—responses whose frequencies of occurrence are controlled by the consequences attached to them. Generally, reinforcers are consequences that we associate with an increase in response frequency while punishers are consequences associated with a decrease in the frequency of responding.

In the conduct of operant studies of stuttering and fluency, the researchers have relied heavily on what has been referred to as the ABA design or some variation thereof. In this type of experiment, which is well suited for the detailed analysis of individual subjects' behavior, the first "A" is used to designate a "baserate" time period. During this segment, the subject under test is simply instructed to speak in monologue or conversation, or perhaps to read aloud. The investigator withholds the reinforcer or punisher and does nothing but carefully count the frequency of occurrence of all behaviors of interest; for example, part-word repetitions, interjections, and/or words spoken fluently. During the "B" (treatment) segment, the experimenter arranges for certain consequences to be applied to a specific aspect of the child's speech behavior. For example, the youngster may receive a token for nonstuttered utterances of a predetermined length, with a certain number of tokens later exchanged for the privilege of bringing a friend along to the treatment sessions (Peters, 1977). Or, points earned for fluent utterances might be removed following moments of stuttering (Ryan, 1971). In some instances, these contingencies are explained to the child beforehand (Shaw & Shrum, 1972)—sometimes the child is even pointedly told, "Try not to stutter"— but explanations and instructions are not typical or mandatory for the success of the treatment. Whatever the case, the child is *not* given instructions such as "talk slowly" or "let some air out" that could aid in speaking more fluently or reducing stuttering by requiring the use of altered speech patterns. The child simply begins talking or reading and the experimenter starts to apply the consequence(s), at the same time noting the frequency of occurrence of the target behavior. If that response is an operant, then it will increase in frequency with the application of the reinforcer, or decrease in frequency with the delivery of a punisher.

In the "A" segment that follows "B," the reinforcer or punisher is removed. This provides the researchers with a chance to observe whether the elimination of the consequence is associated with a reversal of whatever behavior change was noted in "B." Specifically, the experimenter watches to see if the target response returns to its baseline frequency of occurrence. Subsequently, the investigation can be terminated or the consequence reintroduced to see if that step is again associated with some change in the frequency of occurrence of the response of interest. This re-presentation of the consequence creates what has been labeled an ABAB withdrawal design (Herson & Barlow, 1976), which is nothing more than an elaboration on the basic ABA model we have been talking about, but is more rigorous because it requires a replication of the treatment effect and is more appropriate for clinical research because it terminates the experiment in the treatment condition.

The operant studies that have just been described produced two extraordinarily interesting findings. First, neither the application of reinforcers for fluency nor punishers for stuttering has been reported to be associated with any obvious unpleasant emotional reactions among the children tested. Second, in one experiment after another, introduction of reinforcement and/or punishment contingencies has been associated with clinically significant increases in nonstuttered speech and decreases in the frequency of occurrence of stuttering. Taken together, these results demonstrated that direct approaches to the manipulation of fluency and stuttering could be given the most serious consideration rather than rejected out of fear that such straightforward tactics would surely exacerbate the young stutterer's problem (Costello, 1983).

Before concluding this summary, there is one other aspect of the operant research that needs to be mentioned. Specifically, it is noteworthy that the youngsters who served as subjects had not been exposed to a differential assessment prior to their participation in the studies. Therefore, we cannot be sure if these youngsters were in possession of the neurologic, interpersonal, and intrapersonal problems identified by such workers as the Rileys (see p. 9). But let us assume for the moment that any number of these difficulties were present in at least a few of the children. The point to be made here is that it didn't seem to matter. That is to say, in spite of the presumed coexistence of these various complicating conditions and stuttering, the simple process of applying consequences was sufficient to modify the behavior of the children tested. Granted that in some cases this improvement was transient, lasting only until the end of the experiment or shortly thereafter, in most cases treatment effects with young children have been shown to be pervasive and lasting (e.g., Martin, Kuhl, & Haroldson, 1972; Reed & Godden, 1977). Nonetheless, the results of the operant research raise a question that is likely to be hotly debated in the years ahead. That is, is a differential assessment even necessary and must the results from it be used in planning therapy? Costello (1983) embraces the view that stuttering treatment with children should begin with "the basics"—contingent positive feedback for nonstuttered utterances combined with contingent negative feedback for each moment of stuttering—and that only if performance data indicate this simple, direct treatment to be ineffective should "additives" such as rate control, easy onset, or modifications in the language required of the child be introduced into the treatment regimen. She suggests that information gathered during a pretreatment differential assessment would be a good source for pointing the clinician toward potentially facilitating additives, but that ABAB manipulations within the treatment should serve as tests of the actual effectiveness of the selected additive.

Conclusion

It hardly seems arguable that we have made very significant advances in the direct treatment of stuttering in children. Where clinically we used to move with great caution and insecurity, we are now able to proceed with more optimism. Where we once felt lucky if solid fluency was achieved in a minority of our young stutterers, we can now anticipate a much larger number of successful treatment outcomes. This is certainly a happy state of affairs because among stutterers of all ages, it is the afflicted child who possesses the best prognosis for improvement. Indeed, it is the stuttering child who has the best chance of attaining fully normal speech. If that goal once seemed unrealistic, it is now most decidedly within reach.

End Notes

[1] Briefly put, a factor analysis makes it possible to discover commonalities that may exist between 2 or more variables. Such a discovery then "reduces" the set of variables to a single factor. For example, the tasks of following spoken directions and responding appropriately to spoken questions, both tap a common factor—auditory verbal comprehension. The same 2 tasks and the task of repeating a sequence of numbers share the common factor of auditory retention. Once a factor is identified, it is then possible to statistically estimate the extent to which it can account for the variability in a group's responses to tasks.

[2] The term "immediate cause" refers to those forces in the here and now that appear to be triggering the stuttering. Immediate causes are to be contrasted to distal causes (Freeman, 1979). The latter refers to the original instigators of the disorder. Thus, we might say that the immediate cause of a patient's stuttering is difficulty in starting and sustaining voicing. Inquires about the origin of this phonatory defect would direct us toward the distal cause.

[3] This implied slight reduction in the rate of articulation would surely create a modest drop in the number of syllables or words spoken per minute. This point is made because of the growing importance being placed upon decrements in speaking rate as an integral part of stuttering therapy.

[4] The present author has added italics for emphasis.

[5] Ryan's influence here is obvious as Shine clearly notes in his writing (1980).

[6] Shine (1980) has noted that these sorts of formal transfer activities are not needed with many preschool stutterers. Their fluency seems to generalize spontaneously from formal activities like language lotto to more typical verbal exchanges away from the clinic. The present author has made similar observations (Adams, 1980), as have others (Martin, Kuhl, & Haroldson, 1972; Shaw & Shrum, 1972).

Reference Notes

1. Berlin, A. An exploratory attempt to isolate types of stuttering. Unpublished doctoral dissertation. Northwestern University, 1954.

2. Riley, G., & Riley, J. Clinical subtypes of stuttering among 100 children. A paper presented at the Annual Convention of the American Speech and Hearing Association. San Francisco, 1972.

3. Riley, G., & Riley, J. Differential strategies for diagnosing and treating children who stutter. A short course presented at the Regional Convention of the American Speech and Hearing Association, Portland, Ore., 1976.

4. Smith, A., & Daly, D. Neuropsychological assessment: Implications for the treatment of aphasic and stuttering clients. Unpublished manuscript of a paper included within a miniseminar presented at the Annual Convention of the American Speech-Language and Hearing Association. Detroit, 1980.

5. Gregory, H., & Hill, D. Personal communication, 1981.

6. Riley, G., & Riley, J. Personal communication, 1981.

7. Ryan, B., Rustin, L., & Ryan, B. Comparison of speech and therapy of English and American stutterers. A paper presented at the Annual Convention of the American Speech-Language and Hearing Association. Los Angeles, 1981.

8. Mason, D. A follow-up study of fluency training with the young stutterer (ages 2-9 to 8-0 years). Unpublished Master's thesis, East Carolina University, 1981.

References

Adams, M. A clinical strategy for differentiating the normally nonfluent child and the incipient stutterer. *Journal of Fluency Disorders*, 1977, *2*, 141-148.

Adams, M. The young stutterer: Diagnosis, treatment, and assessment of progress. In W. Perkins (Ed.), *Seminars in Speech, Language, and Hearing*, *1*(4), 289-300. New York: Thieme-Stratton, 1980.

Andrews, G., & Harris, M. *The syndrome of stuttering*. London: Heinemann Medical Books, 1964.

Canter, G. Observations of neurogenic stuttering: A contribution to differential diagnosis. *British Journal of Disorders of Communication*, 1971, *6*, 139-143.

Conture, E. *Stuttering*. Englewood Cliffs, N.J.: Prentice-Hall, 1982.

Costello, J. M. Operant conditioning and the treatment of stuttering. In W. H. Perkins (Ed.), Strategies in stuttering therapy. *Seminars in Speech, Language, and Hearing*, 1980, *1*, 311-327. New York: Thieme-Stratton.

Costello, J. M. Current behavioral treatments for children. In D. Prins & R. J. Ingham (Eds.), *Stuttering in early childhood: Treatment methods and issues*. San Diego: College-Hill, 1983.

Curlee, R. A case selection strategy for young disfluent children. In W. Perkins (Ed.), *Seminars in Speech, Language, and Hearing*, *1*(4), 277-288. New York: Thieme-Stratton, 1980.

Davis, D. The relation of repetitions in the speech of young children to certain measures of language maturity and situational factors. *Journal of Speech Disorders*, 1939, *4*, 303-318.

Freeman, F. Phonation in stuttering: A review of current research. *Journal of Fluency Disorders*, 1979, *4*, 79-90.

Gregory H., & Hill, D. Stuttering therapy for children. In W. Perkins (Ed.), *Seminars in Speech, Language, and Hearing, 1*(4), 351-364. New York: Thieme-Stratton, 1980.

Herson, M., & Barlow, D. *Single case experimental designs*. New York: Pergamon, 1976.

Johnson, L. Facilitating parental involvement in therapy for the disfluent child. In W. Perkins (Ed.), *Seminars in Speech, Language, and Hearing, 1*(4), 301-310. New York: Thieme-Stratton, 1980.

Martin, R., Kuhl, P., & Haroldson, S. An experimental treatment with two preschool stuttering children. *Journal of Speech and Hearing Research*, 1972, *15*, 743-752.

Peters, A. D. The effect of positive reinforcement on fluency: Two case studies. *Language, Speech, and Hearing Services in Schools*, 1977, *8*, 15-22.

Prins, D., & Lohr, F. Behavioral dimensions of stuttered speech. *Journal of Speech and Hearing Research*, 1972, *15*, 61-71.

Reed, C. G., & Godden, A. L. An experimental treatment using verbal punishment with two preschool stutterers. *Journal of Fluency Disorders*, 1977, *2*, 225-233.

Rickard, H., & Mundy, M. Direct manipulation of stuttering behavior: An experimental-clinical approach. In L. Ullmann & L. Krasner (Eds.), *Case studies in behavior modification*. New York: Holt, Rinehart, 1966.

Riley, G., & Riley, J. A component model for diagnosing and treating children who stutter. *Journal of Fluency Disorders*, 1979, *4*, 279-294.

Riley, G., & Riley, J. Motor and linguistic variables among children who stutter. *Journal of Speech and Hearing Disorders*, 1980, *45*, 504-514.

Ryan, B. Operant procedures applied to stuttering therapy for children. *Journal of Speech and Hearing Disorders*, 1971, *36*, 264-280.

Ryan, B. *Programmed therapy for stuttering in children and adults*. Springfield, Ill.: Charles C. Thomas, 1974.

Shaw, C., & Shrum, W. The effects of response-contingent reward on the connected speech of children who stutter. *Journal of Speech and Hearing Disorders*, 1972, *37*, 75-88.

Shine, R. Direct management of the beginning stutterer. In W. Perkins (Ed.), *Seminars in Speech, Language, and Hearing, 1*(4), 339-350. New York: Thieme-Stratton, 1980.

Van Riper, C. Experiments in stuttering therapy. In J. Eisenson (Ed.), *Stuttering: A symposium*. New York: Harper & Brothers, 1958.

Van Riper, C. *The nature of stuttering*. Englewood Cliffs, N.J.: Prentice-Hall, 1971.

Williams, D. Stuttering therapy for children. In L. Travis (Ed.), *Handbook of speech pathology*. New York: Appleton-Century-Crofts, 1971.

Williams, D. A perspective on approaches to stuttering therapy. In H. Gregory (Ed.), *Controversies about stuttering therapy*. Baltimore: University Park Press, 1979.

Barry Guitar

Indirect Treatment of Stuttering

Indirect stuttering therapies are those approaches which try to ameliorate a child's stuttering by working on some other aspect of his behavior or environment. An indirect therapy may, for example, work on the child's interactions with parents, on command of language, or on behavior at school. Whatever the focus of treatment, the goal is to decrease the stuttering. The organization of this review is in terms of where the emphasis of the indirect treatment is placed. These include: parent counseling, psychotherapy, drug therapy, control of nonspeech behavior, language-oriented approaches, parent-child interaction, and psychomotor therapy.

There are a variety of reasons for the clinician to select one of these indirect approaches instead of working directly on the child's stuttering. There may be, for example, a reluctance to let the child become aware of his stuttering, for fear it will become worse (Van Riper, 1973). In this case, parent counseling to change the child's environment is typically employed. In other cases, however, a different rationale determines the choice. The clinician may believe that a significant cause of the child's stuttering lies beyond speech production and the child's attitude about speech difficulty. Thus, the nature of the problem may be thought to be beyond the reach of direct therapy. In these cases, an indirect approach—for example, psychotherapy—is chosen according to the clinician's theoretical bent, in accord with what he or she believes to be the significant cause. Still another rationale is both theoretical and empirical. A broad theoretical orientation may lead the clinician to select several variables for experimentation;

then, those that are demonstrated to influence the child's stuttering, empirically, are selected for use in treatment. Parent-child interaction approaches use this rationale.

In this review each of the indirect approaches is described as though it were used as a total treatment package for the child. This is not usually true in practice, however. Sometimes, one indirect approach, such as a language-oriented treatment, may be combined with another indirect approach, such as parent counseling. In other instances, an indirect approach may be combined with a direct approach. Another way in which this review may slightly distort reality is in not including all available indirect approaches. The most readily available published and orally presented reports of indirect treatments have been included, but some worthwhile approaches have undoubtedly been overlooked. Having acknowledged some of the inadequacies of this attempt to present the state of the art, we shall begin with parent counseling.

Parent Counseling

By far the most common indirect approach to treatment is for the speech-language pathologist to counsel the parents of the stuttering child. The goal of this counseling is to help the parent identify and change behaviors which increase the child's stuttering. Inherent in most of the approaches in this category is the assumption that parental feelings and consequent behaviors, while not necessarily the original cause of the stuttering, can worsen the child's stuttering and make it chronic. Thus, in distinction to psychotherapy, parent counseling usually focuses on those behaviors that can be observed to influence the child's stuttering. Feelings are dealt with in the context of how they lead to overt behaviors that aggravate stuttering.

In his book, *Treatment of Stuttering*, Van Riper (1973) describes his own strategies for parent counseling. His approach, taken from several sources and borrowed by many others, aims at reducing parents' feelings of guilt, inadequacy, and ignorance. Another of Van Riper's aims is to help parents manipulate environmental variables influencing their child's stuttering. He advocates that the clinician: (1) maintain a highly accepting attitude toward the parents; (2) help the parents understand what might be influencing the child's stuttering; and (3) create, in the counseling session, a supportive and objective environment in which the parents can discover for themselves which changes in their behavior will reduce the child's stuttering. Specific activities include having the parents keep a daily log of situations in which their child is most fluent and situations in which stuttering occurs a great deal. In addition, Van Riper gradually involves parents in the direct treatment of the child. For Van Riper, parent counseling is usually only an adjunct to direct stuttering therapy for the child. Unfortunately, he has not reported data on the outcome of his combined approach.

Another version of parent counseling is provided by Ainsworth and Gruss (1981) in the most recent edition of *If Your Child Stutters—A Guide for Parents*. This book serves as a paperbound parent counselor by itself. It is probably best used, however, as a supplement to counseling by a speech-language pathologist. Ainsworth and Gruss share the assumption that environmental factors may exacerbate mild disfluency so that it becomes chronic stuttering. The most critical variables, in their estimate, are related to the child's feelings of security and acceptance. Consequently, the book emphasizes ways in which parents can increase their sensitivity to the child's emotional needs. Specific guidelines for parents are given in extended discussions of ways of meeting children's needs. The following suggestions are abstracted from some of the authors' guidelines:

1. decrease criticism;
2. decrease over-control;
3. help the child to release feelings constructively;
4. give the child more attention and support in a crisis;
5. discipline without decreasing the child's sense of security;
6. accept the fact that as other skills are developing, fluency may suffer; and
7. accept disfluencies by realizing that the child is doing the best he can.

Another approach to parent counseling is described in *Understanding Stuttering* by Cooper (1979). This booklet provides information regarding the nature of stuttering and gives parents several suggestions for helping their child. The information section appears to be designed to allay parents' fears that they may have caused the child's stuttering problem, but may also help them realize that their child's stuttering is within the range of normal disfluency (if such is the case). The section on suggestions for parents helps parents to identify their negative feelings toward their child's stuttering and to understand how these feelings may be transmitted to the child. Helpful feelings and responses are suggested. Cooper briefly describes how the child may benefit when parents make responses which:

1. indicate the parent is not angry with the child because of the stuttering;
2. convey that the parent is not blaming the child for the stuttering; and

3.   help the child identify and express personal feelings.

Booklets such as those by Ainsworth and Gruss, Cooper, and others offer several advantages for parent counseling. Among them are: (1) Parents can digest this material at their own pace rather than being required to process it during counseling sessions. (2) The material can be carefully prepared by experienced clinicians to carry a message of acceptance as well as information. (Despite the best intentions, a neophyte counselor may lack a little of both.) (3) The material is always available although a counselor might not be. For small relapses after treatment has terminated, a handy and good booklet may serve as a Band-Aid in place of a major operation involving many trips to a speech pathologist.

Unfortunately, despite the fact that over 100,000 copies of *If Your Child Stutters* and 12,000 copies of *Understand Stuttering* have been distributed, there appears to be little data on their effectiveness. Experimental studies involving counseling with and without a particular booklet are feasible, although control of clinician bias may be difficult. It may also be informative to study parent-child interactions before, during, and after the provision of reading material for parents. Measures of the child's stuttering and parent interactions may reveal what the parents can change via written materials, and to what extent those changes are related to the child's stuttering. In these experiments, clinician counseling of the parents can be administered (and assessed) following a trial of written materials to ensure that parents and child are not deprived of adequate treatment.

Another approach to parent counseling is presented in workshop format for clinicians by Bailey and Bailey (1977; 1982). They advocate modeling of slow, easy, simple speech in a low "time-pressure" context. They also teach Adlerian principles of child rearing that parents can use to help their child feel more competent, more free, and more independent. The Baileys' backgrounds in both speech pathology and counseling place a strong emphasis on parent-child interactions apart from speech. Specific suggestions for parents include:

1.   Tune into the child's feelings as much as possible, encouraging their expression through such techniques as active listening and reflection of the feelings back to the child.
2.   Train the child in those skills you think are important, rather than expecting them to be learned without instruction.
3.   Don't continually teach the child. Allow some things to be learned independently.
4.   Let the child take on as much responsibility—do as much for himself or herself—as possible.

5. Instead of rewards, use encouragement, which implies faith in the child.

The approach described by Bailey and Bailey has not been studied systematically. It would be particularly useful to have data on whether indirect stuttering treatment is any more effective when parents are counseled about child-rearing practices apart from issues regarding their child's speech.

Conture's (1981) indirect treatment approach is specifically designed for cases in which the parents, but not the child, are concerned about the child's stuttering. Conture suggests parent counseling combined with play therapy or general language stimulation for the child. Parent counseling is aimed at helping the parents change environmental influences on the child's speech so that fluency may be increased. Play therapy and/or general language stimulation by the clinician is used as a model from which the parent can learn new styles of interaction. Among the things which are modeled and encouraged are:

1. treating the child with "unconditional positive regard";
2. listening to the content rather than the form of the child's speech;
3. setting down firm rules for the child's behavior;
4. giving the child clear instructions on those tasks that are expected of him or her; and
5. reading slowly and calmly to the child, and allowing the child freedom to interrupt.

Conture implies that once these skills are learned by the parents, they can then proceed on their own to change the child's environment. Conture's implicit position is that if the child is not concerned about stuttering, stuttering will probably be outgrown, so long as environmental conditions are right. Thus, with parents who are concerned about their child's mild disfluencies, a major thrust of treatment is allaying their fears, decreasing unduly high expectations, and increasing the child's sense of security and self worth. Such an approach, like those of Van Riper, Bailey and Bailey, and Ainsworth and Gruss, may or may not be effective. As we have said before, without data it is difficult to estimate which components of these indirect treatments are most effective; without data, it is not clear how many of the children treated with these indirect treatments would not have recovered "spontaneously"; without data, it is not even possible to state how many of the children treated with these indirect treatments recovered at all.

Psychotherapy

Almost all approaches to stuttering therapy with children, direct and indirect, contain a degree of psychotherapy. This section will deal with those that seem to be more psychotherapy than anything else.

In a recent *Smithsonian* (May, 1981), Michael Kernan described the work of Philip Glasner, a psychotherapist who treats stuttering children. Glasner's work, depicted as well outside the mainstream of today's stuttering therapy, appears to be similar to the psychotherapy or play therapy for stuttering advocated by several speech pathologists over the last 25 years (Murphy & FitzSimmons, 1960; Van Riper, 1973; Wyatt & Herzan, 1962). The *Smithsonian* article, however, emphasizes differences between Glasner's approach and any other speech therapy. Glasner apparently sees stuttering as "not a speech disorder at all, but a symptom of far-reaching emotional disturbances" (p. 109). Consequently, his treatment is aimed at reversing the emotional disturbances through parent counseling and, one assumes, play therapy. The example of treatment given in the article suggests Glasner seeks to have the child find understanding and emotional support in the therapist. The same example also suggests that Glasner teaches the child to use loose, easy speech movements. If this is typical of Glasner's approach, it is not pure psychotherapy, but traditional play therapy for stuttering with direct intervention added for good measure. The author of the article quotes Glasner as indicating that "every child patient he has discharged after treatment has not only stopped stuttering but has developed into a far more integrated and better-adjusted person. " No data are available to confirm or deny this optimistic claim.

Van Riper's treatment of the "garden variety" beginning stutterer is another version of psychotherapy combined with direct speech therapy. Van Riper (1973) describes his approach as involving "free and directed play since young children are already experts in this activity" (p. 400). Free play is used to create an emotionally supportive relationship into which a hierarchy of more and more direct speech therapy activities is introduced. Van Riper uses a more truly psychotherapeutic treatment, however, for certain children. This is an approach that has no direct speech therapy, but uses only permissive play activity. Some stutterers with deep emotional conflicts need, in his view, this type of therapy which allows them to "express unacceptable feelings...to utter the unspeakable...to recreate and master many of the stresses that formerly disrupted their lives" (p. 398). Although Van Riper gives few specific guidelines for doing psychotherapy with stuttering children who need it, he excerpts several interesting case examples to illustrate how play therapy might be done.

Van Riper's general approach to psychotherapy with children is similar to the play therapy for young stutterers detailed by Murphy and FitzSimmons (1960). Murphy and FitzSimmons shun the goals of directive speech therapy. Instead, "the clinician is truly nondemanding and nonjudgmental. He respects the child's 'right to stutter, ' his right to express previously forbidden attitudes, his right to resist the therapeutic plan... " (p. 236). Using "permissiveness within realistic limits, " the clinician builds a relationship which allows the child to feel secure and learn to express feelings. This, in turn, is expected to lead to a significant lessening of the stuttering symptoms. Once again, however, we are not given evidence of the effectiveness of treatment, for either Van Riper's or Murphy and Fitz-Simmons' approaches.

In contrast to the above, Wyatt and Herzan (1962) do report outcome data on their approach to psychotherapy with stuttering children. While not rigorous by today's standards, the data-oriented approach is impressive for its time. Wyatt and Herzan's treatment was based on their belief that stuttering is the product of a child's conflict between anger at his mother (for the inevitable separation between mother and child) and fear of further separation. The child's anger is supposedly suppressed because of this fear. Wyatt and Herzan's treatment was carried out by speech pathologists under the advice of a child psychotherapist. The aims were to foster free expression of feeling. While the child was learning to cope with previously unexpressed feelings, impulses, and wishes, the mother was undergoing counseling. She was learning to be aware of, and accept, her feelings. The expression of feelings and acceptance of them was then transferred to the mother-child relationship. The goal of treatment was achieved when the child could feel safe in expressing anger, as the mother learned to accept the anger without feeling threatened.

As additional tools of therapy, Wyatt (1969) also encouraged (a) use of short, simple sentences in talking to the child, (b) setting aside time each day for the mother and child to be alone, and (c) a passive style of interaction on the part of the therapist or mother so that time pressure on the child would be reduced. These latter three aspects of Wyatt's therapy are not uncommon in other indirect therapy strategies. Two of them, the use of short sentences and reduction in time pressure, do not appear to derive directly from the stated goals of psychotherapy. It is problematic, therefore, to attribute improvement in Wyatt's clients simply to psychotherapy. Wyatt's treatment outcome data are difficult to interpret, even apart from contamination by other treatment effects besides psychotherapy.

In their report of treatment outcome, Wyatt and Herzan (1962) present the results of the above treatment for 20 children, discussed as a younger group (12 children, ages 2-6) and an older group (8 children, ages 8-15). The younger children received from 4 to 14 treatment sessions, whereas the older, more confirmed stuttering children received from 10 to 33 sessions. Children were dismissed from treatment "whenever the child had shown normal speech over a period of several months" (p. 650). Evaluation was done at the end of the school year in which the child was treated and again in October of the following school year. Of the 12 children in the younger group, 10 showed marked improvement or spoke with normal fluency. Of the 8 children in the older group, 5 showed marked improvement or a return to normal speech. Elsewhere, Wyatt (1969) has reported that children who were unimproved (in this case, 5 of the 20 children) seemed to be living in family situations which were "emotionally unhealthy" or had high, long-standing stress.

Despite the relatively good success rate (15 markedly improved out of 20), no further study of these techniques has been reported. This apparent lack of interest may be due to the relatively demanding nature of this type of treatment. Few school therapists have the training or time to carry out psychotherapy with both parent and child for 45 minute sessions. Moreover, there is no hard evidence that Wyatt's aggression-anxiety hypothesis about stuttering is valid and that psychotherapy is, therefore, needed.

Drug Therapy

Essentially, there have been no major advances recently in the use of drugs to treat stuttering. An earlier report (Gattuso & Leocata, 1962) on the use of drug *haloperidol* with children had held out some hope. These workers suggested that 80% of the stuttering children treated had completely recovered after a month of treatment. After this optimistic assessment, other workers (Cozzo & Gabrielli, 1965; Prins, Mandelkorn, & Cerf, 1974; Rantala & Petri-Larmi, 1976; Tapia, 1969) followed with studies which examined the effects of haloperidol on both children and adults. This second wave of studies cautiously suggested that some patients showed marked improvement, while many did not. Bloodstein's (1981) summary table of the results of treatment highlights the fact that of all therapy categories, drug therapy has the fewest follow-up measures. Long term benefits after haloperidol treatment is terminated are a particularly valid concern because extended use of the drug is contraindicated by its unpleasant side effects.[1]

Control of Nonspeech Behavior

A relatively recent approach to indirect stuttering treatment is aimed at deviant nonspeech behaviors. Wahler, Sperling, Thomas, Teeter, and Luper (1970) demonstrated that when two sets of parents were taught to control undesirable nonspeech behaviors of their children, the children's stuttering decreased both in the clinic and at home. For one child the target of treatment was "oppositional behavior. " (The child regularly would not follow parental instructions and requests.) For the other child, the targets of modification were constant shifts of activity from one enterprise to another. The researchers point out that although the stuttering decreased concomitantly with the decreases in deviant behaviors, analysis did not show stuttering and deviant behaviors to be linked by stimulus control. Moments of stuttering were not inadvertently directly manipulated by the contingencies delivered for the deviant behaviors. Thus, some third set of variables seems to have been common to both. Luper (Note 1) suggests that the decrease in stuttering may have resulted from the more relaxed, cooperative atmosphere that developed between parent and child once the parents felt they could control their child's behavior. It would be interesting to find out if the behavioral change would work in the other direction. If aspects of the parental behavior critical to maintaining stuttering could be isolated and changed, would the undesirable nonspeech behaviors change as well?

This focus on nonspeech behaviors in stuttering initiated by Wahler et al. has been incorporated into a treatment plan for mild stutterers by Zwitman (1978). The overall aim of Zwitman's approach is to develop consistency in the day-to-day parent-child interaction. Such consistency would seem to do much toward influencing that "third set of variables" alluded to above, which may control both misbehavior and stuttering. The steps in this treatment plan include teaching the parent ways to (1) react to disfluency, (2) improve the child's self-concept and security, and (3) react to misbehavior.

Zwitman's book is designed to be used by clinicians who meet with parents in a group over a period of several weeks. Parents learn new ways of behaving by completing questionnaires and checklists and discussing these in the group. Traditional "parent counseling" suggestions (improving listening skills, structuring conversation in the home to lessen verbal competition, being generous with praise and reassurance) are combined with behavioral management. Parents are taught to respond to misbehaviors by expressing their feelings promptly and using time-out when necessary. Parents are encouraged to give the child clear-cut responsibilities in the home, and to reinforce desirable behavior consistently. Such a broad-spectrum approach, well-structured for step-wise learning, appears to have a good chance of succeeding. Unfortunately, this approach has yet to be systematically researched. Obviously, it is likely that some aspects of this approach are more effective than others. The meetings between parents and clinicians, where feelings are identified and accepted, may be the most powerful aspect of this program. Or, the imposition of a consistent approach to parent-child interactions may be the key. It is also possible that none of this treatment has any positive effect on the speech of the stuttering child. As yet, we don't know.

Language Oriented Approaches

Several studies have suggested that the language development of stuttering or highly disfluent children may be delayed (Andrews & Harris, 1974; Berry, 1938; Kline & Starkweather, 1979; Morley, 1957; Muma, 1971; Murray & Reed, 1977; Wall, 1980; Westby, 1979). There is also evidence that as nonstuttering children are learning new linguistic forms, normal disfluency tends to increase (Colburn, Note 2; Hall, 1977). In light of these findings, a case could be made that stuttering is an outgrowth of difficulty in language acquisition. There are also reports in the literature suggesting that a specific subgroup of stutterers is characterized by language disability (Riley & Riley, 1979; Van Riper, 1982). As evidence of language problems in stutterers accumulates, clinicians are naturally becoming interested in indirect approaches to stuttering which focus on language. There are as yet, however, few published accounts of language-oriented therapy for young stutterers.

Meryl Wall and her colleague Florence Meyers have initiated some language-oriented treatment, following the lead provided by Wall's (1980) finding that a group of stuttering children showed delayed syntax development, compared to their normal peers. Their recent work (Meyers & Wall, 1982; Wall & Meyers, Note 3) has explored ways in which psycholinguistic, psychosocial, and physiological influences on stuttering can be explored in diagnosis and treatment. The psychosocial aspect of their approach employs parent counseling and modeling to help parents reduce social pressures on the child. The physiologic component is used especially when direct treatment is indicated. This component teaches the child loose articulatory contacts, gentle phonatory onsets, and other aspects of "easier talking" similar to Williams (1971) and Dell (1979).

Wall and Meyers combine psycholinguistic information with parent counseling to teach parents ways in which their use of language can facilitate their child's fluency. Slower speaking rate, simpler syntax and semantics, use of open-ended questions, and verbal facilitation of story telling are some of the changes in parent speech and language which may be taught. Meyers and Wall also make use of psycholinguistic principles in their play therapy. They advocate a low-structure situation in which the clinician begins by evoking only brief and syntactially simple responses from the child, gradually working up to more complex responses. As they point out, it is as though the GILCU program (Ryan, 1974) were applied to spontaneous speech. Wall and Meyers' approach combines many techniques from a variety of sources, but is unique in the authors' strong linguistic orientation.

No measurement of treatment effectiveness is yet available, but they have begun to collect data on outcome. Although Meyers and Wall's multifaceted approach may prove beneficial to many children, analysis of the effects of the various components may turn out to be ticklish, if not unmanageable. Analysis of the component contributions is an issue on which all clinical researchers may not agree. Some may be content to know how effective a broad-spectrum approach can be, while others may not be content until they know the relative contributions to successful outcome of each sub-component. Contributions to knowledge regarding theoretical and treatment issues on the role of language variables in the genesis and management of stuttering, however, cannot accrue from this work unless the effect of the language component of treatment is sorted out from the psychological counseling and motor learning treatments that are occurring concurrently.

The indirect treatment strategies used by Riley and Riley (1983) contain a substantial linguistic/cognitive component (although other aspects are addressed, also). At intake, the Rileys evaluate stuttering children in 4 disability categories: (1) attending, (2) oral motor discoordination, (3) auditory processing, and (4) sentence formulation. The children's home environments are examined for 2 potential stressors: (5) communicative stress, and (6) unrealistic parental expectations. A portion of treatment focuses on improving the child's abilities in any of the first 4 disability categories in which the child is found to be weak. Some commercially available materials (e.g., Semel, 1976) are available for some of these categories; others are remediated with the Rileys' own programs. Parent counseling, with the help of *If Your Child Stutters: A Guide for Parents* (Ainsworth & Gruss, 1981) is used to reduce stresses in the environment. In many cases, these indirect strategies are supplemented with direct stuttering modification (using, for example, response contingent stimulation).

Results from the Rileys' treatment (Note 4) have been evaluated for 16 of 19 children, ages 3-9, who were treated using both the Rileys' indirect and direct treatments. Data indicate that for the entire group of 19 children, Stuttering Severity Instrument (SSI) (Riley, 1972) scores were reduced by

57% using the indirect approaches described above to modify contributing and maintaining factors. SSI scores were then reduced an additional 30% using direct stuttering modification. Sixteen of the 19 children were assessed at least 24 months after treatment. Seven were "entirely free" of stuttering, 7 were "almost free" of stuttering, and 2 had regressed. If the "almost free" stutterers are counted as successes, the Riley's combined direct and indirect approach was successful with 88% of the children in the group studied.

Nelson's (Note 5) approach to indirect stuttering treatment also contains a strong psycholinguistic component. In her initial conference with parents, Nelson encourages them to become aware of how their child's fluency varies with a number of psycholinguistic factors. These factors include:

1. abstractness of the topic talked about;
2. immediacy of the event discussed;
3. complexity and familiarity of the language used; and
4. communicative intent of the child's utterances.

Two other nonlinguistic factors which may affect the child's fluency are also brought to the parents' attention:

1. excitement level of the speaking situation;
2. competitiveness of the speaking situation.

In addition to engaging the parents in keeping a log of potential influences on their child's fluency, Nelson also observes the parent-child interaction herself. She notes that the following communicative and psycholinguistic pressures are apt to be placed on the child by the parents via their speech: (a) directing the child's activity, (b) trying to evoke display of child's knowledge, (c) speaking rapidly, (d) using long, complex sentences, and (e) asking about an earlier event.

Nelson's treatment approach is to help the parents—through advising them, modeling for them, and having them practice—decrease some of the above-mentioned communicative pressures on the child. Since this treatment focuses on the nature of the parents' speech and language which is directed toward the child, it can be considered a language-oriented treatment, but it also rings of the earlier-described parent counseling treatment philosophies. The following items are a sample of the ways in which parents would be encouraged to change their own speech and language:

1. slow speech rate—to give the child extra language formulation time as the child's speech rate is developed;
2. no demands for display speech—to lessen demands on memory and language formulation;

3. reduce questions—to reduce social and linguistic pressure on the child;

4. talk in the "here and now" (rather than discussing the past, the future, or abstractions)—to reduce syntactic and conceptual demands;

5. use echo speech (judiciously)—to let the child know his or her message was received;

6. increase attention when the child is talking—to reduce the child's ambivalence about being heard; and

7. speak in simple sentences with many pauses between them (as well as periods of silence during play)—to reduce language comprehension and formulation pressure.

Nelson's treatment approach is to begin with this indirect strategy. If the child does not show some decrease in stuttering in response to 3 weeks of indirect treatment, Nelson uses direct treatment as well (see Nelson, Note 5). Nelson's data indicate that for 7 children (average age, 3; 7), treated with her indirect approach alone and followed up for longer than 6 months postdiagnosis, the outcomes were as follows: 4 children (2 severe, 1 moderate, and 1 mild at diagnosis) were 100% fluent; 1 child (mild) was 90% fluent; 1 child (mild) was 75% fluent; 1 child (mild) was 50% fluent. Of the 7 children, 4 were evaluated at follow-up by the clinician and 3 by parents.

It appears that psycholinguistic approaches are now being explored by an increasing number of clinicians. This may be a particularly productive area, especially in relation to the onset of stuttering. There are, however, many complexities involved in accounting for cause-effect relationships among these variables. Changing one environmental variable (such as parent speech rate, complexity of utterance, or extent of questioning) can affect the child's stuttering in many ways. Changing these variables can physically relax the child, can give a slow mechanism more time to coordinate, and can unburden an overtaxed cognitive capacity. The research-minded clinician, while pleased if such a treatment promotes change in stuttering clients, may be dismayed at the difficulty of knowing which variables are related to success with which children. The contribution of language treatment to therapy outcome may be best assessed when conventional language therapy appropriate to the child is administered alone for a period with a serious effort given to limiting the effects of other treatment variables. Alternatively, a conventional language therapy component may be delivered to a group of child stutterers in the context of another (stuttering) treatment approach, and the long-term outcome compared to that of a similar group who get essentially the same treatment without language therapy. This would assume that both of these groups of children would be assessed as needing some language oriented remediation.

Parent-Child Interaction

First described by Egolf, Shames, Johnson, and Kasprisin-Burelli (1972), parent-child interaction therapy for stuttering seeks to train parents in new ways of talking to their children. This treatment examines parent-child interactions in the clinic. Treatment then focuses on changing neither responses to stuttering, nor management of behavior, but the content and style of the parent-child interaction on the part of the parent. Egolf and his coworkers (Kasprisin-Burelli, Egolf, & Shames, 1972) first demonstrated that parents of stuttering children talked more "negatively" to their children than parents of nonstutterers. Clinicians then modeled for parents a positive, accepting way of interacting. This style produced a greatly reduced frequency of stuttering in the child. Parents then adopted this style of interaction themselves and it was found (in 5 of 9 cases) that their children maintained reduced frequency and severity of stuttering several months after treatment was over. Unfortunately, no data were available to demonstrate the extent to which each parent and clinician changed his or her behavior.

In this study, a relatively large range of positive interactions were modeled for parents. These included: (a) reward and praise for verbal output, (b) attentive listening, (c) open discussion of feelings, especially about stuttering, and (d) noninterruption, among others. Although most of the interactions modeled for the parents were generally more positive and accepting, clinicians tailored their responses to the individual parent-child dyad. That is, the clinicians assessed the parents' style of interacting and modeled an opposite style. This approach probably allowed for individual variations in children's needs to be met more specifically.

Following the lead of Egolf and his associates, Guitar, Kopff, Kilburg, and Conway (Note 6) have also experimented with treatment focused on parent-child interactions. In a single case study, they explored the use of videotaped parent-child play sessions as a stimulus for treatment. The child in this study was a 5-year-old girl whose stuttering frequency at diagnosis was 9.4% syllables stuttered and whose speech rate was 74 syllables per minute. Her blocks were accompanied by eye blinks, facial tension, sighing, head movements, and momentarily stopped articulatory postures. In each therapy session, one of the girl's parents would view new tapes of his or her previous play session with the child. The other parent would experiment with new styles of interaction while being videotaped in play with the child. After several weeks the child became normally fluent and has stayed fluent for 5 years. Posttreatment analysis of the parent-child interactions reveal that as the child gradually became fluent, the parents were changing many aspects of their behavior.

Initial analysis of the tapes indicated that decreases in the mother's speech rate were highly correlated with decreases in the child's stuttering. An analysis of the child's stuttering, which considered primary stuttering separately from secondary stuttering, indicated that primary stuttering appeared more highly correlated with speech rate changes, but secondary stuttering (tension, awareness, avoidance behaviors) was more highly correlated with the proportion of positive, accepting statements in the mother's conversation.

Although this type of treatment and analysis appear to have promise for evaluating and changing factors related to the child's stuttering, a finer-grained examination of the relevant variables should be undertaken. The gross categories of parent speech rate or parental acceptance need to be broken down further. Speech rate includes not only the rate at which sounds are spoken, but also the lengths of pauses between words and phrases (Nelson, Note 5; Starkweather, Note 7; Williams, Note 8). Moreover, as speech rate slows, other aspects of parent behavior may change. Parents may slow their general movements, as well. They may speak with a different voice quality and lower fundamental frequency. There are also myriad changes that may accompany increases in the proportion of parents' positive, accepting statements. They may include changes in body language and vocal inflection. Clinicians are only just beginning careful analysis of those aspects of parent behavior that influence their children's fluency. Perhaps a better understanding of them will lead to better indirect approaches to treatment. Future case studies of this type should also explore the use of single subject designs (e.g., McReynolds & Kearns, 1982) which may permit us to understand the cause-effect relationships between parent behavior and stuttering changes.

Psychomotor Therapy

This review of indirect stuttering therapies leaves out many treatments used abroad because English translations of treatment descriptions are not generally available. Recently, however, a description of some psychomotor strategies used in Europe has become available in English (Versteegh-Vermeij, Note 9). A number of therapists for stutterers in Europe, particularly in the Low Countries, have been experimenting with treatment focused on awareness of body posture, movement, and other aspects of the physical self. This work is an extension of a number of psychomotor therapies which view psychosomatic disorders as the result of emotional blockages. Elizabeth Versteegh-Vermeij, a well known therapist in The Netherlands, has pioneered the use of body-oriented therapy with stuttering children and their parents. In her treatment, parents and children are taught to become aware of the physical feelings of their bodies in isolated movements and then in movements which involve physical touching with others. Versteegh-Vermeij encourages children to develop physical confidence and free, full physical movement in parent-child groups. Her observation is that children (and adults) who gained acceptance and awareness of their physical selves were able not only to make substantial changes in their stuttering, but maintained their fluency after treatment. European therapists do not tend to collect pre- and posttreatment data; consequently, there appears to be little substantiation of the benefit of psychomotor or body-oriented therapies. Clinical researchers in some European stuttering treatment centers are now working to remedy this.

Summary and Conclusions

It is evident, even in this brief account, that the indirect approaches described have much in common. Of the 17 approaches reviewed, 9 advocate encouraging free expression of feeling by the child. Five suggest slowed speech rates by parents and 5 advise parents to increase their attentiveness when their child is speaking. Four encourage clear, firm disciplinary rules, and 3 indicate that parents' use of simple language in their conversation would be helpful. These are timeless remedies; they have probably been suggested for parents for decades. It is noteworthy, though, that all of the suggestions would probably be very beneficial to the nonstuttering as well as to the stuttering child. Thus, most of these approaches are not likely to make a stutterer worse or hurt a misdiagnosed nonstuttering talker. It is our impression, however, that these suggestions (as well as others) are not easy for parents to follow. Busy parents with many more immediate concerns are likely to need a great deal more than suggestions. Hence, programs like those of Zwitman (1978) and of Egolf and his coworkers (1972), which specifically train parents in desired behaviors, seem, on the face of it, more likely to succeed.

But how are we to know which programs do succeed? Recent contributions by Ingham (Ingham & Costello, Chapter 11, this volume; Ingham, Note 10) describe a system of measurement that will allow us to learn a little more about how effective a treatment is. Ingham suggests measuring a child's stuttering (percentage of syllables stuttered and syllables spoken per minute) several times, both in clinic and out, prior to treatment. This provides a baseline of the child's behavior. This measurement, so Ingham advocates, should continue repeatedly during treatment and repeatedly afterwards, for long-term follow-ups, both overt and covert. Although this thoroughness may not be possible for every clinician, careful measurement before and repeated careful measurement after treatment seems a minimum if we are to understand how effective various therapies or their components are.

However, assessment of stuttering frequency and speech rate may not provide enough to determine appropriate treatment. Curlee (1980), in his review of therapy for children, suggests use of direct treatment for those stutterers who show 3 "danger signs, " and an indirect approach for those who don't. Thus, if we are to follow Curlee's advice, we need to find ways of assessing these 3 danger signs: (1) struggling during disfluencies, (2) fear of stuttering, and (3) perceiving speech as a handicap. If these danger signs are related to potential for recovery, a treatment, direct or indirect, which reduced or eliminated these signs might help substantially. Hence, the need for finding reliable measures of "accessory behaviors, " including fear and avoidance of speech. These measures will help us determine which treatments to use for each client, as well as how effective each treatment is.

Effectiveness of treatment is a particularly difficult issue when indirect treatment is being assessed because of the potential for spontaneous recovery. In his review, Curlee points out that spontaneous recovery data show that 75% to 80% of those individuals who ever stuttered recover without treatment. Thus, a tough-minded view would be that if an indirect treatment is doing anything at all, more than 75% of all stutterers treated should recover. Of the 17 treatments described in our review, only 6 provided data on outcome. Two of these, Wahler et al. (1970) and Guitar et al. (Note 6), were essentially single subject studies. They cannot be evaluated as recommended general treatment strategies or considered tests of treatment effectiveness until they have been replicated on more subjects. The Rileys' approach showed a 57% decrease in symptoms via indirect treatment. However, since these children were severe enough to be given direct in addition to indirect treatment, a comparison of their overall outcome (88% of the children appear to have substantially recovered) with other indirect treatments is inappropriate here.

A comparison of the remaining treatments with the spontaneous recovery data must take into account Curlee's (1980) observation that some of the recovered stutterers in the spontaneous recovery literature still stutter in some situations. When we evaluate the reports of Wyatt and Herzan (1962), Egolf et al. (1972), and Nelson (Note 5), we might assume that "substantially improved" stutterers in 2 of these reports are comparable to the "recovered stutterers" in Curlee's figures. In Nelson's report it is a moot point as to whether both the 90% fluent and the 75% fluent (measured at follow-up) children should be called "recovered stutterers. " So we would ask, then, how do these 3 remaining reports stack up against a 75% spontaneous recovery rate? Wyatt and Herzan's data indicate that 75% of their clients recovered. In the Egolf et al. study, only enough data were available to show that 55% recovered. Nelson's data can be interpreted to suggest that either 86% or 71% of her clients recovered. The tough-minded critic would wonder if most of these treatments are accomplishing anything at all.

In our view, this comparison of treatment outcome with 75% spontaneous recovery is unduly harsh on indirect therapies. After all, indirect therapies usually treat stutterers who are severe enough to be of concern to their parents. Many of the spontaneously recovered stutterers probably were not that severe. Moreover, some of the 75% spontaneously recovered stutterers may have been unwitting benefactors of indirect treatments. They may have never known it, because their parents never told them. Recent reviews of the spontaneous recovery literature have also lowered this figure of 75%. Ingham (1983), for example, suggests that for younger children, spontaneous recovery rates may be closer to 50%. Even this 50% recovery is suspected by Ingham to be contaminated by the effects of formal and informal treatment attempts, making recovery not truly "spontaneous."

Despite these doubts, the point must still be made that advocates of indirect treatment have not yet provided data showing that most indirect treatments are more effective than no treatment at all. This conclusion makes a strong case for multiple pretreatment measures (to show that stutterers are not rapidly recovering on their own) and/or control groups of children who are not treated. These control measures are invaluable in showing treatment effectiveness. To be effective, treatments need only demonstrate that treated children improve substantially more than if they were untreated for the same period of time. Even if the untreated children would eventually spontaneously recover, they may be needlessly undergoing years of stuttering. Many adults who have recovered spontaneously in their teen-age years speak with fear and loathing of their childhood stuttering traumas.

How are we to improve treatments? Clinician-researchers are becoming curious about what components of a treatment approach are helpful. This curiosity may lead directly to more effective, more focused treatments. Clinicians are exploring such things as which child-speech variables change when parent behaviors are manipulated. One aspect of this research is analysis of clinician-child or parent-child interactions in natural therapy environments. This will lead toward understanding which particular adult variables seem to be related (directly or indirectly) to a child's stuttering.

This can suggest which, if any, adult variables might be changed to decrease stuttering. Williams (Note 8) discusses some work which deals in this way with rate variables. This work is difficult because it may take considerable training for an adult to change, for example, one speech rate variable (e.g., pause time) without changing another (e.g., articulation rate). But the payoff for this difficult work is great. Only by such experimental manipulation of discrete variables can we really understand what are the more direct antecedents of improvements in a stuttering child's speech.

In summary, the advances we are seeing in indirect approaches have been a quiet whisper amid the tumult of the same old treatments for stuttering children. But it is hoped, as we see an increase in the cries for accountability, the calls for more data by journal editors, and the availability of funding for treatment research, that clinicians will'be examining the subcomponents of their treatments and measuring relevant variables, intent on improving treatment outcome.

End Note

[1] The author once took haloperidol over several weeks, in the interest of science. Fluency improved slightly, but he developed the annoying side effect that the upper half of his body was usually falling asleep, while much of the lower half was in continual, agitated movement.

Reference Notes

1. Luper, H. Personal communication, 1982.
2. Colburn, N. Disfluency behavior and emerging linguistic structures in preschool children. Unpublished doctoral dissertation, Columbia University, 1979.
3. Wall, M., & Meyers, F. *Clinical management of childhood stuttering*. Baltimore: University Park Press, in preparation.
4. Riley, G., & Riley, J. Personal communication, 1982.
5. Nelson, L. Language formulation related to disfluency and stuttering. Paper presented at the Conference on Evaluation of Disfluency, Prevention of Stuttering, and Management of Fluency Problems in Children, Northwestern University, Evanston, Illinois, 1982.
6. Guitar, B., Kopff, B., Kilburg, H., & Conway, P. Parent verbal interaction and speech rate: A case study in stuttering. Paper presented at the Convention of the American Speech-Language-Hearing Association, Los Angeles, 1981.
7. Starkweather, C. W. The development of speech fluency and the definition of a fluency problem. Paper presented at the Conference on Evaluation of Disfluency, Prevention of Stuttering, and Management of Fluency Problems in Children, Northwestern University, Evanston, Illinois, 1982.
8. Williams, D. Emotional and environmental problems in stuttering. Paper presented at the Conference on Evaluation of Disfluency, Prevention of Stuttering, and Management of Fluency Problems in Children, Northwestern University, Evanston, Illinois, 1982.

9. Versteegh-Vermeij, E. Stress and body-oriented therapy. Paper presented at the Speech Foundation of America Conference, St. Petersburg, Florida, 1983.

10. Ingham, R. Evaluation and assessment procedures. Paper presented at the Conference on Evaluation of Disfluency, Prevention of Stuttering, and Management of Fluency Problems in Children, Northwestern University, Evanston, Illinois, 1982.

References

Ainsworth, S., & Gruss, J. F. *If your child stutters—A guide for parents*. Memphis: Speech Foundation of America, 1981.

Andrews, G., & Harris, M. *The syndrome of stuttering*. Clinics in Developmental Medicine, No. 17, London: Spastics Society Medical Education and Information Unit in association with Wm. Heinemann Medical Books, 1964.

Bailey, A. A., & Bailey, W. Workshop on childhood stuttering. Georgia and Tennessee Speech and Hearing Associations Convention, Chattanooga, Tenn., 1977.

Bailey, A. A., & Bailey, W. Workshop on childhood stuttering. Collier County Public Schools, Naples, Florida, 1982.

Berry, M. Developmental history of stuttering children. *Journal of Pediatrics, 1938, 12,* 209-17.

Bloodstein, O. *A handbook on stuttering* (3rd ed.). Chicago: National Easter Seal Society, 1981.

Conture, E. *Stuttering*. Englewood Cliffs, N.J.: Prentice-Hall, 1981.

Cooper, E. *Understanding stuttering*. Chicago: National Easter Seal Society, 1979.

Cozzo, G., & Gabrielli, L. La therapie du begayement avec les butyrophenones. *De Therapia Vocis et Loguelae*, Vol. I. XIII Congress of the International Society of Logopedics and Phoniatry, 1965.

Curlee, R. Assessment and treatment strategies for young stutterers. In L. Bradford & R. Wertz (Eds.), *Communicative disorders: An audio journal for continuing education*. New York: Grune & Stratton, 1980.

Dell, C. *Treating the school-age stutterer: A guide for clinicians*. Memphis: Speech Foundation of America, 1979.

Egolf, D., Shames, G., Johnson, P., & Kasprisin-Burelli, A. The use of parent-child interaction patterns in therapy for young stutterers. *Journal of Speech and Hearing Disorders*, 1972, *37*, 222-232.

Gattuso, R., & Leocata, A. L'Haloperidol nella terapia della balbuzie. *Clinical Otorhinolaryngology*, 1962, *14*, 227-234.

Hall, P. The occurrence of disfluencies in language-disordered school-age children. *Journal of Speech and Hearing Disorders*, 1977, *42*, 364-369.

Ingham, R. Spontaneous remission of stuttering: When will the emperor realize he has no clothes on? In D. Prins & R. J. Ingham (Eds.), *Treatment of stuttering in early childhood: Methods and issues*. San Diego: College-Hill, 1983.

Kasprisin-Burelli, A., Egolf, D., & Shames, G. A comparison of parental verbal behavior with stuttering and nonstuttering children. *Journal of Communication Disorders*, 1972, *5*, 335-346.

Kernan, M. Starting young is a key to working with stutterers. *Smithsonian*, 1981, *12*, 108-116.

Kline, M., & Starkweather, C. Receptive and expressive language performance in young stutterers. *Asha*, 1979, *21*, 797.

Meyers, F., & Wall, M. Toward an integrated approach to early childhood stuttering. *Journal of Fluency Disorders*, 1982, *7*, 47-54.

Morley, M. *The development and disorders of speech in childhood*. Edinburgh: Livingstone, 1957.

Muma, J. Syntax of preschool fluent and disfluent speech: A transformational analysis. *Journal of Speech and Hearing Research*, 1971, *14*, 428-41.

Murphy, A., & FitzSimmons, R. *Stuttering and personality dynamics*. New York: Ronald Press, 1960.

Murray, H., & Reed, C. Language abilities of preschool stuttering children. *Journal of Fluency Disorders*, 1977, *2*, 171-176,

Prins, D., Mandelkorn, T., & Cerf, A. Effects of haloperidol upon stuttering. *Asha*, 1974, *17*, 508.

McReynolds, L., & Kearns, K. *Single-subject experimental designs*. Baltimore: University Park, 1982.

Rantala, S. - L., & Petri-Larmi, M. Haloperidol (Serenase) in the treatment of stuttering. *Folia Phoniatrica*, 1976, *28*, 354-361.

Riley, G. A stuttering severity instrument for children and adults. *Journal of Speech and Hearing Disorders*, 1972, *37*, 314-321.

Riley, G., & Riley, J. A component model for diagnosing and treating children who stutter. *Journal of Fluency Disorders*, 1979, *4*, 279-293.

Riley, G., & Riley, J. Evaluation as a basis for intervention. In D. Prins and R. Ingham (Eds.), *Treatment of stuttering in early childhood*, San Diego, CA: College-Hill, 1983.

Ryan, B. *Programmed therapy for stuttering in children and adults*. Springfield, Ill: Charles C. Thomas, 1974.

Semel, E. *Semel Auditory Processing Program*. Chicago: Follet Educational Publishing, 1976.

Tapia, F. Haldol in the treatment of children with tics and stutterers—and an incidental finding. *Psychiatry Quarterly*, 1969, *43*, 647-649.

Van Riper, C. *The treatment of stuttering*. Englewood Cliffs, N.J.: Prentice-Hall, 1973.

Van Riper, C. *The nature of stuttering* (2nd ed.). Englewood Cliffs, N.J.: Prentice-Hall, 1982.

Wahler, R., Sperling, K., Thomas, M., Teeter, N., & Luper, H. The modification of childhood stuttering: Some response-response relationships. *Journal of Experimental Child Psychology*, 1970, *9*, 411-428.

Wall, M. A comparison of syntax in young stutterers and nonstutterers. *Journal of Fluency Disorders*, 1980, *5*, 321-326.

Westby, C. Language performance of stuttering and nonstuttering children. *Journal of Communication Disorders*, 1979, *12*, 133-145.

Williams, D. Stuttering therapy for children. In L. E. Travis (Ed.), *Handbook of speech pathology*. New York: Appleton-Century-Crofts, 1971.

Wyatt, G. *Language learning and communication disorders in children*. New York: Free Press, 1969.

Wyatt, G., & Herzan, H. Therapy with stuttering children and their mothers. *American Journal of Orthopsychiatry*, 1962, *23*, 645-59.

Zwitman, D. *The disfluent child*. Baltimore: University Park Press, 1978.

Roger J. Ingham
Janis M. Costello*

Stuttering Treatment Outcome Evaluation

Although researchers in stuttering find few areas of agreement, it would seem that today all agree about the importance of systematic measurement in the evaluation of stuttering treatment outcomes. And they would probably agree that over the past decade the management and evaluation of stuttering therapy has been improved by increasing use of measurement methodology. Much of the methodology that has begun to emerge in reports on stuttering therapy is almost wholly attributable to the pervasive influence of behavior therapy principles on stuttering treatment research (Costello, 1982; Ingham, 1983). What researchers still do not agree upon, however, would appear to be the certainty with which current measurement methods adequately account for the constructs implicated in the notion of therapy success or failure. Further, there is no evidence that the measurement methodology described in stuttering research reports has yet invaded the realm of clinical practice (Costello, 1979). The general purpose of this chapter, therefore, will be to offer some considerations on the problems of stuttering treatment outcome evaluation. These considerations will be in two parts: (1) a review of the principal issues in stuttering treatment evaluation, and (2) derivation of a viable clinical format that will assist clinicians and researchers to identify effects of treatment. Both parts will endeavor to identify some of the more important recent developments in the evaluation of stuttering treatment outcome.

*This chapter was prepared while Dr. Costello was Foundation Fellow at Cumberland College of Health Sciences, Sydney.

Stuttering Treatment Evaluation Issues

The clinical validity of the measures and treatment evaluation strategies used in stuttering treatment reports continues to concern researchers and clinicians alike (Gregory, 1978; Sheehan, 1980). Much of this concern can be traced to the absence of agreed upon criteria for evaluating therapy. Some attempts have been made to resolve this problem (Andrews & Ingham, 1972; Ingham, 1981; Ryan, 1974; Silverman, 1981), but none has produced commonly accepted methods for determining the clinical merit of stuttering therapy. Some of the issues that need to be resolved before acceptance is likely were recently summarized by Bloodstein (1981, pp. 386-390). He presented 11 criteria that he believes need to be considered when evaluating stuttering therapy. In what follows, these criteria will be presented (mainly in abridged form) and reviewed for their contribution to the search for clinically suitable measurement methods [2]. This will also provide a useful vehicle for reviewing some recent developments in therapy outcome evaluation.

> *1.   The method must be shown to be effective with an ample and representative group of stutterers. The single-subject design has a place in scientific research. It has been widely misused, however, in the area of research on stuttering therapy, where most single cases written up for publication are apparently chosen for the precise reason that they were successes. This practice produces a distorted picture. In the end we learn little from it beyond what we already know—that somewhere, at sometime almost any therapy can achieve a remarkable result for some stutterers.*

This is not only a criterion, but a recommendation that therapy evaluation should not depend on single-subject research. This is an important recommendation since it challenges the worth of single-subject therapy research designs. Actually the point at issue is the external validity of these designs. Single-subject research designs entered therapy research for a variety of reasons; foremost was the failure of group designs to identify critical aspects of the clinical process (Hersen & Barlow, 1976). Since group trends usually fail to reflect individual treatment response patterns, they also fail to discern the treatment's differential effects on certain individuals and, hence, themselves do not answer Bloodstein's first criterion. Quite obviously, single-subject studies can only show that a treatment has produced some profitable (or unprofitable) results for some stutterers; but that is far from a trivial finding, particularly if the study is internally valid and clearly specifies the treatment's effects. Furthermore, when such findings are replicated on additional subjects, then they not only increase the generality of the findings as Bloodstein would wish, but also strengthen our knowledge about a treatment and highlight relevant considerations for the design of subsequent group studies.

Regarding the concern about reporting only successful treatments, it is worth noting that this tradition probably permeates group research as much as single-subject research.

In the continuing struggle to find reliable treatments, there is increasing evidence that carefully managed time-series investigations are markedly improving clinical knowledge. Bloodstein's claim that a method must be effective across "representative" stutterers may, unwittingly, subscribe to the "uniformity assumption myth" (Kiesler, 1966)—the notion that there should be a uniform treatment suitable for a uniform client. Even treatment techniques promoted as useful for most stutterers, notably the prolonged speech procedures (Andrews, Guitar, & Howie, 1980), have benefited from controlled single-subject investigations (Ingham, 1983).

> 2. *Results must be demonstrated by objective measures of speech behavior such as frequency of stuttering or rate of speech, and by judges' ratings of severity. Such measurements should be made before, during, and after treatment by observers other than the experimenters themselves or without knowledge that might influence their judgment, and due account must be taken of the observers' reliability.*

There are two aspects to this criterion: the types of measures and their reliability. The first refers mainly to the construct validity of measures currently used to assess stuttering behavior. Frequency counts of stuttering and, to a lesser extent, ratings of stuttering severity have become almost *the* descriptive datum for this disorder. Significantly, Bloodstein recommends counts of stutterings, rather than measures of *disfluencies* or *dysfluencies*. Also of interest is the absence of reference to different disfluency categories, a method of measuring stuttering that seems to have faded in its use in treatment. Severity ratings present a number of problems, mainly because there is no agreed-upon method for rating severity. The principal purpose of severity ratings during treatment is to ensure that frequency reduction is not offset by worsening severity. One common method for determining severity is to measure the duration of individual moments of stuttering (Costello, 1981; Costello & Ingham, in press). The difficulty with this measure is that it, too, may lack construct validity, for duration may not be the feature that clinicians or clients regard as stuttering's severity. Speech rate measures, though essential to show that treatment benefits are not simply due to reduced rate, are questionable for similar reasons. At best, syllables per minute (Andrews & Ingham, 1972) or articulation rate scores (Perkins, 1975) only broadly indicate whether the subject is speaking unnaturally fast or slow. And for this reason, there may also be merit in supplementing this measure with perceptual judgments of the naturalness of the subject's speech (see below).

The importance of observer reliability is seemingly self-evident—yet that does not seem to be true for many researchers. A staggering number of treatment reports and experimental studies fail to report relevant reliability data (Ingham, 1983)—a fact that destroys the credibility of much of the current treatment literature. Even when reliability data are provided, they are rarely reported in a way which makes it possible to determine whether a study's reported data trends are also reliable (Hawkins & Dotson, 1975; McReynolds & Kearns, 1982).

One other issue concerns the methods used to obtain stuttering counts and speech rate. There is now a growing body of evidence that clinicians can capably count both of these variables "on line" and reliably (Ingham, 1983).

> 3. *Reports of therapeutic success must be based on repeated evaluations and adequate samples of speech. The great variability of stuttering from time to time and under different conditions is liable to result in assessments that are unrepresentative.*

This criterion is simple to justify, but less simple to prescribe. It is unclear how frequently such evaluations should be made, or what represent adequate samples of speech. Repeated evaluation helps determine whether the variability within and between speaking situations has been unambiguously and significantly modified by treatment. This means that the duration of evaluation cannot always be standardized across individuals—a source of difficulty for the use of group designs in therapy research. The same issue applies to sample size, although there is increasing acceptance of a method used by Ryan (1971; 1974)—that is, 5-minute samples of conversation, monologue, and oral reading. However, the sufficiency and representativeness of this, or any other arbitrarily determined sampling interval, is currently undocumented.

One attempt to derive a methodology that prescribes minimal frequency and sample size parameters will be outlined below. But this attempt is also hindered by the impoverished amount of research into stuttering variability across situations—a surprising circumstance in view of developments in recording technology. The problems involved in recording stuttering in "natural" circumstances have also received insufficient attention (Ingham, 1981). However, the advent of portable microcassette recorders should make it possible to obtain adequate speech samples in representative speaking situations.

The method of choosing "representative" speaking situations has also received very little attention in the treatment literature. One obvious method is to derive these situations from speaking log books prepared by the subject in advance of the treatment study; this would help identify situations that can be regularly used for assessment.

Most treatment research presumes that stuttering variability is largely affected by situational factors. Those may not be the only factors involved. Another feature of variability can be a tendency for time factors to influence variability (Ingham, 1981). The duration of time the subject spends speaking in certain situations, or even the time of day assessments are made, might be worthy areas of investigation.

4. Improvement must be shown to carry over to
speaking situations outside the clinical setting.

This is much related to Criterion 3. Most clinicians are aware that vast differences may occur between clinic and extraclinic speech performance, but evidence showing this difference is surprisingly small. Studies by Ingham and Packman (1977), Resick, Wendiggensen, Ames, and Meyer (1978), and Ingham (1982) go some way towards illustrating this criterion's importance.

Another interesting consideration is the boundary of the "clinical setting." The mere presence of a tape recorder or an assessor in the subject's nonclinic setting may evoke clinic-related speech performance (Ingham, 1981). For example, subjects may be assessed via telephone conversations from home or elsewhere, but the accompanying "assessment variables" may make these telephone conversations atypical (see Ingham, 1981; 1982). The only available solution to this problem would seem to be some form of occasional covert assessment.

5. The stability of the results must be demonstrated
by long-term follow-up investigations. Any number
of methods for making stuttering disappear have been

*known for many years: the great and persistent prob-
lem of stuttering therapy is how to keep the stutterer
from relapsing. Relatively little is known about the
subject of relapse.*

Long-term therapy investigations are becoming more common, despite their technical and conceptual difficulties; not the least of these is the length of time needed to prove that treatment has produced a durable improvement. Some of the issues associated with maintenance of treatment effects have been discussed elsewhere (Ingham, 1981) and will be taken up again later in this chapter.

Bloodstein (1981) suggests that "perhaps eighteen months to two years is the shortest interval after which most experienced clinicians would not feel unduly optimistic in hoping that the improvement was lasting" (p. 387). But their optimism should be tempered by information on what has transpired in that period. Many current treatment programs incorporate strategies for preventing relapse. These include speech practice, routine clinic visits, and continuing interaction with previously treated patients. These may be useful and even crucial techniques for sustaining improvement, but they may also confound the most clinically desirable effect—sustained improvement with the same level of attention to speech that is used by normal speakers. That is not to deny the advantages of "aided" maintenance; it simply suggests that clinicians should recognize that there are different types of sustained improvement. Needless to say, this topic is in dire need of investigation.

Increasing attention is being devoted to both the measurement and management of maintenance (Boberg, 1981). There may be some value in "booster" treatments, and in treatment schedules designed to sustain treatment gains for increasingly longer intervals. Another interesting area of treatment research concerns the use of self-management techniques. There are also numerous suggested approaches to maintenance that need investigation (Boberg, Howie, & Woods, 1979; Hanna & Owen, 1977; Ingham, 1981; Shames, 1981). These mainly include self-help groups, regular speech practice schedules, and the assistance of "significant others. " A large number of other, ostensibly useful, approaches have been reviewed by Stokes and Baer (1977).

One aspect of relapse that has attracted attention is the stutterer's attitude towards communication at the end of treatment. The problem of devising valid measures of attitudes and the shaky foundations of research claiming that poor communication attitudes influence long-term outcome are current concerns (Guitar, 1979, 1981; Guitar & Bass, 1978; Ingham, 1979, 1981; Ulliana & Ingham, in press). Nevertheless, it is highly likely that persons who show little interest in sustaining speech practice or fulfilling treatment requirements will be strong candidates for posttreatment relapse. The complex factors that enjoin patients to seek treatment, wait lengthy periods for treatment to begin, and then complete its often demanding requirements deserve much more research attention. It may well emerge that these are among the most important variables in the success, or otherwise, of the treatment process.

> *6. Suitable control groups or control conditions must be used to show that reductions in stuttering are the result of treatment.*

This criterion highlights the need for treatment designs that overcome threats to their internal validity. The advantage of the within-subject time-series designs (Hersen & Barlow, 1976) is that the effect of most nontreatment-related variables can be identified by the judicious choice of a baserate(s) duration and measurement conditions. The difficulty is to be certain that all validity threats have been controlled before, during, or even after treatment. For instance, one important nontreatment factor that is rarely controlled is the amount and nature of influence that the client is able to exert over stuttering frequency or severity prior to treatment. Certainly a treatment's effects should be independent of the extent and/or duration of such factors.

Group designs as a control procedure can only partially avoid some of the problems of assessing treatment effects since, as was previously mentioned, most fail to identify individual treatment responses. One compromise is a multiple baseline across subjects design wherein treatment is introduced for each subject following nontreatment baselines of differing lengths. Another difficulty with group designs is the choice of an appropriate control group. The best designed group studies presume that roughly matched group mean stuttering frequency, group mean speech rate, and perhaps age and sex, will ensure that the groups have potentially equivalent reactions to the treatment condition. There are literally no data that justify this assumption of uniformity. Even less defensible is the notion that meaningful findings can be derived by merging the differences between subject groups, treatment management techniques, measurement quality, assessment procedures, and treatment time from different therapy studies; but such are the assumptions beneath the use of the "meta-analysis" (Smith & Glass, 1977) technique that Andrews, Guitar, and Howie (1980) used to draw comparisons between different stuttering treatment techniques.

The inherent weakness of meta-analysis for evaluating the effects of a stuttering therapy should be almost self-evident, but it is clearly revealed by examining the foundations of one of the main conclusions reached by Andrews et al. They concluded "that treatments based on training a stutterer in prolonged speech and gentle onset techniques are superior to other types of treatment" (p. 305). While there is evidence to indicate that prolonged speech treatments are indeed successful for many stutterers, the basis for this claim hinges on an investigation that virtually excluded reference to certain treatment techniques and relied upon extremely questionable post-treatment data from others. By necessity, the meta-analysis technique cannot deal with single-subject studies and so almost all reports on response contingent procedures were excluded from their comparison. (The exception was a study by Martin and Haroldson (1969) which was not designed to evaluate therapy outcome). Also, out of the 12 "prolonged speech" studies included for investigation only two reported using beyond-clinic data, and one of these used an extensive uncontrolled maintenance program in the interval when outcome data were collected (Ingham, 1983). It is little wonder that Eysenck (1978) described this method's concern for data quantity rather than quality as an "exercise in mega-silliness" (p. 517), a concern echoed by Sheehan (1980).

Along with suitable designs for discerning stuttering treatment effects there is also a need for clinically viable designs that determine when treatments are impotent, or are no longer needed because their effects have generalized. These phenomena have been identified in some studies through the use of within-session ABA designs, such as that reported by Costello (1975), or multiple baselines (Martin, Kuhl, & Haroldson, 1972). There is also a need to determine the time required to decide when treatment is *not* effective or, conversely, the changes in performance that indicate clinically significant treatment effects.

7. The subjects' speech must sound natural and spontaneous to listeners, and the subjects must be free from the need to monitor their speech.

This criterion has grown in importance in recent years because of therapies that rely on changing the client's speech pattern. Some investigators have measured naturalness by using listeners to rate speech samples either for normalcy or naturalness (Jones & Azrin, 1969; Perkins, Rudas, Johnson, Michael, & Curlee, 1974). Others have tested whether listeners are able to distinguish the stutterer's posttreatment speech from speech samples of normally fluent speakers (Ingham & Packman, 1978; Runyan & Adams, 1978, 1979). Another approach measures aspects of speech, such as vowel duration or rate, in order to relate the subject's speech to normal speech (Metz, Onufrak, & Ogburn, 1979). A different approach to this task is emerging from research by Martin (1981; Martin, Haroldson, & Triden, in press), who found that listeners could rate short speech samples for naturalness on a 9-point scale with high levels of reliability. In consequence, Martin and Ingham are investigating the effects on stuttering and speech quality of feeding back to subjects every 30 seconds a listener's speech naturalness rating of the subject's speech. Preliminary results show that clinicians perform this task with high reliability, and that for some stutterers, providing on-line feedback regarding the naturalness of their speech may positively influence their observed speech quality. Similar endeavors have not been made to measure for "spontaneity" but, in principle, there is no reason why listener judgments could not be used for the same purpose.

Regarding the issue of monitoring, Shames and Florance (1980) reported measuring "monitored" and "unmonitored" speech during their treatment program. Their procedure requires speakers to nominate speaking intervals in which either type of speech will be used. Unfortunately, without independent measures of this variable(s), it is difficult to determine whether speakers can manipulate speech monitoring. But, more importantly, it is not clear how much, or what form of monitoring is desirable for normal speech behavior. Related to this is Webster's (1974) attempt to partially evaluate outcome from the Hollins program by asking listeners on follow-up questionnaires to indicate "how much attention must you pay to the task of speaking fluently?" This may help determine whether posttreatment effects oblige speakers to concentrate excessively on their "fluency. " These preliminary efforts at measuring for monitoring of speech may have some problems, but, at present, no efforts have been made to measure the spontaneity that Bloodstein believes is necessary for normally fluent speech.

> *8. Treatment must remove not only stuttering, but
> also the sense of handicap and the person's self-concept
> as a stutterer.*

This type of criterion is often presumed to present a special challenge to treatments that are mainly concerned with modifying or removing stuttering. It is assumed that a "sense of handicap," or a stutterer's "self-concept" are constructs that either retain the problem or are the essence of the problem. And, more significantly, it is assumed that their removal or alteration is necessary to the treatment's success. However, no data have ever shown that changes in stuttering do *not* also influence the "sense of handicap," or change the talker's concept of himself as a talker. That is not to suggest that patterns of behavior associated with stuttering will readily and immediately change when the disorder is modified. It would be rather surprising, for example, if embarrassing or constantly avoided circumstances were suddenly of no concern when stuttering ceases. Again, no data have shown that the persistence of such reactions is essentially abnormal or prevents normal fluency.

Surprisingly, Bloodstein (1981) partly justifies this criterion by referring to Andrews and Cutler's (1974) claim that the removal of stuttering in one situation was not sufficient to change stutterers' attitudes towards speaking. In fact, Andrews and Cutler's data actually show that when treatment was extended to other situations (in the course of a transfer procedure), the attitude scores showed concomitant and favorable changes. This aligns with findings from a subsequent investigation by Ulliana and Ingham (in press) on the attitude scale (S24) used in Andrews and Cutler's study which shows that the scale's scores are probably strongly influenced by the frequency of stuttering that occurs in situations referenced in the scale's items. In other words, it is highly likely that the "attitudinal factors" measured by the S24 are simply correlates of stuttering frequency. There is no reason to expect that a "sense of handicap," or "self-concept," might not also be related to actual stuttering frequency. In short, there is no evidence (to date) that such variables need particular attention within treatment in order to ensure therapy success.

> *9. The success of a program of therapy should not be inflated by ignoring dropouts.*

Numerous examples of this problem exist in the stuttering treatment literature (Ingham, 1983). This is a problem in almost all areas of treatment research and, when excessive, prevents any meaningful conclusions from a study. The problem may well be much greater than is evident from studies in which large scale dropouts have been reported. For example, in single-subject studies it is very rarely indicated that the treated subjects were the *only* subjects on whom the procedure was tried. This information can be exceedingly important, as is demonstrated by numerous subjects who have dropped out of haloperidol treatment programs (Ingham, 1983). Their response probably reflects the less savory effects of this treatment, and serves to contraindicate haloperidol as a preferred treatment for suttering (Guitar, Chapter 10, this volume). Obviously the true clinical value of many treatments can only emerge when clinical researchers carefully ascertain the reasons for dropouts, and also report on nonresponders in the course of single-subject research.

> *10. The method must be shown to be effective in the hands of essentially any qualified clinician, including those without unusual status, prestige, or force of personality.*

and

11. The method must continue to be successful when it is no longer new and the initial wave of enthusiasm over it has died away.

These are much related criteria that refer to the treatment's replicability and clinical viability. Actually, these criteria appear to have been met by many of the current therapy procedures, although most "replication" studies invariably highlight the contribution of additional treatment factors or therapy variations and are probably conducted by particularly enthusiastic clinicians. At the same time, an increasing number of treatment reports are now being written to reveal both the strengths and weaknesses of certain procedures, especially those using prolonged speech and its variants (Ingham, 1983). This is a vital shift in much stuttering therapy research and meets the spirit of Bloodstein's criterion. At the same time, many of the response contingent and prolonged speech treatment programs are continuing to produce benefits even now that the "initial wave of enthusiasm" has receded.

Bloodstein's (1981) criteria highlight most of the critical issues that need consideration in evaluating stuttering therapy. Some of the criteria seem questionable, most notably Criteria 1 and 8, but in general they are useful guides to stuttering therapy evaluation. Their limitation is that they are relatively nonspecific guides and provide insufficient information to help clinicians evaluate their own therapy endeavors. The purpose of clinical research is not only to design and evaluate treatments but also to improve therapy practice. So, in what follows, an attempt will be made to develop a set of guidelines for measuring treatment efficacy in therapy management. These guidelines will embrace most of Bloodstein's criteria and include a distillation of pertinent findings from recent clinical research.

Towards a Therapy Evaluation System

Introduction

The purpose here is to develop a therapy evaluation system suitable for most stuttering therapy procedures. It is not posed as a "final solution," but draws on the current treatment literature to derive some necessary operations that should accompany therapy. Actually, any search for an all-purpose treatment evaluation design seems to have about as much chance of succeeding as the search for the Holy Grail. Indeed, the problem in such a search is to be able to recognize treatment success. For, if the object of stuttering therapy is to produce normally fluent speech, then that objective continues to be hindered by the absence of measures (or sets of measures) that can be used to describe normal fluency (Starkweather, 1980). But if clinicians are prepared to settle for an assessment strategy that shows when stuttering is changing as a function of treatment, and when some of the presumed relevant features of normal fluency are evident, then perhaps the search will not be fruitless.

One potential impediment to the search is the differing therapy formats among stuttering treatments. There are obvious differences between treatments concerned with directly modifying stuttering and those that treat stuttering by modifying other behaviors. That is not a major impediment, however, since all ultimately aim to modify stuttering, and so their efficacy can probably be related to various speech performance measures. More problematic is whether treatment is delivered intensively or intermittently. Since intensive treatment should produce improved speech more rapidly, the format will need sufficient flexibility to accommodate different expected rates of change. Thus within- and beyond-clinic assessments may need to be made relatively more frequently for intensive programs. Nevertheless, even this problem is surmountable provided the format's principal components and the guidelines for indentifying therapy effects are suitable for both methods. Another difficulty might be the age of clients; there is some indication (Ingham, 1983) that children may be more responsive to certain treatments than adolescents or adults. It is possible that this difference might extend to rates of change, plus any criteria for determining clinically significant improvement. The same arguments could apply to differences in the intellectual level of clients, for there is also some indication that retardates respond more slowly to treatment (Ingham, 1983). The resolution to each of these difficulties is reasonably straightforward if the format is derived empirically. In other words, where data exist that demand exceptional formats, then such formats should be formulated.

Formulating the Evaluation System

The most significant lesson learned from the checkered history of stuttering therapy is that a useful treatment evaluation system should be designed so that it can embrace the known and anticipated variability of stuttering. It must be a system that is capable of demonstrating that therapy progress or outcome is not confounded by the known untreated variability of the subject's stuttering. Treatment evaluation formats that are suitable for this purpose are beginning to emerge from the time-series quasi-experimental designs (Hersen & Barlow, 1976) typically used in within-subject research. They are especially suitable because they not only identify variability, but also help deal with concerns such as accountability, decision making, and outcome evaluation. Furthermore, they are not only the most powerful designs available for determining sources of within-subject variability, but they are also the only ones that will enable the clinician to discern whether therapy is responsible for generalization.

The strength, or internal and external validity, of these designs in a therapy evaluation system depends on data collection within and beyond the therapy setting at clinically relevant intervals before, during, and after treatment. In short, the foundation of the recommended system is an integration of the now familiar multiple baseline and ABA designs. But the clinical viability of this system depends on finding some basis for determining clinically significant frequency, duration, and content of measurement within the system's design. The rationale for one such determination will now be outlined.

The Data Base, or What to Measure

There is probably little argument that an appropriate evaluation system requires access to audio-recorded speech within relevant speaking situations. Perhaps these recordings could be supplemented by video recordings to ensure that the visual aspects of stuttering (especially for severity measurement) are taken into account. In the absence of this facility, there is value in utilizing directly observed performance data.

Perhaps the minimal clinical data would be stuttering frequency counts and syllables (or words) spoken during talking time. They provide the bases for calculating percentages of syllables (or words) stuttered and syllables (or words) per minute—two of the most commonly used indices for recording the speech behavior of stutterers. These measures in turn assist clinicians in gauging changes in stuttering, and the contribution that the amount and rate of speaking make to stuttering variability.

Stuttering counts

The frequency of "moments of stuttering" may not fully depict the extent of disability caused by stuttering. However, this measure has certainly passed the test of time. The virtue of stuttering frequency counts is that they can be integrated with treatment via on-line measurement, while assessing the treatment's success (or otherwise) in removing the crux of the disorder. Most current therapies aim to remove all instances of stuttering, so it is becoming less important that those instances be described as more or less "severe" or as "part-word repetitions," etc. It also makes little sense now to confound stuttering counts with counts of normal disfluencies. There is increasing acceptance that clinicians (and certainly lay observers) are able to distinguish between disfluencies and stutterings (MacDonald & Martin, 1973).[3] This is an important point since there is no obvious advantage in a treatment that removes normal disfluencies but is less successful in removing stutterings. Conversely, a treatment that removes all disfluencies, normal and abnormal, may actually succeed in producing unusual fluency.

There are at least two dangers in relying on frequency counts of stuttering alone in order to evaluate treatment. The first relates to severity. Occasionally, a very low frequency of stuttering may contain exceptionally long moments of stuttering (Ingham, 1981). For this reason, there is good cause to record the duration or visible features of low frequency stuttering. The second reason concerns the role of word avoidance. This must be the least researched stuttering phenomenon, yet one of the best known features of the disorder—especially in adults. Perhaps the only way of measuring its presence is the subject's report and instructional tests for its influence. The latter may be ascertained by asking the subject to try to minimize stuttering for an interval, possibly by "avoiding stutterings" during spontaneous speech, and then comparing this interval with another in which the reverse instruction is given.

Speech rate

The primary reason for measuring speech rate is that it is generally accepted that reduced speech rate may be sufficient to produce reduced stuttering. Of course, reduced speaking as such would have the same effect. Less publicized is the possibility that abnormally fast speech rate may also reduce stuttering (Ingham, Martin, & Kuhl, 1974). However, there is no accepted method for measuring speech rate. One stumbling block is the relationship between existing rate measures and normally fluent speech rate. Speech rate measurement, as Starkweather (1980) has recently pointed out, needs to be much more complex than simple counts of words or syllables per minute. For what is a perceived as "fast" or "slow" turns out to be partially relative, but also dependent upon variables such as sound durations, pause durations, coarticulation, and rate of syllable production. Consequently, the currently used clinical measures of speech rate only approximate what is a perceived rate, or what might be normal rate. In light of this, what options are available?

For some years the senior author and colleagues have used 170 to 210 syllables per minute as a target normal speech rate (Ingham, 1981). But this measure (allowing for its imperfections) is based on a relatively unusual speaking condition: a monologue that is not interrupted by the conversational exchanges typical of most speech behavior; plus it is the speech rate of young adults. Furthermore, these overall syllable-per-minute scores are neither as useful nor, probably, as valid as Perkins's (1975) measure of articulation rate which excludes pauses and occurrences of stuttering. However, in the absence of pertinent speech rate data, both measures probably provide different, but clinically useful, measures of rate during therapy (Costello, 1981; Costello & Ingham, in press).

Another reflection of the need for research in this area is that there is little information on the relevant target speech rates that should pertain to the subject's age. There are some data from school children which indicate that the average syllables-per-minute rates in normal speech progressively increase throughout childhood. Kowal, O'Connell, and Sabin (1975) have shown that in kindergarten years this rate is about 50% of adult rates and rises to near adult rates by around 12 years. At present, those data might provide the best guide for estimating the expected syllable-per-minute rates for different age groups at the end of treatment. Perhaps a better alternative, certainly one worthy of investigation, is the subject's natural speech rate during stutter-free intervals. Admittedly, these intervals (depending on their length) may be influenced by stuttering frequency, but they may also be more appropriate bases for determining the talker's "normally" fluent rate. Actually, the clinician's perceptual judgment of what is an acceptable and normal rate may ultimately translate into the most clinically suitable syllable-per-minute scores for the individual case—especially if speech normalcy or naturalness ultimately emerges as a reliable basis for determining this measure.

There are numerous reasons why speech rate and stuttering frequency measures are necessary, yet incomplete, for assessing speech performance in treatment. The most important is the imperfect connection between zero stuttering at "normal" speech rate and speech that is perceived as normally fluent (Ingham, 1981; Perkins,1981). The need to improve this connection largely stems from the proliferation of treatments that procure "fluency" via unusual speech patterns, such as the variants of prolonged speech. Adams (1982), for example, has been particularly concerned about the need to gain much more information on the indices needed to identify normally fluent speech. Starkweather (1980) also explored these issues and concluded that fluent speech "is the quality of speech that includes rapid and easy, as well smooth production" (p. 195). But, as yet, no known combination of measurement operations quantifies that speech quality.

Speech quality

A number of approaches to the task of measuring speech quality have already been mentioned. These include ratings of naturalness, prosody, rate, and fluency, plus perceptual analyses of differences between speech samples from nonstutterers and treated stutterers. These measures may evaluate the results of treatment but, unfortunately, they cannot be readily integrated with the treatment process in the same fashion as stuttering counts and rate. However, one promising development, as was previously described, is the use of on-line ratings of naturalness, provided it is possible to establish the reliability and validity of such ratings.

In general terms, therefore, measures that have maximum utility in a therapy context are those that yield dual-function data: (1) they provide bases for establishing within- and beyond-clinic treatment effects, and (2) they contribute to treatment operations (i.e., can be used on-line during treatment). Such dual function measures may not aid all therapies, but for most current therapies they should serve the first function. In passing, it is interesting to note the increasing recognition of the value of measures that do more than passively chart the subject's progress through therapy. Indeed, measures that permit decisions about the efficacy of therapy may have an integral role as treatment agents. It is this latter function which is being used lately to assist the transfer and maintenance of therapy effects (Ingham, 1980; 1982).

Where to Collect Data

The crux of the system described herein is the establishment of multiple "standard" measures of the client's speech performance within and beyond the treatment setting. The conditions of such measures should be determined individually for each client so that they provide representative samples to tap the variability inherent in speaking performance within and beyond the clinic. These standard measures would, then, be administered regularly and repeatedly throughout the course of the clinician's (or clinical researcher's) clinical relationship with the client.

Within-clinic measures

It is well known (but not well documented) that stuttering may vary considerably across different speaking tasks and situations (Bloodstein, 1981; Guitar, 1975; Ingham & Packman, 1977; Resick, Wendiggensen, Ames, & Meyer, 1978; Ryan, 1974). A variety of within-clinic measures have been used rather arbitrarily in the literature, their usefulness being determined partly by the information they give regarding relevant parameters of the client's speech performance and, partly, by the convenience they offer to the clinician. What should be regarded as necessary? The most obvious contenders are converstional speech, monologues, and oral reading, since they are useful not only for assessment but are typically treatment activities as well. Oral reading is included mainly because of its utility in certain therapies; otherwise, it seems strange that so many stuttering assessment procedures recommend a task that is rarely performed in the natural environment (except occasionally in the school setting). Nevertheless, it does have the presumed advantage of controlling for word avoidance. Clinician-client conversations and telephone conversations, both heavily laced with questions, are obviously good choices. The latter task is especially useful because of its suitability for beyond-clinic treatment and assessment as well. The ideal duration for each task is yet another "unknown," but in the context of demands on clinician time, perhaps each should be three minutes.

Beyond-clinic measures

The choice of the situations in which the subject's speech should be measured will be conditioned by the recordability of the situation as much as its validity. The recording process has been greatly assisted by the availability of exceedingly small, good quality microcassette recorders that should be within the resources of a clinic or a client. They can be worn comfortably and equipped with remote hand controls that simplify recording in most situations.

The choice of recordable assessment situations presents some complicated, but not unsolvable, difficulties. There are some logical choices: parents or spouse, peers, and significant others, and a reasonable cross-section of regularly occurring occasions where the client talks. The frequency and variety of talking situations occurring for individual stutterers could be derived with reasonable precision from logs kept by the client (or the client's parent) previous to enrollment in the treatment program (Darley & Spriestersbach, 1978). The number of beyond-clinic measures regularly obtained for each client will differ according to the breadth and frequency of a given client's talking occasions. The goal is that the clinician's (or experimenter's) beyond-clinic samples reflect the variability that would be found were it possible to have data on all of the client's speech throughout every day. (See Ingham & Packman, 1977, for an example of such continuous and complete measurement.) Typical beyond-clinic measures for children might contain standard samples of talking with the family during dinner, with a sibling during playtime, with the mother while riding in the car, and at school during "show and tell," and reading group.

The typical adult client might provide recordings of speech from typical work situations, frequently occurring social situations, and conversations with his or her spouse at home.

The validity of the selected situations may be aided by two other considerations: use of the client's self-judged "difficult" (but recordable) situations, and the relative frequency with which these situations occur. These additional considerations should certainly be included within the decision base for choosing samples from the client's environment. A logical starting point for deciding the length each sample should be is that it reflects the client's typical talking time in similar settings. For example, if a child's speech with a parent occupies, say, 50% of his or her estimated talking time, then recordings of similar talking should account for about 50% of the beyond-clinic data collected for that client.

When to Collect Data

Reaching an agreeable decision about the frequency and duration of samples in a repeated measures assessment design involves at least three considerations: identifying variability, establishing that a treatment is "working," and managing data. However, taking account of these considerations in a generally acceptable therapy format is like putting together a jigsaw puzzle that has its pieces shaped by special interest groups whose members can never agree—arguably one common characteristic in this field. Nevertheless, there may be some parts of the puzzle that can be solved using compromise pieces.

Perhaps the first puzzle piece—identifying variability—should come from the ranks of clinical researchers. The difficulty is that these persons also offer little guidance on the minimum number of data points needed to reflect variability. For compromise purposes, therefore, perhaps the much-referenced text by Hersen and Barlow (1976) should be a guide. They recommend at least three "data points" in any phase of an evaluation design employing data trend comparisons, although many of their text's examples use four or more data points for this purpose. Perhaps, therefore, the seemingly small number of four is an acceptable starting point. But does this translate into measuring relevant behavior for four consecutive days, once every four weeks, or perhaps, once every four months? This piece of the puzzle should probably come from two interest groups: practicing clinicians and the editors of journals reporting treatment studies, for it relates to the frequency with which treatment is offered, and the interval of time needed to convince peers that treatment efficacy has been established. The factors involved in constructing this piece will be deferred for the moment.

The third, and most overlooked factor, is the sheer task of data collecting from audio recordings, and the subject's ability to obtain such recordings.

Determining a Treatment Effect

Once a suitable measurement schedule has been determined and introduced during the pretreatment period, it is continued throughout the instatement and transfer phases of the program. The next task is to find a suitable time frame that can be used to decide whether or not the therapy procedures are beneficial. This could lead to a veritable Pandora's Box—comparing different therapies and their effects. Fortunately, the interior of the box is not as daunting as might be expected. We can at least take advantage of a body of therapy literature to gain some idea of the rate of change in target behaviors from successfully treated clients. Indeed, if that literature cannot be used for this purpose, then it has virtually no external validity (Birnbrauer, 1981). At the very least, it should show the expected rate of change in stuttering if a client responds to a particular treatment. For example, if the chosen treatment was one of the response contingent procedures, then perhaps a less dramatic decline in stuttering frequency should be expected when compared with rhythm or any of the numerous variants of prolonged speech. On the other hand, the relevant target behavior for these speech pattern techniques is usually eventual restoration of normal speech rate , thus extending the time needed ultimately to determine treatment responsiveness.

There is no reason to skirt the "treatment effect time" issue with generalities since much of the reviewed treatment literature—at least that which provides single-subject data—is able to be summarized for this purpose. Tables 11-1 and 11-2 provide summaries of the treatment studies that permit estimates of the treatment time required for stuttering or disfluencies (sometimes "dysfluencies") to decrease by at least 50% relative to baserate. The term "successful outcome" is used in a very broad sense. It refers to those subjects who were reported, at the end of their treatment, to have reduced stuttering by at least 50% without decreased speech rate (when these data are reported). A 50% reduction in stuttering is certainly far from absolute treatment success, but, in the spirit of compromise, it is regarded as evidence that a substantial change in performance has been achieved by the treatment. The successfully treated subjects have been divided into children, those 12 years of age or younger (see Table 11-1), and adults (see Table 11-2). This is for no special reason, other than the recurring suggestion in the literature that children appear to respond more rapidly to some treatments than adults. Generally the tables confirm that children do respond a shade more rapidly to most treatment procedures, particularly the response

TABLE 11-1

This table summarizes the results of a survey of stuttering treatments involving children 12 years of age or younger. The survey was designed to identify studies in which it was possible to discern the treatment time needed for individual subjects to reduce stuttering or disfluencies by more than 50% relative to pretreatment performance. That point was established when the target behavior reached the 50% reduction level on two assessment occasions. In the case of the "Gradual Increase in Length and Complexity of Utterance" (GILCU), the 50% reduction level was regarded as equivalent to half the time required to achieve the designated treatment target. For the speech pattern procedures, the 50% reduction level was regarded as equivalent to half the time required to complete the treatment's instatement phase.

METHOD	PROCEDURE	STUDY	HOURS REQUIRED FOR 50% REDUCTION IN TARGET BEHAVIOR	NUMBER OF SUBJECTS/ AGE RANGE
Response Contingent	GILCU	Costello (1980)	15.50	1/11
		Johnson, Coleman, & Rasmussen (1978)	10.50	1/6
		Ryan (1974)	3.30–30.05	6/7–9
		Mowrer (1975)	5.00	1/10
	Positive Reinforce-ment	Peters (1977)	0.60	2/8
		Shaw & Shrum (1972)	0.67	3/9–10
	Combined Punishment and Reinforce-ment	Ryan (1974)	1.00–6.00	2/9

Category	Method	Study		
	Punishment	Martin & Berndt (1970)	0.67	1/12
		Martin, Kuhl, & Haroldson (1972)	1.33–2.00	2/3–4
		McDermott (1971)	1.20	1/9
		Reed & Godden (1977)	1.33–1.67	2/3–5
Masking	Continuous	MacCulloch, Eaton, & Long (1970)	6.00	4/11.9
Speech Pattern	Rhythmic Stimulation	Herscovitch & Le Bow (1973)	2.00	2/12
	MCSR	Brady (1971)	4.00	1/12
	DAF/ Prolonged Speech	Ryan (1971)	2.00	1/8
		Ryan (1974)	5.65–20.25	2/8–12
		Turnbaugh & Guitar (1981)	4.50	1/12
Speech Pattern	Regulated Breathing	Hee & Holmes (1976)	1.50	1/10
	Shadowing	Ottoni (1974)	1.00	1/9
Traditional	Programmed	Ryan (1974)	2.30	1/10

TABLE 11-2
Table incorporates the same information as Table 11-1 but for subjects older than 12 years.

METHOD	PROCEDURE	STUDY	HOURS REQUIRED FOR 50% REDUCTION IN TARGET BEHAVIOR	NUMBER OF SUBJECTS/ AGE RANGE
Response Contingent	GILCU	Mowrer (1975) Ryan (1974)	5.00–9.75 5.25–19.30	2/23,31 3/16–35
	Punishment	Costello (1975) Ryan (1974)	1.83 3.05–5.15	1/18 2/15,20
	Self- management	James (1981) La Croix (1973)	23.00 1.00	1/18 2/?
Anxiety Reduction	Reciprocal Inhibition	Boudreau & Jeffrey (1973)	12.00	4/16–22

Speech Pattern		Study		
Speech Pattern	Rhythmic Stimulation	Brady (1971)	5.00–31.00	17/14–53
	Prolonged Speech	Andrews (1973)	5.00	1/?
	DAF/ Prolonged Speech	Boberg & Fong (1980)	15.00	1/19
		Goldiamond (1965)	3.08	2/40,?
		Ingham & Andrews (1973)	1.63–4.60	11/18–56
		Ryan (1974)	1.00–88.60	23/14–45
		Webster (1970)	5.00–20.00	8/15–47
Biofeedback	EMG	Guitar (1975)	2.67	1/32
Traditional	Programmed	Ryan (1974)	1.45–12.05	9/14–43

contingent techniques. The rate of response to the GILCU and speech pattern techniques are more difficult to translate since there is no clear indication of the time taken to reach 50% improvement. For this reason, half the treatment time, or talking time, required to reach the final target behavior was judged equivalent to 50% improvement. This is probably the main reason why these treatments appear to take longer to reach the "treatment effect" criterion.

Resolving the Treatment Design Puzzle

The next task is to translate the preceding information into solution pieces for the treatment design puzzle. The first issue must be the frequency with which baseline and subsequent measures during and after treatment should be made. Andrews and Harvey (1981) have gathered data that they suggest show that pretreatment speech measures from adult stutterers do not show improvement over a 6-week nontreatment period. Thus, the most conservative treatment design might incorporate up to 6 weeks of weekly recordings of the subject's speech within and beyond the clinic prior to the initiation of treatment. The least conservative, though possibly the most practical, approach might utilize the 4-data point principle, with a minimum of, say, once weekly recordings of all selected within- and beyond-clinic speech samples. This would seem to provide adequate sampling of the existing variability in the client's stuttering across settings and time.

Clinicians should be aware that this recommended 4-week base rate data collection interval is not necessarily a period of clinical inactivity. It is during this period that the clinician might train the client's spouse or parents not only to collect appropriate beyond-clinic recordings but also to score these recordings reliably. Also, in some instances the authors have found that the base rate recording procedure, per se, appears to have produced "treatment effects", thus influencing subsequent intervention decisions. Finally, the base rate period can be used to organize the format of treatment procedures. The methods for choosing these procedures are considered in more detail by Costello and Ingham (in press).

Tables 11-1 and 11-2 suggest that the treatment phase for almost all current data-based treatments should not exceed about 12 treatment hours for children or 23 hours of treatment for adults, before a decision is made as to whether the chosen treatment should be continued or changed. Actually, quite discernible trends in relevant data should be expected by the fifth hour if some treatments are likely to be beneficial. Of course, this does not mean the treatment will be ultimately successful, since it is likely that many treatment failures showed evidence of responsiveness within the suggested time frames. On the other hand, relatively few successful treatments demonstrated responsiveness over longer intervals.

If treatment is progressing appropriately, at some point within-clinic and beyond-clinic data will begin to converge until speech performance under all conditions has reached criterion. At this point, the clinician will need to make some decision about the number of data collection occasions that are needed to verify that change and thus indicate the appropriateness of termination of the establishment-transfer phase of treatment. The simple fact is that there are almost no data that can be used to address this issue. Perhaps the sole exception occurs in a single-subject study by Ingham and Packman (1977). Obviously, more data are needed to address this issue, one research area in which group data would be useful. In the absence of those data, the clinician might be best advised to rely on the data collection intervals used thus far throughout baseline and treatment. These will provide at least one source for determining whether clinically significant changes have resulted from treatment. Perhaps, therefore, the client's performance pattern over four beyond- and within-clinic data collection points, while treatment has ceased, might be one rational basis for deciding whether maintenance procedures should be introduced to the therapy process. However, there are more complex issues associated with assessing treatment outcome that will be discussed later.

Dismantling Therapy

It may well be that a number of treatments are tried before a therapy strategy is found that will achieve within- and beyond-clinic treatment gains. These will be strategies that establish and transfer treatment gains. It is, therefore, necessary for the assessment process to incorporate strategies that will indicate when the initial phase of treatment (i.e., establishment and, if necessary, transfer) should be replaced by maintenance strategies.

There is general agreement that active maintenance strategies are necessary components of the therapy process, although that is often difficult to believe considering the slight amount of research they have attracted. There are some very limited data available that demonstrate the efficacy of some maintenance techniques (Boberg, 1981; Boberg, Howie, & Woods, 1977; Ingham, 1980, 1981, 1982), though they give no guidance on how to choose assessment procedures for this phase. To some extent, that task has been eased by some useful data that suggest that when beyond-clinic generalization occurs in the treatment of preschool children, then unassisted maintenance will follow (Ingham, 1983; Prins & Ingham, 1983). But the evidence is certainly not so persuasive in the case of older-aged children.

As mentioned earlier, repeated beyond- and within-clinic assessments at the end of treatment should continue over at least four data collection points. This should provide a reasonable basis for estimating the initial stability of these gains. However, the dismantling of the therapy process may also blend with treatment and assessment procedures. One internally valid method of establishing when treatment should be withdrawn is to use a period when the beyond/within-clinic data collection scores (i.e., nontreatment scores) and therapy-controlled measures of speech performance begin to merge. Martin, Kuhl, and Haroldson (1972) demonstrated the prospects of this strategy when they compared treatment and nontreatment setting performance of two preschool stutterers treated by contingency arrangements. Costello (1975) used this strategy during therapy sessions by comparing nontreatment and treatment intervals over contingency-managed therapy sessions.

A strategy used by the senior author in recent years (Ingham, 1980; 1981; 1982) involves systematic withdrawal of regular assessment sessions contingent upon sustained performance, plus comparisons with intermittent covert assessments. This is also an example of how beyond-clinic (or within-clinic) assessments can serve dual functions; that is, they decrease the contact frequency with the client but remain a useful source of speech control.

The above-mentioned method for continuing maintenance and evaluation illustrates how maintenance and outcome evaluation strategies may be gradually integrated. In this procedure the subject is required to return to the clinic initially for two once-weekly assessments, and if the target behavior (0% syllables stuttered at between 170 and 210 SPM) is maintained in all within- and beyond-clinic assessments, then the subject "earns" a 2-week rest from assessments. If these 2-week-apart assessments achieve the target behavior, then the subject earns a 4-week rest from assessments. This systematic and performance-contingent withdrawal of assessment continues until two 32-week-apart assessments are passed successfully. If the subject fails on any assessment (that is, has one stuttering or departs from the target speech rate on any task), then the weekly assessments are reinstated. Recently this procedure was successfully used in conjunction with a self-management technique (specifically, self-evaluation training) in order to shift the responsibility for conducting this performance-contingent assessment strategy to the subject (Ingham, 1982). These procedures have been mainly used with adults, but they have also been useful with older-aged children (Ingham, 1980). Of most relevance here is the fact that the data from these studies have been supplemented by nonperformance-contingent assessments made in beyond-clinic conditions, thereby establishing the point when the data from the nontreatment-related assessments blend with those from the treatment-related assessments. They have also been supplemented by a wide variety of covert assessments that have shown, in some cases, that data gained from overt and covert assessments differ markedly. Generally, these concurrent assessments indicate that the maintenance strategy may be phased out well before the 32-week-apart assessment point.

Covert assessment

Undoubtedly, covert assessment procedures are among the most contentious assessment techniques used in stuttering therapy. Some recent group studies (Howie, Woods, & Andrews, 1982; Andrews & Craig, 1982) have questioned their worth by finding that covert and overt group data are not significantly different 6 months or more after treatment. But studies on individuals (Ingham, 1980; 1982) have shown that the data from both sources may be quite different well after the initial phase of treatment has ceased. In consequence, covert assessments certainly have the potential of providing the most clinically valid treatment assessment data, particularly when used in conjunction with relevant overt assessment data. Their claim to validity, however, is only as strong as their claims to be unobtrusive—and these claims are often difficult to defend. There are various types of covert and perhaps not-so-covert assessment techniques that might be relatively free of the reactive features of overt assessment, features that many clinicians suspect produce "artificial" posttreatment data. Perhaps the most useful is the "unplanned telephone call," made, ideally, by a person not associated with the treatment. Other relevant information may be obtained from the subject's associates, and can then be validated by carefully arranged recordings. Admittedly, this all sounds uncomfortably unethical, but it need not be. In the case of older-aged children, adolescents, and adults, it is unlikely that the assessment's validity will be threatened if, before treatment, the client agrees that such assessments will only be used to test the treatment's worth. The authors have often used this procedure over the past decade, and have yet to meet one client who found it to be unacceptable. More importantly, it has often provided an immensely useful clinical service. For instance, if repeated unobtrusive assessments yield evidence of poorer performance compared to other, more directly obtained measures, then the consequent trend of performance scores can be used to determine the merit of continuing an extraclinic treatment procedure. When the extraclinic covert data fail to show improvement, then it may be necessary to integrate such data with treatment. For example, in the current applications of the above-described maintenance schedule , clinicians intermittently telephone subjects. If the clinician detects stuttering, then, regardless of whether the subject "passed" the previous assessment, the subject automatically fails that assessment and returns to the initial step in the maintenance schedule.

How should covert assessments be organized within an assessment schedule? Like all other assessment decisions, the decision to use covert assessment should be guided, where possible, by treatment and evaluation considerations. However, the difficulty with this form of assessment is that its "cover" is vulnerable if it is used too frequently. This type of assessment probably carries adequate treatment and assessment value if it occurs on at least four occasions during the transfer phase and on another four occasions during the immediate posttreatment assessment phase. This allows the clinician to decide whether the subject's assessed speech performance is reflected in less stimulus-bound conditions. Probably the most practical procedure for this purpose is an unannounced telephone conversation with a person unconnected with the treatment. It is up to the clinician to decide how the data should be obtained, but there is no reason why it cannot be assessed on-line by a trained clinician. The frequency with which covert assessments should be made during the maintenance phase largely depends on the duration of that phase. Of course, in turn, this raises the issue of time spans for posttreatment assessments, the final phase of this suggested format.

Follow-up Assessment

To date, our literature has little information that could be used to justify the use of certain prescribed follow-up intervals or follow-up assessments. The typical recommendations are that posttreatment assessments should occur at intervals ranging from a few weeks to five years (Silverman, 1981). What this reflects is yet another area of confusion, this time about the function of posttreatment evaluation. The primary purpose of the follow-up evaluation is surely to establish whether the client is unimproved, improved, or free of his or her problem after a period in which variables likely to influence the problem have had every opportunity to occur. The fact that a subject shows improvement, or otherwise, at follow-up may have very little to do with treatment. Quite clearly, the longer the interval between cessation of treatment and follow-up evaluation, the more likely it is that this interval will be filled with variables of far more relevance to current performance than the original treatment. Unfortunately, there is also little information available on the nature of these variables, but there are some logical contenders: practice regimes, "significant others," self-control of speech performance, and even additional treatment are good prospects for consideration.

At best, it would appear that follow-up evaluation may give the clinician and client knowledge about the current state of the disorder and some useful hypotheses about the durability of the treatment's effects. For this reason, perhaps the most practical guideline for follow-up evaluation is to schedule intermittent assessments over the following year. This will probably accommodate a clinic's annual time-tabling arrangements, and is consistent with the intervals used in many clinical studies.

The frequency of follow-up assessments presents another imponderable. Perhaps the logical solution is to use the "four-data-point" principle from the previously mentioned therapy assessment format. This means that follow-up assessments should occur at 3-month intervals. And in order to determine the validity of this trend, perhaps these assessments should be interspersed with another four covert assessments.

The content of these posttreatment assessments deserves additional comment. The logical contenders are the within- and beyond-clinic assessments used over the initial therapy phases. Perhaps the most practical option for covert assessment is a 3-to-5 minute surprise telephone call involving a question-answer conversation with a stranger. But at least two other assessments may be important: some form of assessment of the subject's speech quality (discussed above) and a questionnaire similar to those devised by Webster (1974) and Perkins (1981). The main value of Webster's questionnaire, for instance, is that it solicits the subject's judgment on the extent of attentiveness or self-monitoring required to continue to speak fluently. At present, no other means are available for determining the extent to which therapy gains are sustained at the cost of unusual levels of attention to speaking. Once again, there are no available norms for this part of Webster's questionnaire, but it might be expected that over the follow-up period there should be some evidence that the subject's level of attention to his speech declines in concert with sustained improvements. That would seem to be one final clinically valid indication of treatment success.

Conclusions

Let us now try to put together all the pieces of our therapy assessment puzzle. It begins when we have established the subject's suitability for therapy. This followed by a base rate period containing repeated within- and beyond-clinic recorded assessments. There should be at least four once-weekly within- and beyond-clinic assessments over the base rate period which would, therefore, extend for four weeks. These assessments continue at this frequency during the establishment and transfer phases of therapy. When data from all within- and beyond-clinic measures show criterion performance for four consecutive assessments, formal treatment could be terminated. Thus, at the end of the establishment or transfer phase, beyond-

and within-clinic assessments should continue for the same duration as the base rate in order to establish performance stability, or otherwise. The subsequent maintenance phase may include decreasingly frequent assessments that might also be tied to the treatment process. The pattern of maintenance assessments should continue until they occur at 3-month intervals. At this point, they should fade into follow-up assessments made at 3-month intervals over a year.

The overt within- and beyond-clinic assessment procedure throughout the preceding format should be supplemented by at least four unobtrusive or covert assessments made during both the treatment and transfer phases, plus another four assessments during the immediate posttreatment phase. In addition, perhaps covert assessments (of one form or another) should be made at regular intervals over the maintenance and follow-up periods. The content of the overt assessments should include representative speech samples from the client's natural environment, plus oral readings, monologues, and telephone conversations within the clinic.

The minimum data used in assessments should be syllables per minute and/or articulation rate, and percentage of syllables (or words) stuttered. These data should be supplemented by ratings of speech quality, especially during the final part of the treatment phase. The posttreatment phase of therapy might also include a questionnaire which solicits the subject's estimate of the extent to which it is necessary to "control" speech performance.

We hope that this suggested therapy management system will be given serious consideration as one means of shifting stuttering therapy towards a reasonably common pattern of assessment. This might help achieve a clearer understanding of the therapy process—an understanding that will be of immense benefit to all concerned with this disorder. There is an almost desperate need for a data base from field clinicians on the outcome of current stuttering therapy procedures. If clinicians could be encouraged to gather and report data within the suggested system, then the profession should be considerably advanced in solving that need, for only clinicians can show the strengths and weaknesses of these treatments in the field, rather than in the research laboratory. At the same time, the use of this system would go some distance towards meeting Bloodstein's (1981) therapy evaluation criteria. Finally, it should be mentioned that the suggested therapy management system has already been used successfully in clinical conditions. Ingham and Onslow (1983) have prepared a Stuttering Treatment Evaluation Manual which incorporates guidelines on the use of the previously described procedures. There is every indication from the trial use of this manual with various clinicians in diverse settings that the procedures can be easily implemented.

End Notes

[1] The content of this chapter takes as a starting point some ideas about stuttering treatment outcome evaluation that were first presented in Ingham (Note 1) and further developed in Ingham (1983).

[2] The interested reader is urged to read Bloodstein's justification for each criterion.

[3] Less decisive findings have been reported by Curlee (1981).

Reference Note

1. Ingham, R. J. Towards a therapy assessment procedure for treating stuttering in children. Paper presented at the Conference on Evaluation of Disfluency, Prevention of Stuttering, and Management of Fluency Problems in Children. Northwestern University, Evanston, IL 1982.

References

Adams, M. R. Fluency, nonfluency, and stuttering in children. *Journal of Fluency Disorders,* 1982, *7,* 171–185.

Andrews, G. Stuttering therapy: How simple can an effective treatment programme become? *Australian Journal of Human Communication Disorders,* 1973, *1,* 44–46.

Andrews, G., & Craig, A. Stuttering: Overt and covert measurement of the speech of treated subjects. *Journal of Speech and Hearing Disorders,* 1982, *47,* 96–99.

Andrews, G., & Cutler, J. Stuttering therapy: The relation between changes in symptom level and attitudes. *Journal of Speech and Hearing Disorders,* 1974, *39,* 312–319.

Andrews, G., Guitar, B., & Howie, P. Meta-analysis of the effects of stuttering treatment. *Journal of Speech and Hearing Disorders,* 1980, *45,* 287–307.

Andrews, G., & Harvey, R. Regression to the mean in pretreatment measures of stuttering. *Journal of Speech and Hearing Disorders,* 1981, *46,* 204–207.

Andrews, G., & Ingham, R. J. An approach to the evaluation of stuttering therapy. *Journal of Speech and Hearing Research,* 1972, *15,* 296–302.

Birnbrauer, J. S. External validity and experimental investigation of individual behavior. *Analysis and Intervention in Developmental Disabilities,* 1981, *1,* 117–132.

Bloodstein, O. *A handbook on stuttering* (3rd ed.). Chicago: National Easter Seal Society, 1981.

Boberg, E. *Maintenance of fluency.* New York: Elsevier, 1981.

Boberg, E., & Fong, L. Therapy program for young retarded stutterers. *Human Communication,* 1980, *2,* 95–102.

Boberg, E., Howie, P., & Woods, L. Maintenance of fluency: A review. *Journal of Fluency Disorders,* 1979, *4,* 93–116.

Boudreau, L.A., & Jeffrey, C.J. Stuttering treated by desensitization. *Journal of Behavior Therapy and Experimental Psychiatry,* 1973, *4,* 209–212.

Brady, J. P. Metronome-conditioned speech retraining for stuttering. *Behavior Therapy,* 1971, *2,* 129–150.

Costello, J. M. The establishment of fluency with time-out procedures: Three case studies. *Journal of Speech and Hearing Disorders,* 1975, *40,* 216–231.

Costello, J. M. Clinicians and researchers: A necessary dichotomy? *Journal of the National Student Speech and Hearing Association,* 1979, *7,* 6–26.

Costello, J. M. Operant conditioning and the treatment of stuttering. In W. H. Perkins (Ed.), *Strategies in stuttering therapy. Seminars in Speech, Language and Hearing, 1,* New York: Decker, 1980.

Costello, J. M. Pretreatment assessment of stuttering in young children. *Communicative Disorders: An Audio Journal for Continuing Education.* New York: Grune & Stratton, 1981.

Costello, J. M. Techniques of therapy based on operant theory. In W.H. Perkins (Ed.), *Current therapy of communication disorders.* New York: Thieme-Stratton, 1982.

Costello, J. M., & Ingham, R. J. Assessment strategies for child and adult stutterers. In W. Perkins & R. Curlee (Eds.), *Nature and treatment of stuttering: New directions.* San Diego: College-Hill, in press.

Curlee, R. F. Observer agreement on disfluency and stuttering. *Journal of Speech and Hearing Research,* 1981, *24,* 595-600.

Darley, F. L., & Spriestersbach, D. C. *Diagnostic methods in speech pathology.* New York: Harper & Row, 1978.

Eysenck, H. J. An exercise in mega-silliness. *American Psychologist,* 1978, *33,* 517.

Goldiamond, I. Stuttering and fluency as manipulatable operant response classes. In L. Krasner & L. P. Ullmann (Eds.), *Research in behavior modification.* New York: Holt, Rinehart, & Winston, 1965.

Gregory, H. H. (Ed.) *Controversies about stuttering therapy.* Baltimore: University Park Press, 1978.

Guitar, B. Reduction of stuttering frequency using analog electromyographic feedback. *Journal of Speech and Hearing Research,* 1975, *18,* 672-685.

Guitar, B. E. A response to Ingham's critique. *Journal of Speech and Hearing Disorders,* 1979, *44,* 400-403.

Guitar, B. E. A correction to "A response to Ingham's critique." *Journal of Speech and Hearing Disorders,* 1981, *46,* 440.

Guitar, B., & Bass, C. Stuttering therapy: The relationship between attitude change and long term outcome. *Journal of Speech and Hearing Disorders,* 1978, *43,* 392-400.

Hanna, R., & Owen, N. Facilitating transfer and maintenance of fluency in stuttering therapy. *Journal of Speech and Hearing Disorders,* 1977, *42,* 65-76.

Hawkins, R. P., & Dotson, V. A. Reliability scores that delude: An Alice in Wonderland trip through the misleading characteristics of interobserver agreement scores in interval recording. In E. Ramp & G. Semb (Eds.), *Behavior analysis: Areas of research and application.* Englewood Cliffs, NJ: Prentice-Hall, 1975.

Hee, J. C., & Holmes, P. A. Elimination of stuttering by a regulated breathing approach. *Journal of Communication Pathology,* 1976, *8,* 40-44.

Herscovitch, A., & LeBow, M. D. Imaginal pacing in the treatment of stuttering. *Journal of Behavior Therapy and Experimental Psychiatry,* 1973, *4,* 357-360.

Hersen, M., & Barlow, D. H. *Single-case experimental designs.* New York: Pergamon, 1976.

Howie, P. M., Woods, C. L., & Andrews, G. Relationship between covert and overt speech measures immediately before and immediately after stuttering treatment. *Journal of Speech and Hearing Disorders,* 1982, *47,* 419-422.

Ingham, R. J. Comment on "Stuttering therapy: The relation between attitude change and long-term outcome." *Journal of Speech and Hearing Disorders,* 1979, *44,* 397-400.

Ingham, R. J. Modification of maintenance and generalization in stuttering treatment. *Journal of Speech and Hearing Research,* 1980, *23,* 732-745.

Ingham, R. J. Evaluation and maintenance in stuttering treatment: A search for ecstasy with nothing but agony. In E. Boberg (Ed.), *Maintenance of fluency.* New York: Elsevier, 1981.

Ingham, R. J. The effects of self-evaluation training on maintenance and generalization during stuttering treatment. *Journal of Speech and Hearing Disorders,* 1982, *47,* 271–280.

Ingham, R. J. *Stuttering and behavior therapy: Current status and experimental foundations.* San Diego: College-Hill, 1983.

Ingham, R. J. & Andrews, G. An analysis of a token economy in stuttering therapy. *Journal of Applied Behavior Analysis,* 1973, *6,* 219–229.

Ingham, R. J., Martin, R. R., & Kuhl, P. Modification and control of rate of speaking by stutterers. *Journal of Speech and Hearing Research,* 1974, *17,* 489–496.

Ingham, R. J., & Onslow, M. *Stuttering treatment evaluation manual.* Sydney: Cumberland College of Health Sciences, 1983.

Ingham, R. J., & Packman, A. Treatment and generalization effects in an experimental treatment for a stutterer using contingency management and speech rate control. *Journal of Speech and Hearing Disorders,* 1977, *42,* 394–407.

Ingham, R. J., & Packman, A. Perceptual assessment of normalcy of speech following stuttering therapy. *Journal of Speech and Hearing Research,* 1978, *21,* 63–73.

James, J. E. Behavioral self-control of stuttering using time-out from speaking. *Journal of Applied Behavior Analysis,* 1981, *14,* 25–37.

Johnson, G. F., Coleman, K., & Rasmussen, K. Multidays: Multidimensional approach for the young stutterer. *Language, Speech, and Hearing Services in Schools,* 1978, *9,* 129–132.

Jones, R. J., & Azrin, N. H. Behavioral engineering: Stuttering as a function of stimulus duration during speech synchronization. *Journal of Applied Behavior Analysis,* 1969, *2,* 223–229.

Kiesler, D. J. Some myths of psychotherapy research and the search for a paradigm. *Psychological Bulletin,* 1966, *65,* 110–136.

Kowal, S., O'Connell, D. C., & Sabin, E. F. Development of temporal patterning and vocal hesitations in spontaneous narratives. *Journal of Psycholinguistic Research,* 1975, *4,* 195–207.

LaCroix, Z.E. Management of disfluent speech through self-recording procedures. *Journal of Speech and Hearing Disorders,* 1973, *38,* 272-274.

MacCulloch, M. J., Eaton, R., & Long, E. The long term effect of auditory masking on young stutterers. *British Journal of Disorders of Communication,* 1970, *5,* 165–173.

MacDonald, J. D., & Martin, R. R. Stuttering and disfluency as two reliable and unambiguous response classes. *Journal of Speech and Hearing Research,* 1973, *16,* 691–699.

Martin, R. R. Appercus. In E. Boberg (Ed.), *Maintenance of fluency.* New York: Elsevier, 1981.

Martin, R. R., & Berndt, L. A. The effects of time-out on stuttering in a 12 year old boy. *Exceptional Children,* 1970, *36,* 303–304.

Martin, R. R., & Haroldson, S. K. The effects of two treatment procedures on stuttering. *Journal of Communication Disorders,* 1969, *2,* 115–125.

Martin, R. R., Haroldson, S. K., & Triden, K. A. Stuttering and speech naturalness. *Journal of Speech and Hearing Disorders,* in press.

Martin, R. R., Kuhl, P., & Haroldson, S. K. An experimental treatment with two preschool stuttering children. *Journal of Speech and Hearing Research,* 1972, *15,* 743–752.

McDermott, L. D. Clinical management of stuttering behavior: A case study. *Feedback,* 1971, *1,* 6–7.

McReynolds, L. V., & Kearns, K. P. *Single-subject experimental designs in communicative disorders.* Baltimore: University Park Press, 1982.

Metz, D. E., Onufrak, J. A., & Ogburn, R. S. An acoustical analysis of stutterer's speech prior to and at the termination of therapy. *Journal of Fluency Disorders,* 1979, *4,* 249–254.

Mowrer, D. An instructional program to increase fluent speech of stutterers. *Journal of Fluency Disorders,* 1975, *1,* 25–35.

Ottoni, T. M. Uso de la tecnica delineamento del habla para cambiar la conducta verbal. *Revista Interamericana de Psicologia*, 1974, *8*, 3-4.

Perkins, W. H. Articulatory rate in the evaluation of stuttering treatments. *Journal of Speech and Hearing Disorders*, 1975, *40*, 277-278.

Perkins, W. H. Measurement and maintenance of fluency. In E. Boberg (Ed.), *Maintenance of fluency*. New York: Elsevier, 1981.

Perkins, W. H., Rudas, J., Johnson, L., Michael, W. B., & Curlee, R. F. Replacement of stuttering with normal speech: III. Clinical effectiveness. *Journal of Speech and Hearing Disorders*, 1974, *39*, 416-428.

Peters, A. D. The effect of positive reinforcement on fluency: Two case studies. *Language, Speech, and Hearing Services in Schools*, 1977, *8*, 15-22.

Prins, D., & Ingham, R. J. *Treatment of stuttering in early childhood: Methods and issues*. San Diego: College-Hill, 1983.

Reed, C. G., & Godden, A. L. An experimental treatment using verbal punishment with two preschool stutterers. *Journal of Fluency Disorders*, 1977, *2*, 225-233.

Resick, P. A., Wendiggensen, P., Ames, S., & Meyer, V. Systematic slowed speech: A new treatment for stuttering. *Behaviour Research and Therapy*, 1978, *16*, 161-167.

Runyan, C. M., & Adams, M. R. Perceptual study of the speech of "successfully therapeutized" stutterers. *Journal of Fluency Disorders*, 1978, *3*, 25-39.

Runyan, C. M., & Adams, M. R. Unsophisticated judges' perceptual evaluations of the speech of "successfully treated" stutterers. *Journal of Fluency Disorders*, 1979, *4*, 29-38.

Ryan, B. P. Operant procedures applied to stuttering therapy for children. *Journal of Speech and Hearing Disorders*, 1971, *36*, 264-280.

Ryan, B. P. *Programmed therapy for stuttering in children and adults*. Springfield, IL: Charles C. Thomas, 1974.

Shames, G. H. Relapse in stuttering. In E. Boberg (Ed.), *Maintenance of fluency*. New York: Elsevier, 1981.

Shames, G. H., & Florance, C. L. *Stutter-free speech: A goal for therapy*. Columbus: Charles E. Merrill, 1980.

Shaw, C. K., & Shrum, W. F. The effects of response-contingent reward on the connected speech of children who stutter. *Journal of Speech and Hearing Disorders*, in W. H. Perkins (Ed.), *Strategies in Stuttering Therapy*. 1972, *37*, 75-88.

Sheehan. J. G. Problems in the evaluation of progress and outcome. *Seminars in Speech, Language, and Hearing, 1,* New York: Decker, 1980.

Silverman, F. H. Relapse following stuttering therapy. In N.J. Lass (Ed.), *Speech and language: Advances in basic research and practice* (Vol. 5). New York: Academic Press, 1981.

Smith, L. M., & Glass, G. Meta-analysis of psychotherapy outcome studies. *American Psychologist*, 1977, *32*, 752-760.

Starkweather, C. W. Speech fluency and its development in normal children. In N.J. Lass (Ed.), *Speech and language: Advances in basic research and practice* (Vol. 4). New York: Academic Press, 1980.

Stokes, T. F., & Baer, D. M. An implicit technology of generalization. *Journal of Applied Behavior Analysis*, 1977, *10*, 349-367.

Turnbaugh, K. R. & Guitar, B. E. Short-term intensive stuttering treatment in a public school setting. *Language, Speech, and Hearing Services in Schools*, 1981, *12*, 107-114.

Ulliana, L., & Ingham, R. J. Behavioral and nonbehavioral variables in the measurement of stutterers' communication attitudes. *Journal of Speech and Hearing Disorders*, in press.

Webster, R. L. Stuttering: A way to eliminate it and a way to explain it. In R. Ulrich, T. Stachnik, & J. Mabry (Eds.), *Control of human behavior* (Vol.2). Glenview, IL: Scott Foresman, 1970.

Webster, R. L. *The Precision Fluency Shaping Program: Speech reconstruction for stutterers*. Roanoke, VA: Hollins Communication Research Institute, 1974.

AUTHOR INDEX

A

Adams, J. A., 133, 135, 136, 141, 149, 150
Adams, M., 234, 239, 248, 262, 264, 265, 271
Adams, M. R., 232, 239, 242, 320, 327
Adams, R. E., 98
Ainsworth, S., 293, 301
Albert, M., 176
Alfrey, A. C., 246
Allen, G., 55, 56, 57
Alper, J., 238
Aman, L. A., 169
American Speech-Language-Hearing Association, 93
Ames, S., 317, 328
Anderson, S., 62
Andrews, G., 234, 239, 240, 241, 242, 244, 245, 248, 249, 250, 267, 300, 314, 315, 316, 319, 321, 335, 336, 339
Angle, E. H., 204
Ansberry, M., 4
Aram, D. M., 167, 168, 169, 171, 173, 181
Archambault, P., 98
Arndt, W., 6, 16, 139, 140, 142, 143, 144, 151
Aslin, R., 34, 56
Atkinson-King, K., 56, 65
Ayres, A. J., 182
Azrin, N. H., 320

B

Baer, D. M., 318
Bailey, A. A., 294
Bailey, W., 294
Baker, W., 58, 59
Bangert, J., 151, 152
Bankson, N., 16, 20, 50, 129, 138, 143, 147, 149, 150, 152
Bar, A., 251
Barlow, D., 286, 314, 319, 325, 330
Barton, D., 55, 60, 61
Bashir, A. S., 178
Bass, C., 318
Bates, E., 40
Baughman, C. H., 167
Beech, H. R., 239
Beecher, R., 205
Beilin, H., 65
Bell, A., 27
Bell, J., 239
Bennett, S., 21
Benson, D. F., 245
Berger, K. W., 95
Berko, J., 58
Berlin, A., 267
Berlin, C. I., 176
Berliner, K. I., 100
Berndt, L. A., 333
Bernstein, M., 205
Bernstein, N., 148
Bernthal, J., 14, 50, 129, 138, 147, 150, 152
Berry, M. F., 242, 300
Besner, D., 66
Bilodeau, I., 150
Birnbrauer, J. S., 331
Bishry, Z., 242
Bjerkan, B., 235
Blakeley, R. W., 174
Blankenship, J., 238
Bloch, E. L., 244
Blood, G. W., 242
Bloodstein, O., 234, 236, 238, 239, 240, 241, 244, 245, 246, 299, 314, 318, 321, 323, 328, 342
Bloom, K., 37
Bloomer, H. H., 202, 204, 205, 214, 215

SUBJECT INDEX

Date Due